Centrifugation in Density Gradients

Centrifugation in Density Gradients

C. A. PRICE

Waksman Institute of Microbiology
Busch Campus
Rutgers University
New Brunswick, New Jersey

With contributions by Eric F. Eikenberry

1982

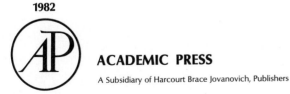

ACADEMIC PRESS

A Subsidiary of Harcourt Brace Jovanovich, Publishers

New York   London
Paris   San Diego   San Francisco   São Paulo   Sydney   Tokyo   Toronto

ACADEMIC PRESS, INC.
111 Fifth Avenue, New York, New York 10003

United Kingdom Edition published by
ACADEMIC PRESS, INC. (LONDON) LTD.
24/28 Oval Road, London NW1 7DX

Library of Congress Cataloging in Publication Data

Price, C. A. (Carl Arthur), Date.
  Centrifugation in density gradients.

  Includes bibliographies and index.
  1. Centrifugation, Density gradient. 2. Biology--
Technique. I. Title.
QH324.9.D46P74   574.87'028   81-12693
ISBN 0-12-564580-5   AACR2

PRINTED IN THE UNITED STATES OF AMERICA

82 83 84 85   9 8 7 6 5 4 3 2 1

Dedicated to Norman G. Anderson

Contents

vii

Appendix A: Some Useful Units, Values, and Conversions

Appendix B: Properties of Particles

Appendix C: Properties of Gradient Materials

Appendix D: Gradient Shapes

Appendix E: Zonal Rotors

Appendix F: Chemical Resistance of Various Plastics   418

Appendix G: Addresses of Some Manufacturers   420

Index   **423**

Foreword

Living cells are the most complex systems with which modern science deals. Centrifuges have become indispensable tools for the disassembly and analysis of cells, and for the separation of different cell types. This work describes admirably the history and present status of this field.

Basic tools are generally taken for granted, especially so because they reach the user almost entirely (and correctly so) through commercial channels. However, progress is almost completely limited by the tools available, so that with the development of each—whether for microscopy, histochemistry, radioautography, x-ray diffraction, centrifugation, chromatography, electrophoresis, or enzyme kinetics—a new wave of concepts and results appear. Because tools are absolutely basic to continued advancement, it is not unlikely that we do not now possess the basic tools required to solve the cancer problem, for example, even if we knew what questions to ask. Thereby hangs, in part, the answer to a singular puzzle in the biomedical sciences, namely, why the organized support mechanisms have assiduously avoided providing adequate (or even minimal) support for the development of the tools which experience suggests will be required. For nearly all research one must proceed with what one has—to consider a present problem to be unsolvable because tools are lacking must operationally and in the mass be looked on as evidence of research incompetence. Thus in proposals and other writings the opposite must always be made to appear to be the case; i.e., we do not lack the requisite tools. The short-term, episodic nature of most research funding tends to discourage sober contemplation of the basic underlying problems. In addition the nonquantitative nature of most biological research prevents precise definitions both of limits and of advances. Thus, in marked contrast to the physical sciences where there is often general agreement on basic tool development, there has been little in the biomedical sciences. While arguments may exist relative to so-called "big" science vs "little" science, a feature of large scientific programs which have been successful is identification of barriers to the solution of core problems, and the mobilization of interdisciplinary efforts to solve them. It is for this reason that no counterparts of the large-scale and successful efforts in nuclear energy and in space exist in biology. If they did, or were contemplated, then careful attention would have to be given to the tools required. The space and nuclear energy programs were both deeply concerned with the theoretical and experimental basis on which they rested. A serious, mature attempt to solve some of the remaining biomedical problems—transplantation, cancer, many of the degenerative diseases—would have to face directly the simple fact that we are not prepared for the complexity involved. It is essential, therefore, to encourage as much as possible the development of the tools of future exploration—of which the gradient or zonal centrifuge is an important one.

A word about the problem to be solved. A complete picture or positional representation of cellular constituents down to the atomic level is essential but insufficient. Cellular substructures are self-assembling. The rate of replacement and the mechanisms by which it occurs have been examined only in the most preliminary way. The strangest thing about it is that some sort of feedback appears to occur such that protein synthesis is sensitive in detail to requirements—thus when part of a unicellular organism is extirpated, just the synthesis to replace the missing organelles occurs. In contrast, in other instances when a surface protein is bound to antibodies, the gene for that protein appears to be shut off. The exquisite responsiveness of the genes and their associated synthetic machinery to internal and external signals remain almost entirely unexplored. On a larger scale, the orchestration of development with the precise phasing of many sets of genes turned on and off in sequence is even more dimly seen. Yet our curiosity about these problems is what drives us. In each instance, when we attempt to approach these problems experimentally we find that asking the right question is insufficient without a favorable biological model, and without the proper tools.

Norman G. Anderson
MOLECULAR ANATOMY (MAN) PROGRAM
OAK RIDGE NATIONAL LABORATORY
OAK RIDGE, TENNESSEE

Preface

Density gradient centrifugation has reached a gratifying state of maturity in which the art, science, and technology are in harmony. It is possible to analyze or to separate substantial quantities of virtually any kind of biological particle, intact, and in as high degree of purity as desired. It not only works well but, for particles down to the size of the largest macromolecules, is typically the method of choice.

This monograph is intended for those who need to separate biological particles. Although the underlying principles and much of the technology are equally applicable to nonbiological particles, our examples are drawn from the biological universe and we give only passing reference to such topics as nonaqueous gradient materials, which are important for the separation of mineral particles.

The book is divided into nine chapters plus an extensive appendix. Those interested in the history of science may turn to Chapter 2; although density gradient centrifugation is barely 30 years old, its roots and development involved questions that were also pivotal to the development of modern biochemistry and cell biology. Chapter 3 provides a nonrigorous treatment of the physical basis of density gradient centrifugation; readers who remember something of college calculus and physics should have no trouble with it. Chapter 4, written by Eric F. Eikenberry, is a more rigorous treatment that is fully consistent with physical and chemical theory. Chapters 5–7 deal with the nuts and bolts of density gradient centrifugation, the composition and construction of gradients, the properties and operation of centrifuge systems, and certain arcane but highly useful procedures, such as reorienting gradient centrifugation. Chapter 8, also by Eric Eikenberry, is concerned with density gradient centrifugation in the analytical ultracentrifuge. Chapter 9 is a collection of protocols for separating particles ranging in size from whole cells to macromolecules. It includes procedures for both swinging bucket and zonal rotors. We hope that readers will find the appendix particularly useful. We have tried to assemble there all of the tabular information that we have ever required for experimental work in this field.

I want to acknowledge several people who influenced me strongly during my involvement with density gradient centrifugation. Anyone concerned with the development of analytical biochemistry is in debt to the creative imagination, the remarkable combination of insights into physical, biological, and engineering principles, and the organization skills of Norman G. Anderson. He not only fathered the zonal centrifuge, but contributed to numberless conceptual and methodological advances in the analysis of biological components. I am grateful to be one of many who were infected with his spirit of excitement and enthusiasm. For these reasons I dedicate this book to Norman Anderson.

For several years I enjoyed the collaboration of Eric Eikenberry. I particularly admire his ability to formulate physical models of biological processes, and I would not have undertaken this monograph without his collaboration.

My concern with the development of density gradient centrifugation grew out of a desire to study the biochemistry of organelles under conditions where they could be treated as ideal multimolecular systems: homogeneous, pure, and intact. In the case of the larger organelles, however, even density gradient centrifugation yielded preparations that were often impure or inactive or both. Håkan Pertoft realized that the high osmotic potential of sucrose gradients was the likely villain and, through his studies on the use of silica sols as gradient materials, extended the full benefits of density gradient centrifugation to membrane-bound particles. A culmination of these efforts was his invention of "Percoll."

Following the example of Pertoft, Jean-Jacques Morgenthaler in my laboratory developed a method for the isolation in silica sol gradients of exceptionally pure, intact, and active chloroplasts. Leticia Mendiola–Morgenthaler subsequently demonstrated that chloroplasts isolated in this way were ideal subjects for the study of protein synthesis in plastics. I am grateful to Norman Anderson for drawing me into the development of density gradient centrifugation, but I am also grateful to Håkan Pertoft, Jean-Jacques Morgenthaler, and Lettie Morgenthaler for perfecting the methodology to the point where I could return to studies of the biochemistry and molecular biology of organelles confident that the particles could be obtained in an optimum state. I have not been disappointed.

I want to thank Mary Lou Tobin for toiling over the early drafts of this book in an era before word processors; numerous students and associates who contributed ideas, criticism, and data; and my wife and children who endured with surprising cheerfulness the boredom of having me write another book. I also want to acknowledge the advantages afforded by the superb collection of periodicals of the Marine Biological Laboratory and the Woods Hole Oceanographic Institution.

C. A. Price

1

Particle Abstraction in Biology — An Introduction

Most biologists and chemists regard the world as being composed of molecules, and in particular they regard the biological world as being composed principally of organic molecules. As with most successful abstractions, we are rarely aware that this view *is* an abstraction. While the more philosophically oriented researcher distinguishes with some acerbity between the components of a bacterium and the *Ding Ansicht* (the notion of the thing itself), those with a molecular orientation plunge onward from one triumph to another in their accounting of biological functions to the properties of molecules.

My prejudices in this discussion are clear, but one must admit that this molecular view of the world, now dominant, *is* an abstraction and, no matter how clever molecules are proved to be, it is but one among many possible abstractions (forces, fields, systems, populations, potentials, to list only a few). The notion of a particle is offered as an alternate abstraction that can help organize one's thoughts about biological systems at a variety of levels and is nicely complementary to the notion of molecules.

In this view the organism is composed of particles; indeed, whole organisms can be usefully thought of as particles. The cell is a particle, as are the nuclei, mitochondria, chromosomes, lysosomes and all the other "somes," nucleic acids, and proteins; macromolecules, micromolecules, and multimolecules; cell walls, plasma membranes, inner membranes, outer membranes, membranes rough and smooth; particles on particles and particles within particles; not to mention virus particles.

The beauty of particles, and their advantage over molecules for present purposes, is that particles have physical properties that are measurable and exploitable even when we are innocent of the chemical composition. Particles have size, mass, density, shape, charge, surface, hydration, and some have osmotic properties. At a time when biologists are becoming ever more ambitious, the notion of particles provides an occasion for quantitative treatment and unambiguous designations of unknown aggregations; it also provides a magnificent strategy for separation and for purification.

Four principal properties of biological particles have been exploited for their separation and purification. Centrifugation relies principally on size and density (but is also influenced by shape and response to osmotic pressure). Electrophoresis uses charge and mass. Finally, the phase separation techniques rationalized and popularized by Albertsson (1972) exploit surface properties.

Although we shall be concerned exclusively with centrifugation, one should be aware that other physical properties can and should be exploited as additional and independent parameters for the characterization of particles.

Rationale of Density Gradient Centrifugation

A fundamental equation of centrifugation (Eq. 1.1) (cf. Chapters 3 and 4), says that sedimentation velocity is related to the sedimentation coefficient s, which is mostly a function of particle size, and the density of the particle ρ_p.

$$\frac{dr}{dt} = sr\omega^2 \frac{\eta_w}{\eta_m} \frac{\rho_p - \rho_m}{\rho_p - \rho_w} \tag{1.1}$$

where r is the distance of the particle from the axis of rotation, ω the angular velocity, η the viscosity, p particle, w water at 20°C, and m the medium.

In ordinary centrifugation carried out in tubes, suspensions of particles are spun until the particles pellet against the bottom of the tubes. In this case the rate of sedimentation or the combination of speed and time required to pellet is almost wholly dependent on the size of the particles. Specifically, such separations depend on s. If the suspension contains a mixture of particles, we can fractionate the mixture by first pelleting at low speeds followed by higher speeds or longer times (Fig. 1.1). This method of *differential* or *fractional* centrifugation has been enormously useful; however, because small particles that are initially near the bottom of the tube will be collected in the pellet of large particles, it has inherently poor resolution. There is, moreover, a tendency for particles to strike the tube wall and subsequently move more rapidly along the wall as aggregates than they would in free suspension or, the reverse, become stuck to the wall and move less rapidly.

A quite different aspect of particles and of Eq. (1.1) is exploited by biochemists seeking to separate and characterize lipoproteins of blood serum. The sera are centrifuged in solutions of different densities (Fig. 1.2) where-

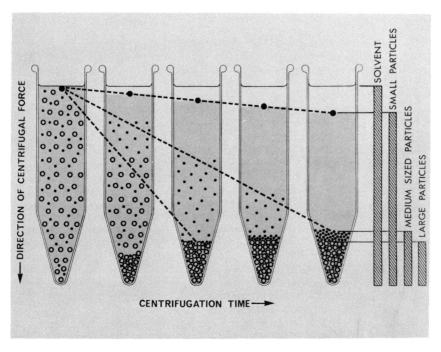

Fig. 1.1. Differential centrifugation. Separations in differential or fractional centrifugation are based principally on differences in the size of particles; larger particles are sedimented most rapidly followed progressively by smaller particles. Courtesy of Oak Ridge National Laboratory.

upon some proteins are seen to float in solutions in excess of some limiting densities. We can see this mathematically from the factor $(\rho_p - \rho_m)$; if this quantity is less than zero, the particles must float.

Density gradient centrifugation (Fig. 1.3) is used to separate particles on the basis of s and ρ (size and density) by employing a medium of graded densities. One can visualize from Fig. 1.4 that a band containing different sizes and densities of particles is layered over a density gradient. During a relatively short or slow centrifugation, particles separate according to size, the larger particles sedimenting farther than smaller ones. During a long, fast centrifugation, particles move to positions in the gradient where the density of the medium is the same as the particle density; $(\rho_p - \rho_m) \to 0$. Thus, a small, dense particle (small solid circles) initially sediments less rapidly than a large particle of low density. The large particles reach their position of equilibrium density early, while the small, dense particles slowly pass through the large particle zone and ultimately take up an equilibrium position deeper into the gradient.

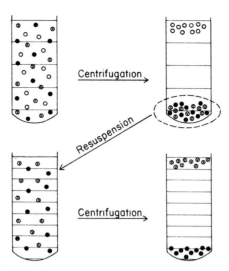

Fig. 1.2. Differential flotation. By centrifuging in media of progressively increasing density, one can separate particles of different densities. As the density of the medium increases, particles of higher and higher densities float to the surface during centrifugation.

We see that density gradient centrifugation offers two types of separation: (1) rate or s-rate separations based primarily on the sedimentation coefficient or size of particles and (2) equilibrium density or isopycnic separations based on the densities of particles.*

A fundamental advantage of rate separations in density gradients over differential centrifugation is that density gradients permit particles with quite small differences in s values to be resolved from one another (see Chapter 3). Similarly, resolution in isopycnic separations is at least an order of magnitude better in density gradients compared to differential flotation.

Anderson (1966), after a decade of contemplating the sedimentation behavior of biological particles, pointed out that different particles have unique combinations of s and ρ values.† He then proposed a Cartesian coordinate system with sedimentation coefficient and particle density as the ordinates (Fig. 1.4). A class of particles could be represented as a region (rarely a point) in s–ρ space. Anderson especially noted that most viruses fall into a region of s–ρ space bounded top and bottom by endoplasmic reticulum and ribosomes, which he called the "virus window."

---

* The densities of real particles, and especially membrane-bound particles, are sometimes unpredictable, but depend in predictable ways on the composition of the medium.

† The densities of particles suspended in aqueous systems are greatly affected by their hydration, which may vary in complicated ways with the composition of the medium. This is especially true for membrane-bound particles.

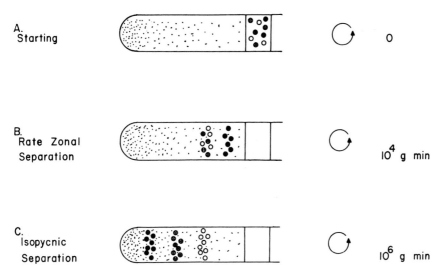

Fig. 1.3. Density gradient centrifugation, in its original and simplest form, is a mixture of particles layered over a medium whose density increases from top to bottom (A). In a short or slow centrifugation large particles sediment more rapidly than small particles (B). During prolonged centrifugation particles migrate to a position of equilibrium density, which is independent of particle size (C).

The major role of s–ρ space has been as a visual aid to biologists. However, biologists as a group tend to think with images (rather than the mathematical symbols endemic to the physical sciences), and this one has been of substantial and continuing significance.

s–ρ Space as a Strategy for Particle Separation

Many kinds of particles have overlapping s or ρ values, but, as we see in Fig. 1.4, rarely the same combination of s and ρ. For example, the densities of mammalian mitochondria and lysosomes overlap almost completely, whereas the s values of mitochondria and peroxisomes overlap. The three particles can be largely resolved from one another and from other cell components by two separation steps (Fig. 1.5). Fractions in an s-rate separation correspond roughly to a vertical slice of s–ρ space (Fig. 1.6). Lysosomes are in one slice and mitochondria and peroxisomes in the next. The fractions of interest from the rate separation are then subjected to a second centrifugation in a second gradient, and the particles sedimented to equilibrium (Fig. 1.6). The mitochondria are then separated from the peroxisomes. The fractions in an isopycnic separation can be thought of as horizontal slices in s–ρ space (Fig. 1.6).

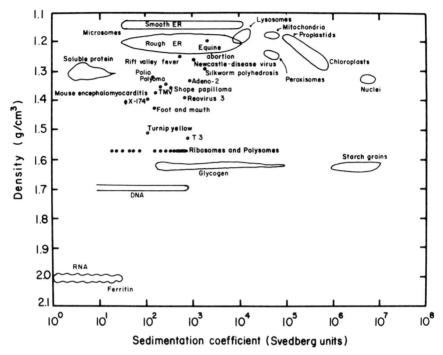

Fig. 1.4. Subcellular particles can usually be assigned specific sedimentation coefficients and equilibrium densities (s–ρ space). Anderson (1966) pointed out that these can be taken as coordinates in a two-dimensional space. Note that the actual values for real particles are dependent on the nature of the medium.

Characterization of Particles by s–ρ Coordinates

The terms 70 S* and 80 S ribosomes, of 16 S and 23 S RNA, and of 7 S and 9 S macroglobulins are well known. Nuclear DNA is accepted as having a density of 1.703 and a satellite band of 1.695. These separate coordinates of s–ρ space are used routinely to characterize and identify biological particles.

A logical extension of this practice would be to employ s and ρ values as identifying coordinates. This has rarely been done, but it offers the advantages of quantitation and, provided the centrifugation media are defined, permits an unambiguous reference for other workers. One should be able to say, for example, that a preparation of mitochondria (in such-and-such medium) had $s = 30,000 \pm 1750$ and $\rho = 1.16 \pm 0.05$ with a minor contaminant at $s = 18,000$, $\rho = 1.17$. It is high time that biochemists, who have

---

* The units of s are the Svedberg (S); S $= 10^{-13}$ sec (0.1 ps).

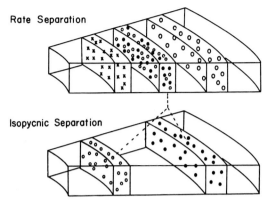

Fig. 1.5. *s*–*ρ* separation. Particles may be fractionated in a rate separation (upper drawing) and these fractions recentrifuged in a fresh, denser gradient to their equilibrium densities. In this way most particle mixtures can be resolved into homogeneous components.

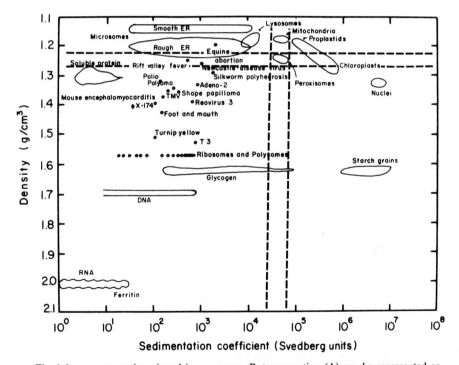

Fig. 1.6. *s*–*ρ* separation viewed in *s*–*ρ* space. Rate separation (A) can be represented as vertical slices of *s*–*ρ* space; isopycnic separation (B) as horizontal slices. The vertical slices curve toward larger values of *s* because the density factor in the equation for rate sedimentation becomes an increasingly important factor as the density of the medium approaches that of the particle (cf. Eq. 3.10).

long demanded chromatographic purity from their micromolecules and homogeneity from their macromolecules, apply similar standards to the larger subcellular assemblies.

Development as a Migration in s–ρ Space

It has long been known that glycogen is a heterogeneous polymer; it was widely assumed that such was one of the crosses to be borne by polymer

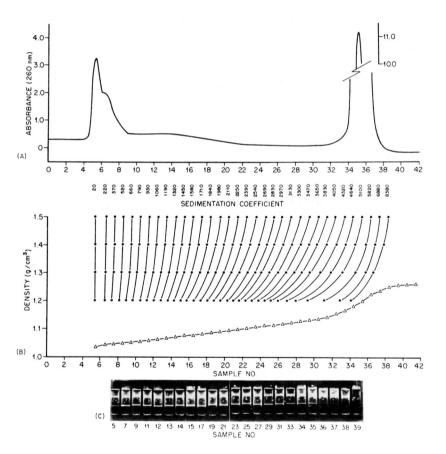

Fig. 1.7. *s–ρ* separation of glycogen (Barber *et al.*, 1966). (A) The absorbance profile of a crude preparation of glycogen from liver, (B) the observed density gradient (△) and a computer plot of the equivalent sedimentation coefficients of particles of different theoretical densities. For example, a particle of 1.6 which had migrated to fraction 36 would have an equivalent sedimentation coefficient of 5300 s. (C) A photograph of the fraction sedimented to equilibrium in CsCl. This shows that glycogen of widely varying *s* values has the same density.

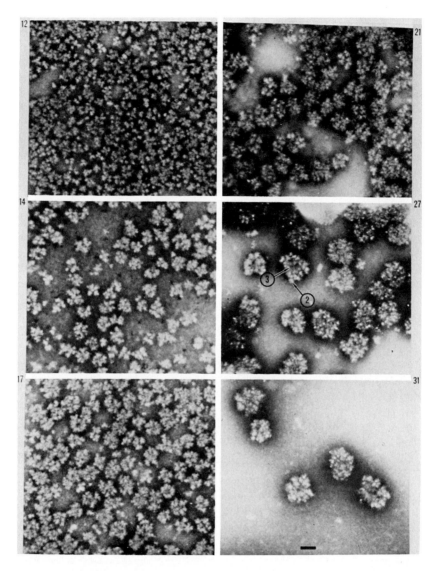

Fig. 1.8. Electron photomicrographs of glycogen fractionated by rate sedimentation (Barber *et al.*, 1966). Fractions 12 through 31 from Fig. 1.7 show progressively larger aggregations. The increasing equivalent sedimentation coefficients are therefore due to increasing particle size. Arrows labeled 2 and 3 in the photomicrograph of fraction 27 identify β and α particles, respectively, which are different aggregation states of glycogen.

chemists. When, however, the glycogen of rat liver was subjected to an $s-\rho$ analysis, the heterogeneity was seen to consist entirely in s; ρ was constant (Barber *et al.*, 1966).

It was then found that the rate fractions of glycogen corresponded to a graded and specific sequence of size and complexity (Figs. 1.7 and 1.8), and that the larger, more complex molecules were almost certainly derived from the smaller. As a macromolecule glycogen demonstrates a much more general phenomenon of particles such that the development of subcellular structures frequently can be followed as a change in their s and ρ coordinates; that is, particles "migrate" in $s-\rho$ space as precise and repeatable functions of their development.

We showed, for example, that yeast mitochondria, as they emerge from catabolite repression, follow changes in both size and density that correspond to ultrastructural changes (Neal *et al.*, 1971). The precision is such that one can select out particles at a specified stage of development from a population undergoing exponential or random growth. This type of analysis appears to be valid even though mitochondria obtained by cell disruption are almost certainly the fragments of much larger, lobed structures *in situ* (Hoffmann and Avers, 1973).

The general method of analyzing development from changes in s and ρ can also be fruitful at the level of whole cells (cf. Cartledge and Lloyd, 1972).

Density gradient centrifugation is worth a close look from several points of view: it is a striking chapter in the history of science; its fundamental principles can be deduced in a most satisfying manner from physical theory; and the art is complex but rewarding. We shall explore these several aspects in the remainder of this volume.

Immediately following is a list of general references: monographs and reviews on density gradient centrifugation which complement and supplement material presented in this volume.

REFERENCES

This list includes some general references not cited in the text.

Albertsson, P. -A. (1972). "Partition of Cell Particles and Macromolecules," 2nd ed. Wiley, New York.
Anderson, N. G. (1966). Zonal centrifuges and other separation systems. *Science* **154**, 103–112.
Anderson, N. G. (1968). Preparative particles separations in density gradients. *Q. Rev. Biophys.* **1**, 217–263.
Barber, A. A., Harris, W. W., and Anderson, N. G. (1966). Isolation of native glycogen by combined rate-zonal and isopycnic centrifugation. *Natl. Cancer Inst. Monog.* **21**, 285–302.
Birnie, G. D., ed. (1972). "Subcellular Components, Preparation, and Fractionation." Butterworth, London.

Brakke, M. K. (1960). Density gradient centrifugation and its application to plant viruses. *Adv. Virus Res.* **7,** 193–224.

Browning, P. M., compiler (1969). "Preparative Ultracentrifuge Applications." Beckman Instruments, Palo Alto, California.

Cartledge, T. G., and Lloyd, D. (1972). Subcellular fractionation by zonal centrifugation of glucose-repressed anaerobically grown *Saccharomyces carlsbergensis. Biochem. J.* **127,** 693–703.

Chervenka, C. H., and Elrod, L. H. (1972). "Manual of Methods for Large Scale Zonal Centrifugation." Beckman Instruments, Palo Alto, California.

de Duve, C., Berthet, J., and Beaufay, M. (1959). Gradient centrifugation of particles. Theory and applications. *Prog. Biophys. Biophys. Chem.* **9,** 325–369.

Hinton, R., and Dobrota, M. (1976). "Density Gradient Centrifugation." North-Holland Publ., Amsterdam.

Hoffman, H. -P., and Avers, C. J. (1973). Mitochondrion of yeast: Ultrastructural evidence for one giant, branched organelle per cell. *Science* **181,** 749–751.

Neal, W. K., II, Hoffman, H. -P., and Price, C. A. (1971). Sedimentation behavior and ultrastructure of mitochondria from repressed and derepressed yeast, Saccharomyces cerevisiae. *Plant Cell Physiol.* **12,** 181–192.

Schumaker, V. N. (1967). Zone centrifugation. *In Adv. Biol. Med. Phys.* **11,** 245–339.

Reid, E., ed. *Adv. Biol. Med. Phys.* **11,** 245–339. "Methodological Developments in Biochemistry," Vol. 3. Longmans, Green, New York.

Vinograd, J., and Hearst, J. E. (1962). Equilibrium sedimentation of macromolecules and viruses in a density gradient. *Fortschr. Chem. Org. Naturst.* **20,** 372–422.

2

Origins of Density Gradient Centrifugation

Bei kleinen Partikeln, wie sie bei der Zell- und Gewebetrennung in allgemeinen in Frage kommen, muss zentrifugiert werden, um einen Bestandteil in die Zone gleichen spezifischen Gewichtes zu bringen.

M. Behrens, 1938

Mention to a biochemist the terms ribosome, virus, membrane, or mitochondrion, and he will conjure images of multimolecular arrays articulating structure and function. Whether or not any one of these images is an accurate reflection of reality, collectively they have become a feature of growing importance in modern biochemistry.

Until about 1940, physical structure was regarded as appropriate enough to cytology, but rarely admitted to be proper to biochemistry. At the same time chemical composition had not been demonstrated to be of crucial significance to the understanding of classical cytology. The events that brought about the mutually profitable merger of biochemistry and cytology comprise an interesting chapter in the history of biology and led to the development of density gradient centrifugation.

As noted in Chapter 1, biochemistry was inspired and continues to be dominated by a captivating abstraction that organisms are collections of molecules. The promise of this idea has been that when the properties of all the molecules in an organism are understood then functions and behavior of the organism will be understood. This abstraction has served biology admirably; I am persuaded that most of those biological generalizations with real predictive value (as opposed to mere extensions of catalogs) derive from this single, broad abstraction. At the same time it has produced in biochemists a certain amount of rifle vision, if not downright arrogance. Until the early 1950s the criteria in classical organic chemistry which permitted molecules to be characterized applied exclusively to small molecules that could be brought into true solutions and purified by crystallization.

Thus, the professional disdain that inorganic chemists had earlier reserved for organic chemists was transferred to those who dared to work on such poorly characterized or characterizable entities as proteins and nucleic acids. The larger and less soluble the structure, the less attractive it appeared to biochemists.

On the other side cytologists during this period devoted themselves to what could be seen in the light microscope. They invoked thin sectioning, a myriad of stains, and ingenious optics, but the limit of resolution remained of the order of 0.1 μm, or two orders of magnitude larger than the largest molecule subject to detailed chemical analysis. In this state of the arts the cytologists were unable to visualize objects of acute interest to the biochemist, and the findings of biochemists contributed little to the understanding of cell structure. One can understand how it was that in 1940 neither discipline was of much significance to the other.

A few soldiers marched to a different drummer. Bensley (1943) throughout his long career was concerned with the compositional basis of cell structure. In 1934, Bensley and Hoerr announced the first isolation of mitochondria, although Warburg had separated them in 1913 under the term "respiring granules" (*atmende Körnchen*). Later studies (e.g., Hoerr, 1943) included some chemical characterization. Although Bensley, who was very influential among cytologists, legitimized a concern for the composition of subcellular structures, neither he nor any of his school created the paradigm needed to demonstrate the power of biochemical thinking in cytology. Part of the problem, as seen in retrospect, was that mitochondria prepared according to Bensley's recipe were neither sufficiently pure nor intact to manifest their unique role in respiration. Claude (1943; cf. also de Duve, 1971), with whom Bensley's group sparred desultorily, found succinic dehydrogenase in mitochondria, and declared them to be the "power plants" of the cell. As prophetic as this description was, it could be contested, because activities and components were distributed in an inconclusive manner between mitochondria, microsomes, and soluble fractions. Similarly, Mirsky and Pollister's historic report (1943) that deoxyribonucleoprotein was limited to nuclei was greeted with undisguised skepticism. Neither cytology nor biochemistry was ready to accept the idea of biochemical localization within the cell. To illustrate the paucity of interest in intracellular fractionation, the report of Mirsky and Pollister (1943) is only the third in the history of science to deal with isolated nuclei.*

In 1938, Granick published the results from his doctoral dissertation on the

---

* The first was Ackermann's (1904) isolation of nuclei from avian erythrocytes in a milk centrifuge and the second was Stoneburg's (1939) description of the method adopted by Mirsky and Pollister involving citric acid extraction.

isolation and composition of chloroplasts. In addition to his insistence on correspondence between the microscopic appearance of his isolated particles with that of chloroplasts *in situ*, Granick's report marked the first use of an osmoticum in the extraction medium (he recommended glucose or sucrose).* Menke (1939) had sought independently to isolate chloroplasts, but he had followed the procedure of his mentor Noack (1927), which started with the pressed sap of spinach. Without protection from the vacuolar sap, the chloroplasts were quickly denatured.

Despite these measured successes, the general indifference to intracellular fractionation might have continued for some time because biologists are, with few exceptions, intensely practical people. Neither theory nor rational appeal will displace them from their appointed laboratory routines as long as these continue faithfully to generate notebooks full of data. They wait for a paradigm, a model that demonstrates some principle with particular elegance; then hesitantly at first, but with a rush of enthusiasm as the paradigm's star brightens, they seek extensions and parallels to the new principle. Sumner's demonstration of the proteinaceous nature of urease guided the isolation of a hundred enzymes; the elucidation of glycolysis by Embden, Meyerhof, and Parnas implied all metabolic pathways; and Wendell Stanley's identification of TMV as a nucleoprotein foretold the story of virus isolation for 40 years to come.

Within the clutch of publications from Albert Claude,† his collaborators, and successors, one in particular set the course for the succeeding 20 years of intracellular fractionation. This was by Hogeboom *et al.* (1948). The thesis that mitochondria contain succinic dehydrogenase and cytochrome oxidase had been stated before, but for the first time, the three authors brought to bear three sets of criteria to prove their case: (1) enzymological, in that the enzyme assays be enzyme limited, (2) chemical, in that the quantities in the cell brei be recovered among the individual fractions, and (3) cytological, in that the separated mitochondria show all of the classical properties, including reversible staining with Janus Green B. A nontrivial ingredient in the success of Hogeboom *et al.* was their adoption of Granick's strategem of employing sucrose as an osmoticum to stabilize the organelles.

The paradigm that emerged was simple and immensely attractive: mitochondria are the principal if not the sole loci of the enzymes of electron

---

* It is curious how many historic developments started (and stalled) with plant material. In the subject at hand the earliest studies on the effects of centrifugal fields on subcellular structures were on plants (Mottier, 1899; Andrews, 1903) as was the first use of centrifuges with living organisms (Knight, 1806).

† Although Claude's specific findings were of relatively transitory significance, the Nobel Prize Committee in 1974 identified Claude as the fountainhead for the new paradigm of organelles.

transport and they can be isolated intact and functioning from the cell. The fractionation scheme of Hogeboom *et al.*, shown in Fig. 2.1, produced fractions that we now know to be grossly impure, but the power of their paradigm was sufficient that this same scheme with minimal variations remains the standard to the present day.

The success of the mitochondrial paradigm was due in no small part to

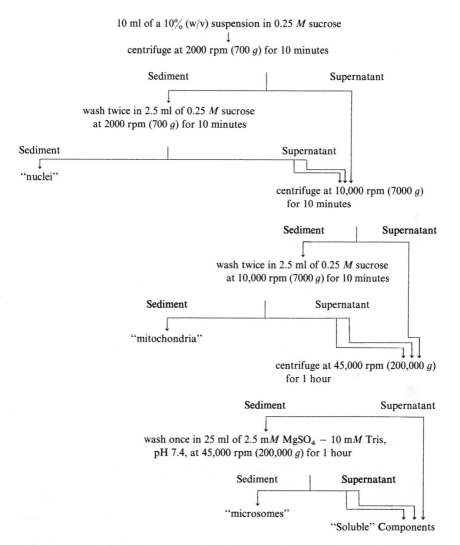

Fig. 2.1. A scheme of cell fractionation adopted by Hogeboom and Schneider for the separation of particles from rat liver (adapted from Schneider, 1972).

the other idols of the time: Krebs had just completed his masterful proof that the citric acid cycle accounted almost wholly for the oxidative consumption of pyruvate in minced pigeon breast muscle; Keilin's scheme of electron transport among the cytochromes was being latched firmly to the web of oxidative dehydrogenation; and Lipman's ATP had surfaced as the universal unit of energy currency and had been demonstrated to be formed in tandem with respiration. What a convergence of vital functions to be found packaged in a single structure! Ironically, Hogeboom and Schneider, hewing carefully to their insistence that all cell fractions be examined before judgment be passed on enzyme localization (cf. Hogeboom et al., 1953), were skeptical that the citric acid cycle was limited to the mitochondria. It was Green (1952), a latter-day convert from "cyclophorase," who claimed this activity for mitochondria, along with most of the metabolism of the cell. With pauline enthusiasm, Green also derided claims for other organelle systems; microsomes were dismissed as "comminuted mitochondria."

The discovery of mitochondria by biochemists had profound consequences. The simplistic model of the cell as a bag full of enzymes was banished forever. (It had hardly ever been more than a strawman for the antireductionists.) More positively, biochemists saw the possibilities of studying enzyme systems in fixed physical arrays on or within membranes; the remarkable efficiency of energy conversions in respiration could now be examined as phenomena in the solid state or at least two-dimensional state. More generally, parallels to the mitochondrial paradigm could be sought in all areas of metabolism; perhaps every segment of metabolism was physically compartmented. If there is an organelle for respiration, and one for photosynthesis, there could be one for the synthesis of lipids, proteins, etc. Biochemistry would never again be the same.

Meanwhile, two additional developments in the late 1940s and 1950s served to bring the studies of structure, composition, and function closer together and to loosen the continuing domination of biochemistry by the abstractions and methodology of organic chemistry.

The first was the steady progress in the physical characterization of macromolecules at first by sedimentation and electrophoresis and later by molecular exclusion (gel filtration), X-ray diffraction, optical rotatory dispersion, and light scattering. Sanger's brilliant solution in 1952 to the problem of deciphering the primary amino acid sequences of proteins gained chemical legitimacy to macromolecules, but even apart from the sequencing of macromolecules, biological progress permitted one to characterize discrete particles weighing many millions of atomic mass units and measuring tens of nanometers in diameter.

The second event was the development of electron microscopy. Almost at one stroke the limit of resolution was lowered two orders of magnitude.

Mitochondria were no longer merely small blobs that turned from green to red in Janus Green B, but had a striking and unique ultrastructure (Palade, 1953). Membranes were seen to consist typically of three layers, each on the order of 3 nm thick. Virus particles could be seen and their internal structure described. Controversy would continue over what was fact and what was artifact, but the significance of these twin developments was that from the early 1950s on, macro- and multimolecules could be studied and characterized at every level from slices of the intact cell to that of homogeneous solutions. Cytology, biophysics, and biochemistry had become part of a biological continuum.

Differential Centrifugation and a Need for Something Better

The scheme of cell fractionation adopted by Hogeboom and Schneider is straightforward differential centrifugation (Fig. 2.1). As such it has the advantages of simplicity and large capacity and the disadvantage of poor resolution. Although differential centrifugation can measure sedimentation rates with surprising precision (Anderson, 1968; Schumaker and Rees, 1969), one can separate particles cleanly only when they sediment at rates differing by at least a factor of 10. The reason for this is illustrated in Fig. 1.1 (p. 3). In order to obtain a firm pellet of large particles including those that are initially at the top of the tube, one must centrifuge long and hard enough to pellet smaller particles that are initially near the bottom of the tube.

Although differential centrifugation produced only crude organelle fractions, few workers concerned themselves with fundamental improvements in resolution. First, the method can provide multigram quantities of the major cell organelles. Second, most biochemists were unaware of or indifferent to the purity of their material. Because of the 50-year accumulation of professional idols, biochemists were unprepared to adopt morphological criteria of identification or purity; they were not suddenly to begin looking through microscopes. Consequently a curious inversion occurred: organelles came to be identified primarily by their enzymatic activities or chemical composition; mitochondria became a centrifugal fraction with cytochrome oxidase activity or, better, oxidative phosphorylation; chloroplasts were particles centrifuged at low speed and contained chlorophyll; and ribosomes, for which biochemists at least had the priorities of discovery, were named after their content of RNA.

It was and is a practical and largely consistent system, but the failure of many biochemists not to demand the same standards in preparations of organelles that they routinely applied to micro- and macromolecules, and their failure to combine their talents and resources with those of cytologists led to a number of missteps and misconceptions. With the benefit of hindsight, we see that the method of preparing chloroplasts by differential centrifugation in saline solutions, a standard procedure through the 1950s, despite Granick's clear example (1938) to the contrary, yields particles which are green and 5–15 μm in diameter; unfortunately, after several pelletings they are not chloroplasts but rather the lamellae or internal membranes of chloroplasts and largely devoid of the soluble proteins and ribosomes normally present (Jacobi and Perner, 1961). Again, the activities of catalase and α-hydroxyacid oxidases, originally ascribed to mitochondria and chloroplasts, are in fact due to peroxisomes, particles of comparable size but distinguishable in ultrastructure and separable by their different densities.

From the beginning of the era of cell fractionation there were, of course, the "lumpers" and the "splitters,*" but until the early 1950s biochemists found no difficulty in explaining away reports of heterogeneity. Then Novikoff *et al.* (1953), using unexceptionable methods, showed that the activities of succinic dehydrogenase, uricase, phosphatase, and esterase were sedimented from a cell brei at overlapping but measurably different rates. The prospect of heterogeniety within the mitochondrial fraction, the possibility that their might be a multiplicity of organelles with different enzyme complements and different functions, stirred several laboratories to seek something better than differential centrifugation. Several groups (Wilbur and Anderson, 1951) experimented with centrifuging a layer of cell brei through an underlying dense layer of sucrose (Fig. 2.2A) but the strategem was successful only when the underlay was sufficiently dense to float contaminating particles. Otherwise, as Brakke (1951) observed, the sediment will contain a complete mixture of particles. He noted that parts of the overlaid sample are carried to the bottom of the tube by a curious phenomenon, which he called droplet sedimentation (cf. Fig. 2.2B,C). We shall return to this in Section 3.2.4. Instead Brakke (1951) proposed the following.

> A thin layer of the suspension to be fractionated is floated on a solution having a density gradient. If the suspended particles sediment ideally, i.e., as discrete entities, during subsequent centrifugation, those of each sedimentation rate will travel down the tube as a separate zone. Centrifugation may be continued until the particles reach density equilibria, yielding a separation dependent on particle density only. If centrifugation is stopped earlier, a separation dependent on the sedimentation rates of the particles may be obtained. Theoretically, the latter variation should have the higher resolving power since for two particles to have the same sedimentation rates throughout a tube with a density gradient, their densities and ratios of mass to frictional constant must be identical. In addition to the density gradient, aqueous systems will usually have an osmotic pressure gradient. Then for two particles to sediment at the same rate throughout the tube they must not only fulfill the above criteria, but must also change hydration at the same rate with changing osmotic pressure.

---

* In 1947, Chantrenne inferred a continuum of particle types from the spread of enzyme activities among centrifugal fractions.

Time of Centrifugation →

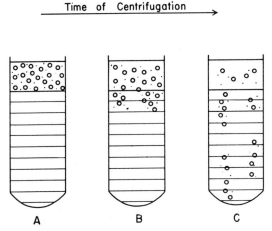

A   B   C

Fig. 2.2. Sedimentation through a discontinuous gradient. When a suspension of particles in a light medium is layered over a uniform, denser medium, the system is initially stable (A), but over the course of time droplets begin to descend into the denser medium (B and C). Following centrifugation the sediment will contain a mixture of all of the particles in the original suspension.

In this single, remarkable paragraph Brakke succinctly described the principles that were to guide a decade of development in density gradient centrifugation. Brakke himself (1953 *et seq.*) continued to demonstrate the utility of rate zonal sedimentation in the purification and characterization of viruses.

Actually, Brakke was first to describe rate zonal separations. Isopycnic separations, the other principal kind of density gradient centrifugation, were first employed by Behrens (1938) in his studies on nonaqueous methods of cell fractionation. Again, Vallee *et al.* (1947) described how leukocytes could be separated from whole blood in a step gradient of albumin. Even earlier, the Harvey's had used density gradients in their classical studies on centrifugal stratification of the eggs of marine invertebrates (Harvey, 1932). Brakke (1951) and Kahler and Lloyd (1951), who independently described isopycnic separations, were either unaware of the earlier work or did not recognize that the principles were identical.

Thomson and Mikuta (1954) and Thomson and Moss (1956), applying Brakke's method to the problem of heterogeneity of the mitochondrial fraction, converted sedimentation rates to equivalent radii of ideal spheres. They found, in elegant support of Novikoff *et al.* (1953), that succinic dehydrogenase particles sedimented as if they were three times as large as uricase particles. A group from the Carlsberg laboratories reported both rate (Ottesen and Weber, 1955) and density (Holter *et al.*, 1953) heterogeneity within the mitochondrial fraction.

However, for reasons which have still not been completely sorted out (cf. Sections 3.2.1, 3.2.2), rate zonal separations of particles of mitochondrial size were never very satisfactory in either angle rotors or in swinging-bucket rotors. Each experiment was something of a *tour de force*, separations were only marginal, and the yields were quite inadequate for biochemical characterization of the recovered particles.

Isopycnic separations were distinctly better and for many years density gradient centrifugation was commonly assumed to mean isopycnic separation. Schneider and Kuff (1954) reported the isopycnic separation of Golgi bodies, and Kuff and Schneider (1954) showed that the heterogeneity of enzymatic activities within the mitochondrial fraction also corresponded to density differences.

The happy ending to the chapter on mitochondrial heterogeneity was provided by de Duve and his group at Louvain. De Duve declared (1963) that the acid hydrolases were contained in a membrane-bound particle to be called *lysosomes*. This concept was enormously successful in organizing a growing body of data and has subsequently proven to have substantial predictive value. A second class of organelles with catalase and α-hydroxy-acid oxidase activities was subsequently dissected out of the mitochondrial fraction and named *peroxisomes* (de Duve and Baudhuin, 1966); this concept is proving equally successful.

De Duve and his group ultimately became strong champions of density gradient centrifugation and contributed substantially to its theoretical development (de Duve *et al.*, 1959).

It must not be thought that the development of density gradient centrifugation proceeded linearly from the clear directions provided by Brakke (1951). For one thing, high-speed, swinging-bucket rotors and centrifuges to drive them were not widely available; the revolutionary SW-39 rotor capable of centrifuging three 4-cm^3 tubes at 39,000 rpm was introduced by Spinco in 1953 (Hogeboom and Kuff, 1954). Other technical impediments included a general innocence of means for the construction of gradients and of the recovery of gradients from tubes.

Perhaps equally important was the existence of a collateral principle of density gradient centrifugation, one highly regarded by the cognoscenti, but virtually unknown today. It originated with Pickels (1943), but its roots lay with the analytical ultracentrifuge, which had been developed a generation earlier by Svedberg. In the analytical ultracentrifuge sedimentation is followed optically as a moving boundary (Fig. 2.3). Although molecular species could be characterized by their sedimentation velocity, there was no provision for physical recovery of separated species, nor was there any means of detecting species in dilute or complex mixtures.

Pickels (1943) asked if one could obtain sedimentation analysis in pre-

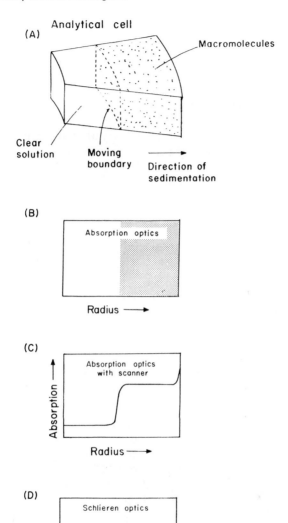

Fig. 2.3. Moving boundary analysis in the analytical ultracentrifuge. (A) The centrifuge cell, initially filled with a uniform suspension of a macromolecule. During centrifugation the particles sediment toward the edge of the cell, leaving a particle-free solution. The distribution of particles may be observed with absorption optics (B and C) or schlieren optics (D), which detects the change in refractive index at the moving boundary.

parative centrifuges, where one could hope to identify sedimenting species by performing chemical and biochemical analyses on the separated zones. Because the only high-speed rotors then available were angle rotors, Pickels had to contend with rather complex fluid dynamics including centrifugal movement of particles, the movement of particle-rich solvent downward along the outer wall of the centrifuge tube, and the convective backflow of particle-poor solvent upward along the inner wall (Fig. 2.4). In the course of his studies Pickels observed that concentrated, but not dilute solutions of proteins maintained a stable boundary during sedimentation. He reasoned that the concentration gradient formed by the moving boundary corresponded to a density gradient and, in the case of concentrated solutions, the

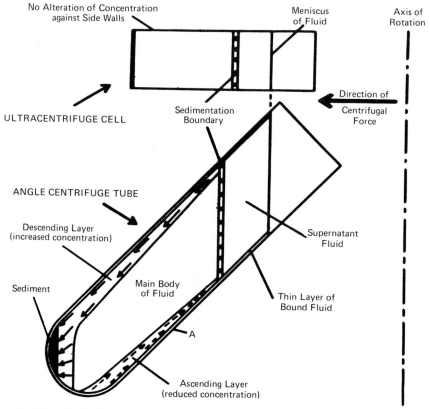

Fig. 2.4. Moving boundary sedimentation in angle rotors. Pickels (1952) visualized that the sedimentation boundary of particles moved in angle rotors very much as in the cell of the ultracentrifuge, except that a circulation of particle-rich fluid down the outer wall and of particle-poor fluid up the inner wall perturbed the boundary.

density gradient was sufficient to counteract convective forces. He confirmed this by stabilizing dilute solutions with an imposed density gradient of sucrose (Fig. 2.5).

Pickels had substantial scientific influence,* so that his strategem for stabilizing sedimenting systems was rather widely (and successfully) employed (Schlesinger, 1950; Kahler and Lloyd, 1951; Hogeboom and Kuff, 1954; Kuff *et al.*, 1956). Although Pickels' gradients are really a modification and improvement over conventional differential centrifugation, and are correspondingly inferior in resolution to rate–zonal centrifugation, they do represent an interesting historical link with analytical centrifugation. The thread, moreover, continues to the present day in analytical differential centrifugation (Anderson, 1968; Schumaker and Rees, 1969).

The evolution of density gradient centrifugation set in motion by both Pickels and Braake was inspired by the hope that preparative centrifugation could physically separate particles with the same resolution as one could see in the analytical cell, but by the mid-1950s it became evident that density gradient centrifugation was in principle superior to the moving boundary method employed in the analytical ultracentrifuge. One important factor was that interaction among different particle populations, which was known to affect sedimentation rates, was eliminated as soon as particle zones were separated from one another.

Moreover, swinging-bucket rotors became larger and faster. A photograph of one of the modern rotors is shown in Fig. 2.6.

Meselson *et al.* (1957) at Caltech repaid part of the debt to the analytical ultracentrifuge by demonstrating separations on the basis of density in the analytical cell. Their method (cf. Sections 5.3 and 8.2.3) consists of allowing the solute–solvent system to reach an equilibrium of sedimentation and diffusion over an interval of several days. Within the dimensions of the analytical cell such an equilibrium distribution will correspond to a linear density gradient. Macromolecules within the system will seek narrow Gaussian distributions about their own equilibrium densities. This procedure has proven enormously valuable in the characterization of DNA in gradients of CsCl.

The balance of the debt was repaid by the same laboratory in 1963, when Vinograd *et al.*, devised the technical means and part of the supporting theory to measure rate–zonal centrifugation in the analytical cell.

Thus by 1960 density gradient centrifugation had come of age. It had become firmly established in the biological armamentarium for both prepara-

* Following a fruitful career at the Rockefeller Institute, he founded Spinco (Specialized Instruments Corporation, now a division of Beckman Instruments). The Model E and L ultracentrifuges were principally his design (Pickels, 1952).

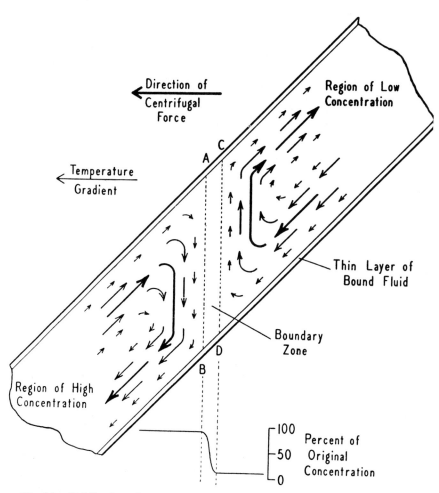

Fig. 2.5. Stabilization of a moving boundary by imposition of a step gradient of sucrose (Pickels, 1952). Pickels proposed that a step gradient of sucrose, imposed on an otherwise uniform suspension of particles, would restrict convective movements to each region of uniform density and thus stabilize the movement of a sedimenting boundary. A continuous density gradient would stabilize the boundary throughout the tube.

tion and analysis and its technical and theoretical limitations, many and severe, were soon to be swept away.

Development of zonal centrifuges. Anderson (1956) of the Oak Ridge National Laboratories published a searching critique of problems of subcellular fractionation. A man of catholic biological interests, Anderson brought to biology an exceptional appreciation of physical and engineering

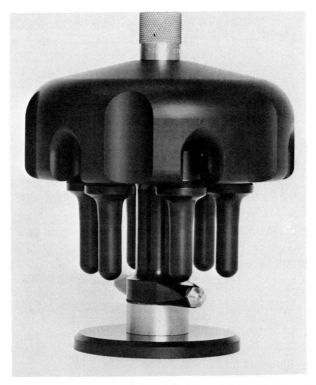

Fig. 2.6.   The SW 56 Ti swinging-bucket rotor (Spinco Division/Beckman Instruments). This rotor will swing six 4-ml tubes at a speed of 56,000 rpm.

principles. Almost uniquely among his colleagues he perceived that the string-and-beeswax tradition of biological research was at best a quaint virtue and at worst an inexcusable waste of talent in an era when electronics, computers, and modern metallurgy offered such brave, new promises.

For several years Anderson (1955, 1956) occupied himself with some of the first direct analyses of the sedimentation behavior of particles in the preparative centrifuge. Convinced that only density gradient centrifugation would provide the resolution sufficient for the separation of pure, intact subcellular particles, Anderson identified the conventional centrifuge tube as the principal villain: it was too small, and it invited wall effects.

In 1962, Anderson described the design of a radically new rotor, the zonal rotor. In effect, the lateral walls of a swinging-bucket tube are extended through 2π to form a bowl or cylinder (Fig. 2.7). The replacement of lateral walls with incomplete, radial septa minimizes the adverse effects of walls on resolution and, in addition, stress analysis of cylinders rotating on their

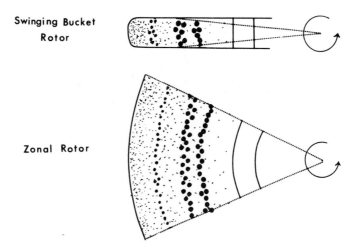

Fig. 2.7. Evolution from swinging-bucket to zonal rotors. The zonal rotor may be thought of as a tube in which the lateral walls extended through 360°.

axes offers more than tenfold increases in volume for a given speed as compared to swinging buckets (Table 2.1).

The most critical problem was in assuring a means for filling and emptying the rotor. The solution came in the design of a two-way fluid seal (Fig. 2.8 and 2.9). A current zonal rotor is shown in Fig. 2.10.

The subsequent evolution of zonal rotors, most of it in Anderson's laboratories, has led to rotor systems that are no more complicated to operate

Table 2.1. **Comparison of Speeds and Volumes of Some Swinging-Bucket and Zonal Rotors**[a]

Rotor type	Speed (rpm)	g^{max}	Volume (cm³)
HL 8[b] swinging bucket	3,700	3,720	8 × 100
Z-8[c] zonal	8,000	9,000	1,250
SW 27[d] swinging bucket	27,000	131,000	6 × 38.5
B-29[c] zonal	35,000	121,100	1,670
SW 41 Ti[d] swinging bucket	41,000	286,000	6 × 13
B-30[c] zonal	50,000	186,500	659
SW 65L Ti[d] swinging bucket	65,000	420,000	3 × 5

[a] More complete lists of the properties of these rotors are presented in Tables 6.1 and 6.2.
[b] Ivan Sorvall/Du Pont.
[c] IEC/Damon.
[d] Spinco/Beckman.

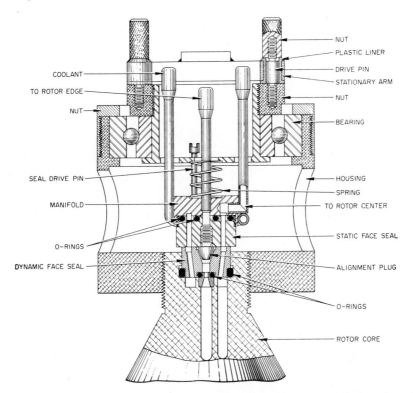

Fig. 2.8. A-type seal for zonal rotors (Oak Ridge National Laboratories). A static seal made of chrome-plated steel contains an axial and peripheral channel; it fits into a rotating seal of rulon.

than swinging-bucket rotors, run at speeds suitable to the separation of particles ranging in size from whole cells to macromolecules, in quantities up to many grams, and with resolution not inferior to that obtained with swinging buckets.

Design of gradients.   Prior to 1960, density gradients were invoked in rate separations to stabilize the movement of particle zones against convection; in this sense they played a passive role. Several workers (Kuff *et al.*, 1956; Thomson and Mikuta, 1954) employed complicated and admittedly inexact formulas to relate sedimentation rates to some kind of idealized sedimentation coefficients, but in 1959, Harrison and Nixon turned the tables and described a gradient in which sedimentation rate was independent of the distance migrated. Martin and Ames (1961) devised a similar gradient shape in which the enzymes catalyzing steps in the tryptophan pathway migrated in approximate proportion to their sedimentation coefficients.

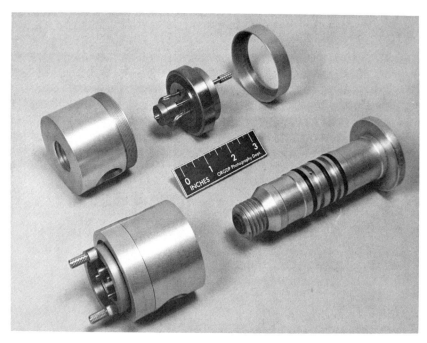

Fig. 2.9. A-type seal disassembled (Oak Ridge National Laboratories).

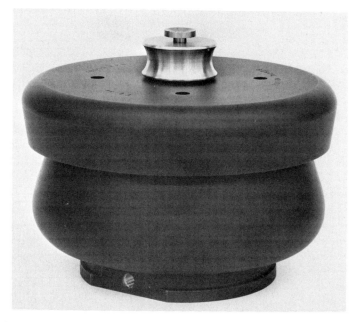

Fig. 2.10. The B-XV type of zonal rotor (Spinco Division/Beckman Instruments). The Ti 15 will spin 1675 ml at 32,000 rpm.

De Duve *et al.* (1959) had also proposed a similar tactic. This important principle, evidently discovered independently by three groups, was important in that the shape of the gradient (in this case a simple exponential) was employed to optimize the behavior of particle zones. Later Noll (1967) formalized the tactic with a whole family of gradient shapes, which he called isokinetic (cf. Section 3.2.3).

The idea of exploiting the shape of gradients prospered and led to gradients with improved capacity and resolution (Berman, 1966; Spragg and Rankin, 1967; Schumaker, 1966; Eikenberry *et al.*, 1970; Spragg *et al.*, 1969; Pollack and Price, 1971). The quest for theoretical models that will yield advantageous gradient shapes remains one of the strong contemporary trends in the field.

REFERENCES

Ackermann, D. (1904). Zur Chemie der Vogelblutkerne. *Hoppe-Seyler's Z. Physiol. Chem.* **43**, 299–304.

Anderson, N. G. (1955). Brei fractionation. *Science* **121**, 775–776.

Anderson, N. G. (1956). *Phys. Tech. Biol. Res.* **3**, 299–352.

Anderson, N. G. (1962). The zonal ultracentrifuge. A new instrument for fractionating mixtures of particles. *J. Phys. Chem.* **66**, 1984–1989.

Anderson, N. G. (1968). Analytical techniques for cell fractions. VIII. Analytical differential centrifugation in angle-head rotors. *Anal. Biochem.* **23**, 72–83.

Andrews, F. M. (1903). Die Wirkung der Zentrifugalkraft auf Pflanzen. *Jahrb. Wiss. Bot.* **38**, 1–40.

Behrens, M., (1938). Zell-und Gewebetrennung. *In* "Handbuch der biologischen Arbeitsmethoden" (E. Abderhalden, ed.), Vol. V (10-II), pp. 1363–1392. Urban u. Schwarzenberg, Munich.

Bensley, R. R. (1943). Chemical structure of cytoplasm. *Biol. Symp.* **10**, 323–334.

Bensley, R. R., and Hoerr, N. L. (1934). Studies on cell structure by the freezing-drying method. VI. The preparation and properties of mitochondria. *Anat. Rec.* **60**, 449–455.

Berman, A. (1966). Theory of centrifugation: Miscellaneous studies. *Natl. Cancer Inst. Monogr.* **21**, 41–76.

Brakke, M. K. (1951). Density gradient centrifugation: A new separation technique. *J. Am. Chem. Soc.* **73**, 1847–1848.

Brakke, M. K. (1953). Zonal separations by density-gradient centrifugation. *Arch. Biochem. Biophys.* **45**, 275–290.

Chantrenne, H. (1947). The heterogeneity of the cytoplasmic granules of mouse liver. *Biochim. Biophys. Acta* **1**, 437–438.

Claude, A. (1943). Distribution of nucleic acids in the cell and the morphological constitution of cytoplasm. *Biol. Symp.* **10**, 111–129.

de Duve, C. (1963). The separation and characterization of subcellular particles. *Harvey Lect.* **59**, 49–87.

de Duve, C. (1971). Tissue fractionation: Past and present. *J. Cell Biol.* **50**, 20D–55D.

de Duve, C., and Baudhuin, P. (1966). Peroxisomes (microbodies and related particles). *Physiol. Rev.* **46**, 323–357.

de Duve, C., Berthet, J., and Beaufay, H. (1959). Gradient centrifugation of cell particles. Theory and applications. *Prog. Biophys. Biophys. Chem.* **9**, 325–369.

Eikenberry, E. F., Bickle, T. A., Traut, R. R., and Price, C. A. (1970). Separation of large quantities of ribosomal subunits by zonal ultracentrifugation. *Eur. J. Biochem.* **12**, 113–116.

Granick, S. (1938). Quantitative isolation of chloroplasts from higher plants. *Am. J. Bot.* **25**, 558–561.

Green, D. E. (1952). Organized enzyme systems. *J. Cell Comp. Physiol.* **39**, Suppl. 2, 75–111.

Harrison, B. D., and Nixon, H. L. (1959). Separation and properties of particles of tobacco rattle virus (potato stem mottle virus) with different lengths. *J. Gen. Microbiol.* **21**, 569–581.

Harvey, E. B. (1932). The development of half and quarter eggs of Arbacia puntulata and of strongly centrifuged whole eggs. *Biol. Bull.* (*Woods Hole, Mass.*) **62**, 155–167.

Hoerr, N. L. (1943). Methods of isolation of morphological constituents of the liver cell. *Biol. Symp.* **10**, 185–231.

Hogeboom, G. H., and Kuff, E. L. (1954). Sedimentation behavior of proteins and other materials in a horizontal preparative rotor. *J. Biol. Chem.* **210**, 733–751.

Hogeboom, G. H., Schneider, W. C., and Palade, G. E. (1948). Cytochemical studies of mammalian tissues. I. Isolation of intact mitochondria from rat liver: Some biochemical properties of mitochondria and submicroscopic particulate material. *J. Biol. Chem.* **172**, 619–636.

Hogeboom, G. H., Schneider, W. C., and Striebich, M. J. (1953). Localization and integration of cellular function. *Cancer Res.* **13**, 617–632.

Holter, H., Ottesen, M., and Weber, R. (1953). Separation of cytoplasmic particles by centrifugation in a density gradient. *Experientia* **9**, 346–348.

Jacobi, G., and Perner, E. (1961). Strukturelle und biochemische Probleme der Chloroplastenisolierung. *Flora* (*Jena*) **150**, 209–226.

Kahler, H., and Lloyd, B., Jr. (1951). Sedimentation of polystyrene latex in a swinging-tube rotor. *J. Phys. Colloid Chem.* **55**, 1344–1350.

Knight, T. A. (1806). On the direction of the radicle and germen during the vegetation of seeds. *Philos. Trans. R. Soc. London* **99**, Part I, 218–220 (abstr.).

Kuff, E. L., and Schneider, W. C. (1954). Intracellular distribution of enzymes. XII. Biochemical heterogeneity of mitochondria. *J. Biol. Chem.* **206**, 277–685.

Kuff, E. L., Hogeboom, G. H., and Dalton, A. J. (1956). Centrifugal, biochemical and electron microscopic analysis of cytoplasmic particulates in liver homogenates. *J. Biophys. Biochem. Cytol.* **2**, 33–53.

Martin, R. G., and Ames, B. N. (1961). A method for determining the sedimentation behavior of enzymes: Application to protein mixtures. *J. Biol. Chem.* **236**, 1372–1379.

Menke, S. W. (1939). Untersuchungen über das Protoplasma grüner Pflanzenzellen. I. Isolieruug von Chloroplasten aus Spinatblättern. *Hoppe-Seyler's Z. Physiol. Chem.* **257**, 43–48.

Meselson, M., Stahl, F. W., and Vinograd, J. (1957). Equilibrium sedimentation of macromolecules in density gradients. *Proc. Natl. Acad. Sci. U.S.A.* **43**, 581–588.

Mirsky, A. E., and Pollister, A. W. (1943). Fibrous nucleoproteins of chromatin. *Biol. Symp.* **10**, 247–260.

Mottier, D. M. (1899). The effect of centrifugal force upon the cell. *Ann. Bot.* (*London*) **13**, 325–363.

Noack, K. (1927). Der Zustand des Chlorophylls in der lebenden Pflanzen. *Biochem. Z.* **183**, 135–152.

Noll, H. (1967). Characterization of macromolecules by constant velocity sedimentation. *Nature* (*London*) **215**, 360–363.

Novikoff, A., Podber, E., Ryan, J., and Noe, E. (1953). Biochemical heterogeneity of the cytoplasmic particles isolated from rat liver homogenate. *J. Histochem. Cytochem.* **1,** 27–46.

Ottesen, M., and Weber, R. (1955). Density-gradient centrifugation as a means of separating cytoplasmic particles. *C. R. Trav. Lab. Carlsberg* **29,** 417–434.

Palade, G. E. (1953). An electron microscope study of the mitochondrial structure. *J. Histochem. Cytochem.* **1,** 188–211.

Pickels, E. G. (1943). Sedimentation in the angle centrifuge. *J. Gen. Physiol.* **23,** 341–360.

Pickels, E. G. (1952). Ultracentrifugation. *Methods Med. Res.* **5,** 107–113.

Pollack, M. S., and Price, C. A. (1971). Equivolumetric gradients for zonal rotors: Separation of ribosomes. *Anal. Biochem.* **42,** 38–47.

Schlesinger, R. W. (1950). Incomplete growth cycle of influenza virus in mouse brain. *Proc. Soc. Exp. Biol. Med.* **74,** 541–548.

Schneider, W. C. (1972). Methods for the isolation of particulate components of the cell. *In* Manometric and Biochemical Techniques" (W. W. Umbreit, R. H. Burris, and J. F. Stauffer, eds.), 5th ed., pp. 196–212. Burgess Publ., Minneapolis, Minnesota.

Schneider, W. C., and Kuff, E. L. (1954). On the isolation and some biochemical properties of the Golgi substance. *Am. J. Anat.* **94,** 209–224.

Schumaker, V. N. (1966). Limiting law for boundary spreading in zone centrifugation. *Sep. Sci.* **1,** 409–411.

Schumaker, V. N., and Rees, A. (1969). Theory of different centrifugation in angle-head rotors. *Anal. Biochem.* **31,** 279–285.

Spragg, S. P., and Rankin, C. T., Jr. (1967). The capacity of zones in density gradient centrifugation. *Biochim. Biophys. Acta* **141,** 164–173.

Spragg, S. P., Morrod, R. S., and Rankin, C. T., Jr. (1969). The optimization of density gradients for zonal centrifugation. *Sep. Sci.* **4,** 467–481.

Stoneburg, C. A. (1939). Lipids of the cell nuclei. *J. Biol. Chem.* **129,** 189–196.

Thomson, J. F., and Mikuta, E. T. (1954). Enzymatic activity of cytoplasmic particulates of rat liver isolated by gradient centrifugation. *Arch. Biochem. Biophys.* **51,** 487–498.

Thomson, J. F., and Moss, E. M. (1956). The intracellular distribution of a bound acid phosphatase of rat liver as studied by gradient centrifugation. *Arch. Biochem. Biophys.* **61,** 456–460.

Vallee, B. L., Hughes, W. L., and Gibson, J. G. (1947). A method for the separation of leukocytes from whole blood by flotation on serum albumin. *Blood* **1,** 82–87.

Vinograd, J., Bruner, R., Kent, R., and Weigle, J. (1963). Band-centrifugation of macromolecules and viruses in self-generating density gradients. *Proc. Natl. Acad. Sci. U.S.A.* **49,** 902–910.

Warburg, O. (1913). Über sauerstoffatmende Körnchen aus Leberzelle und über Sauerstoffatmung in Berkefeld-Filtraten wässriger Lebenextracte. *Pfluegers' Arch. Gesamte Physiol. Menschen Tiere* **154,** 599–617.

Wilbur, K. M., and Anderson, N. G. (1951). Studies on isolated cell components. I. Nuclear isolation by differential centrifugation. *Exp. Cell Res.* **2,** 47–57.

3

Sedimentation Theory:
A Semiquantitative Approach

3.1 BEHAVIOR OF PARTICLES IN CENTRIFUGAL FIELDS

We shall examine the factors controlling the behavior of particles in centrifugal fields, first in analogy with gravitational fields. We shall then develop the basic equations of sedimentation.

3.1.1 Analogy with Gravitational Fields

We are accustomed to living in a gravitational field. At all points near the surface of the earth, objects experience a downward acceleration of $1\ g$, which is equal to 980 cm/sec^2.

A centrifugal field is similar to a gravitational field; however, its intensity may be thousands of times greater. In a modern centrifuge the magnitude of this field is under our control. To a particle the two fields are qualitatively indistinguishable,* and one may usefully compare the behavior of particles in centrifuges to those in simple gravitational fields.

The centrifugal field F experienced by an object is a function of the distance from the axis of rotation r and the angular velocity ω.

$$F = r\omega^2 \tag{3.1}$$

If r is in cm and ω in radians† per second, F will be in cm/sec^2, which is exactly

---

* Pilots caught in a tailspin at night may be totally unaware of the spin unless they happen to observe the wild gyrations of their instruments.

† A radian is $1/2\pi$ of a circle. The speed of a centrifuge is usually reported in revolutions per minute (rpm); so that radians/sec = rpm $\cdot\ \pi/30$. Therefore, 78 rpm = 8.17 radian/sec.

comparable to the units of acceleration due to gravity. Equation (3.1) may be used to calculate the centrifugal field on a particle of dust 14.7 cm from the center of a phonograph disk turning at 78 rpm (Fig. 3.1)

$$F = 14.7 \text{ cm} \left[\frac{78\pi \text{ radians}}{30 \text{ sec}} \right]^2 = 980 \text{ cm/sec}^2 = 1 \, g$$

In this example the particle will indeed experience an acceleration of $1 \, g$ toward the edge of the record, but it will probably not move. Resistive forces (friction or electric charges) hold the particle in place.

A useful general equation relating the centrifugal field* measured in gravities to the rotational speed and distance from the axis of rotation is

$$F_g = 1.118 \times 10^{-5} r_{cm} (\text{rpm})^2 \qquad (3.2)$$

Before exploring centrifugal fields further, let us consider some examples of particles moving in a gravitational field: Galileo's weights falling from the tower of Pisa, snowflakes drifting lightly in still air, and finely divided silt settling out of a river. These objects are all subject to the same acceleration, although their velocities may differ by orders of magnitude. We recognize that the differing rates of sedimentation in the three systems are attributable to different effects of friction and buoyancy in the medium.

Galileo determined that the velocity of v of the weights falling from the

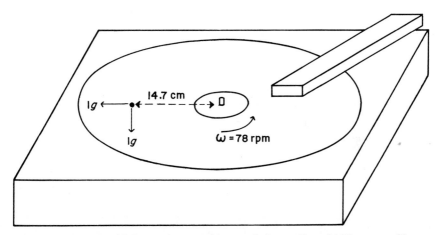

Fig. 3.1. Centrifugal field on phonographic record. At a radius of 14.7 cm on a 78 rpm phonograph record, a particle will experience a centrifugal field in magnitude equal to that of the gravitational field.

* Also known as "relative centrifugal force" or RCF. This is a misnomer since a force is always mass × acceleration, not acceleration alone.

tower increased progressively with time t. We should now write

$$v = gt$$

which is to say that velocity of an object starting from rest is proportional to the product of the acceleration g due to gravity and time.

We all know that snowflakes behave quite differently: they waft down at a slow, constant rate, which we may call their *terminal velocity*. In general, large, compact snowflakes fall more rapidly than small, frilly ones. Stokes identified the factors controlling the *viscous drag* of ideal, spherical objects in his Law

$$F_\eta = 3\pi\eta_m dv_T \tag{3.3}$$

where F_η is the viscous drag or Stokes resistance expressed in the units of force, η_m the viscosity of the fluid, d the diameter of the particle, and v_T the terminal velocity. Terminal velocity will be reached in this case when the viscous drag equals the gravitational force on the particle, which equals mass × gravity (Fig. 3.2). Therefore, when the particle reaches terminal velocity

$$MG = F_\eta = -3\pi\eta_m dv_T \tag{3.4}$$

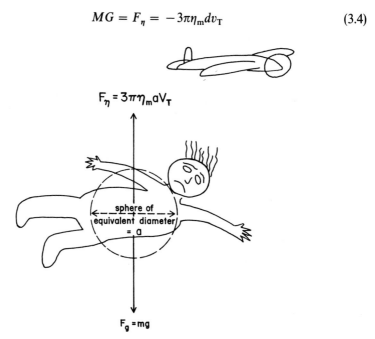

$$F_\eta = 3\pi\eta_m a V_T$$

sphere of
equivalent diameter
= a

$$F_g = mg$$

Fig. 3.2. Terminal velocity of a falling object. A spherical object falling in a viscous medium will reach a terminal velocity when viscous drag equals the force of gravity on the object.

The effect of buoyancy can be seen in the case of a particle of sand suspended in water. If the particle is spherical, its mass will be equal to its density times volume

$$M = \rho_p \frac{\pi d^3}{6}$$

where ρ_p is the density of the particle (Fig. 3.3). However, the particle, having displaced an equal volume of water, will act as if its mass has been reduced by the Archimedian buoyancy, which is the mass of displaced water M_w.

$$M_w = (\rho_w \pi d^3)/6$$

We can therefore think of the particle as having a "reduced density" $(\rho_p - \rho_w)$ and a "reduced mass" M'.

$$M' = (\rho_p - \rho_w)\pi d^3/6$$

Alternatively, we can think of the buoyant force F_b due to the difference in pressure P between the top and bottom of the particle

$$F_b = -v_p \Delta P$$

In either case the net downward force F_d on the particle will be less than it would have been in air (or in a vacuum).

$$F_d = (\rho_p - \rho_m)\pi d^3 g/6$$

At the terminal velocity this will be equal and opposite to the viscous drag. Combining

$$3\pi \eta_m dv_T = (\rho_p - \rho_m)\pi d^3 g/6$$

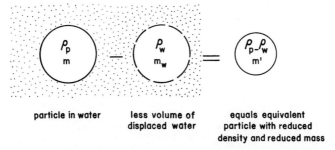

particle in water   less volume of   equals equivalent
                      displaced water   particle with reduced
                                              density and reduced mass

Fig. 3.3. Notion of reduced or buoyant density and reduced mass. The effective density and mass of a particle in water can be thought of as the actual density and mass diminished by the density of water and the mass of the displaced volume of water.

so that the terminal velocity v_T is

$$v_T = (\rho_p - \rho_m)d^2g/18\eta_m \tag{3.5}$$

3.1.2 Sedimentation Coefficient

We stated at the outset that centrifugal and gravitational fields were analogous. Now consider a narrow, sectorial zone of particles in a centrifuge rotor; the particles are suspended in a suspending fluid or medium (Fig. 3.4). The presence of the medium has two consequences. First, its simplest function is to transfer angular momentum from the whirling centrifuge to the particles so that the particles are always moving at very nearly the same angular velocity as the centrifuge. Second, the fluid is the source of forces (arising from viscosity and buoyancy) that affect the actual rate of sedimentation.

We may substitute in Eq. (3.5) the centrifugal field $F = r\omega^2$ [Eq. (3.1)] for the gravitational field g and obtain the rate of sedimentation, that is, the terminal radial velocity v_r of an ideal spherical particle in a centrifugal field

$$v_r = (\rho_p - \rho_m)d^2r\omega^2/18\eta_m \tag{3.6}$$

where ρ_p is the density of the particle, ρ_m density of the medium, d diameter of the particle, r distance from the axis of rotation, ω angular velocity, and η viscosity of the medium (cf. Fig. 3.3). Note that the square of the diameter

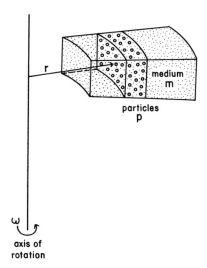

Fig. 3.4. Acceleration of particles in a centrifugal field. Particles at a distance of r from the axis of rotation experience a centrifugal field of $r\omega^2$ and reach a terminal velocity dr/dt described by Eq. (3.6) or, more generally, by Eq. (3.10).

of the particle appears in Eqs. (3.5) and (3.6). Since the volume of a sphere varies with the cube of the diameter, it follows that the sedimentation rate varies with volume$^{2/3}$.

The sedimentation rate of an ideal, spherical particle in a fluid whose density and viscosity are known can be readily predicted from Eq. (3.6). The reverse is also true: one can predict the diameter of such a particle from measurements of its sedimentation rate and density. It is convenient to refer all sedimentation rates to standard conditions, that is, water at 20°C. We specifically define the sedimentation coefficient $s_{20,w}$ of a particle in water at 20°C by Eq. (3.7), although we might never actually centrifuge anything under these conditions; $s_{20,w}$ has the dimension of seconds and the usual unit is the Svedberg (S $= 10^{-13}$ sec) named after Thé Svedberg. Therefore, $s_{20,w}$ in Svedbergs is

$$s_{20,w} = (\rho_p - \rho_w)d^2/18\eta_w \tag{3.7}$$

Correspondingly

$$d = \left(\frac{18\eta_w s_{20,w}}{\rho_p - \rho_w}\right)^{1/2} \tag{3.8}$$

where d is in nanometers and $s_{20,w}$ is in Svedbergs.

3.1.3 Generalized Sedimentation Equation

From Eqs. (3.6) and (3.7) the sedimentation rate of an ideal particle in water at 20°C is

$$v_r = s_{20,w} r\omega^2 \tag{3.9}$$

We may correct for the differences in viscosity and buoyancy in media other than water at 20°C by adding two factors to Eq. (3.9)

$$v_r = s_{20,w} r\omega^2 (\eta_w/\eta_m)(\rho_p - \rho_m/\rho_p - \rho_w) \tag{3.9a}$$

From here on, we shall be speaking mostly of sedimentation in density gradients in which the viscosity η_m and the density of the medium ρ_m both vary along the radius. The velocity of the particles also varies. Therefore, Eq. (3.9a) we should rewrite so that the density and viscosity of the medium are functions of radius

$$dr/dt = s_{20,w} r\omega^2 (\eta_w/\eta_m(r))[\rho_p - \rho_m(r)]/(\rho_p - \rho_w) \tag{3.10}$$

where dr/dt is the instantaneous radial velocity of the particles, $s_{20,w}$ the sedimentation coefficient of the particles, r the distance from the axis of rotation, ω the angular velocity, η refers to viscosities, and ρ refers to densities:

the subscript p refers to particles, m to medium, and w to water at 20°C. Equation (3.10) is referred to frequently in later sections.

3.1.4 Ideality and Nonideality of Particles

Shape

The Stokes equation for viscous drag [Eq. (3.3)] was deduced for spheres. The expression $3\pi\eta_m d$ in the Stokes equation is called the *frictional coefficient* f_0 of a sphere. Bodies having other shapes have different frictional coefficients (Appendix B2)

$$f = \theta f_0 \tag{3.11}$$

where θ is the *frictional ratio*. To accommodate particles of other shapes one may apply θ to Eq. (3.6)

$$dr/dt = (\rho_p - \rho_m)d_e{}^2 r\omega^2/18\eta_m\theta \tag{3.12}$$

where d_e is the diameter of a sphere whose volume is equal to that of the particle. It should be noted that all departures from the spherical result in slower sedimentation; the extreme case is shown by filamentous molecules such as DNA. Another way of looking at frictional ratios is that the non-spherical particle sediments as if it were a sphere of volume less than the actual volume of the particle (Fig. 3.5).

Interaction with the Medium

Hydration.   Biological particles are typically hydrated and the extent of hydration is affected by the medium: its osmotic potential, concentration of

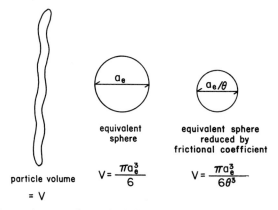

Fig. 3.5. Sedimentation rate of nonspherical particles. A filamentous particle behaves in a centrifugal field as if it were a sphere whose volume is the same as that of the actual particle reduced by the frictional coefficient.

salts, polymers, etc. The extent of hydration may affect in turn the effective size and the density of the particle.

Osmotic potential.   An extreme case of differential hydration occurs in the case of particles with osmotic properties. Imagine, for example, the case of a microbial cell sedimenting into a gradient of sucrose (Fig. 3.6). The existence of a membrane around the cell impermeable to sucrose results in a progressive loss of water from the cell as it moves into higher and higher concentrations of sucrose. In order to maintain osmotic equilibrium the cell shrinks and (usually) becomes more dense. Consequently there are drastic changes in the sedimentation coefficient and ρ_p. Not only do these changes greatly complicate the sedimentation behavior of the particle, but extensive dehydration and shrinkage may result in irreversible changes in the structure of the cell. Subcellular organelles, such as mitochondria, lysosomes, and chloroplasts appear to be especially sensitive to osmotic pressure.

De Duve *et al.* (1959) deduced equations* for the sedimentation behavior

* Their equations were developed from the following model:

V_p, M_p, and ρ_p are the volume, mass, and density of the particle.

V_d, M_d, and ρ_d are the volume, mass, and density of the particle entirely deprived of solvent.

α is the concentration of osmotically active substances inside the particle calculated on the mass of particle deprived of solvent.

ρ_w is the density of the solvent (water).

ρ_s is the density of the solutes in the solution.

$\overline{V}_s$ is the partial molal volume of the solutes.

C_m is the molal concentration of the solutes in the solvent.

C_s is the molar concentration of the solute; in the solvent.

Osmotic equilibrium is obtained when the concentration of water is the same inside and outside the particle. This will occur when

$$V_p = V_d[1 + (\rho_d \alpha / \rho_w C_m)]$$

$$M_p = M_d[1 + (\alpha / C_m)]$$

$$\rho_p = \rho_d \rho_w[(\alpha + C_m)/\rho_d \alpha + \rho_m C_m]$$

provided that the particle membrane exerts no appreciable hydrostatic pressure. The density of the medium is

$$\rho_m = \rho_w(1 + \rho_d \overline{V}_s C_m)/(1 + \rho_w \overline{V}_s C_m)$$

Combining the last two equations, we obtain for the equilibrium density of the particle

$$\rho_{eq} = \rho_d(1 + \rho_s \overline{V}_s \alpha)/(1 - \rho_d \overline{V}_s \alpha) \tag{3.13}$$

The sedimentation equation in terms of the particle deprived of solvent then becomes

$$s = (V_d/f)(1 - \rho_d \alpha \overline{V}_s)(\rho_e - \rho_m) \tag{3.14a}$$

$$dr/dt = r\omega^2(V_d/f)(\rho_e - \rho_m) \tag{3.14b}$$

Time of centrifugation ⟶

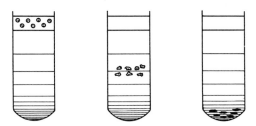

Fig. 3.6. Shrinkage of osmotically sensitive particles in a gradient of sucrose. As the particle sediments farther into the gradient where the osmotic potential is higher, the particle loses water, shrinks, and becomes more dense.

of "perfect osmometers" in density gradients, including calculations for changes in the sedimentation coefficient. They then elaborated the model further to include the common case of organelles having one compartment permeable to a solute such as sucrose and a second compartment impermeable to it. The data of Tedeschi and Harris (1955) on the swelling of mitochondria appear to conform nicely to the elaborated equations.

Using a similar set of assumptions but adding considerations of permeant and fixed charges, Steck *et al.* (1970) asked how the resolution of two or more membrane-bound vesicles could be optimized in isopycnic sedimentation. They concluded that resolution would be favored in gradients with minimum osmotic and ionic activities and under conditions which also minimize the fixed charges on the membranes.

The simple equations should be used with extreme caution, since few biological particles are composed of a single, differentially permeable compartment, although over narrow regions of osmotic potential they may behave superficially as if they were. Also, the presence of multiple variables in a mathematical model increases the probability that it will correspond to a multiplicity of physical models. Finally, because of the large probability that high osmotic potentials will work anomalous and sometimes irreversible changes (cf. Day *et al.*, 1970), it is by far preferable to employ gradients of constant osmotic potential in which the size and shape of the particle can be expected to remain constant. These *isosmotic gradients* can be formed with D_2O or with polymers of negligible osmotic potential, such as silica sols or Ficoll. The use of polymers for isosmotic gradients is discussed in Sections 5.1.2 and 5.1.3.

Charge.   The presence of charged species in the medium can be guaranteed to interact with changes on the surface of the particle. In some cases this alters the hydration of the particle. DNA, for example, has a density of about 1.7 in CsCl but only about 1.4 in sucrose. High concentrations of salt can strongly alter even nonosmotic particles. Ribosomes, for example, when exposed to concentrated CsCl lose about one-half of their proteins to become so-called "core particles," composed of RNA and tightly bound, residual proteins. The nature of the counterion can strongly affect the sedimentation coefficient of highly charged species. The sedimentation rates of nucleic acids, for example, increase by 10% and 50–90% when sodium ions are replaced by potassium or cesium ions, respectively. The behavior of proteins on the other hand is only slightly affected by these substitutions (Doppler-Bernardi and Duane, 1969).

Low concentrations of some salts are essential to the stability of some organelles. Nuclei typically require Ca^{2+} at a level of about 0.1 mM. However, the addition of divalent cations to other organelles can be disastrous. Mg^{2+} often causes severe aggregation of subcellular particles and may permanently alter the composition of membrane fragments.

Surface effects. Components of the medium may interact with the surface of a particle in ways which may be difficult to quantitate but nonetheless have dramatic effects on its sedimentation behavior. For example, a wide variety of polymers [proteins, polyvinylpyrrolidone (PVP), Ficoll, etc.] in relatively low concentrations can reversibly change the form of mitochondria from spherical to rod shaped (Novikoff, 1957: Laties and Treffry, 1969).

The mechanism for such "surface effects" may well be analogous to the partition effects described by Albertsson (1972). A polymer in the presence of a solute (which may be a second polymer) and solvent tends to form two phases in which solvent, solute, and polymer are unequally partitioned. For example, the system of Ficoll–PVP–water will form two phases within certain concentration ranges. The Ficoll-rich phase will also be rich in water and the PVP-rich phase will be poor in water. In the same way a polymer may form a three-membered system with water and the surface of a particle to form a solvent-poor phase on the particle surface. The result would appear similar to partial dehydration, though no corresponding changes in the colligative properties of the solution would be detected.

Pertoft (1966 *et seq.*) has added a variety of polymers to silica sols in order to alter the sedimentation behavior of the silica particles for the self-generation of density gradients (Sections 5.3 and 9.2.1).

Particle–Particle Interaction

A substantial concentration of particles (e.g., proteins) may measurably decrease the activity coefficient of the particles but increase the viscosity of a medium. These local effects are one of several factors that may cause the sedimentation rate of particles to be less at high concentrations of particles than at low concentrations (Fig. 3.7). It is customary therefore to report sedimentation coefficients extrapolated to infinite dilution $s^\circ_{20,w}$. For most proteins the sedimentation rate at concentrations of 0.1 mg/ml is within 1% of the rate at infinite dilution.

Proteins and other particles will often form dimers, trimers, and larger aggregates. The sedimentation coefficient of the aggregates will be larger than that of the single unit and the tendency to aggregate will be concentration dependent. Thus two particles can interact to form a dimer

$$p + p \leftrightarrows p - p$$

or a polymer

$$np \rightleftarrows p_n$$

These associations may follow simple association kinetics

$$[p_n]/p^n = K_n$$

or may show strong cooperativity up to some favored oligomer.

It follows that the sedimentation behavior of a zone of associating particles may be quite complex; particles near the center of the zone may sediment more rapidly than particles near the edge of the zone because of association or less rapidly because of the effects of particle concentration on viscosity and activity.

As an example of the high probability of interaction among sedimenting

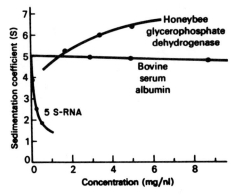

Fig. 3.7. Dependence of sedimentation rate on particle concentration (Van Holde, 1971). The sedimentation coefficients of most molecules decrease with concentration because of mutual interference; this is especially so with long, thin molecules, such as nucleic acids. However, sedimentation coefficients can increases with concentration when particles associate reversibly, as in the case of avian glycerophosphate dehydrogenase.

particles, we calculated (Eikenberry *et al.*, 1970) that ribosomes at 20 mg/ml would be separated by less than 3 particle diameters and at 64,000 g the particles were sedimenting at a velocity of 200 diameters/sec. The probabilities of particle–particle interaction under these conditions are prodigious.

Because of all of the possibilities for nonideal behavior and difficulties in measuring $s_{20,w}^{\circ}$ for impure particles, one may wish to hedge one's bets by reporting an *equivalent sedimentation coefficient* as s,* which is defined as the sedimentation coefficient of an equivalent, ideal particle.

3.2 RATE SEPARATIONS

We saw in Eq. (3.6) that the rate of sedimentation of a particle was related to its size (specifically, the square of the diameter d or volume$^{2/3}$). It follows that two particles of the same shape and density ρ_p but of different size should sediment at different rates (Fig. 3.8). Particles of the same shape and size but of different densities will also sediment at different rates, since ρ_p also figures in the equation for sedimentation velocity [Eq. (3.6)]. The contribution of the ρ_p term is apt to be underestimated, because the usual estimates of ρ_p, made by isopycnic sedimentation in gradients of sucrose or CsCl, yield a value corresponding to a lower hydration and hence a higher density than the particle would have under the more moderate conditions of osmotic potential or ionic strength commonly encountered in gradients employed for rate separations. Examination of Eq. (3.6) shows furthermore that the value of the density correction factor ($\rho_p - \rho_m$) becomes particularly sensitive to differences in ρ_p the nearer ρ_p approaches ρ_m.

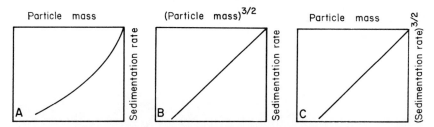

Fig. 3.8. Dependence of sedimentation rate on particle size. For a given class of particles of the same density and shape (polysomes for example), the sedimentation rates under otherwise identical conditions are proportional to the volume$^{2/3}$ or mass$^{2/3}$ of the particles. (A) is a plot of sedimentation rate and mass each to the first power. (B) and (C) show how this relation can be plotted as linear functions (cf. Fig. 3.20).

3.2.1   Rate Separations in Tubes

Imagine first that we have loaded a centrifuge tube with a gradient of sucrose over which we place a small quantity of particles (Fig. 3.9). As the particles are centrifuged they will move outward along radial lines. Those particles initially near the lateral walls of the tube will strike the walls, while those in an elliptical zone near the center will sediment unhindered toward the bottom of the tube. The particles striking the wall will not necessarily move at the same speed as those fully in the solution: thus the width of the sedimenting zone may become progressively broadened. This artifact, known as wall effect, substantially complicates the theory of rate separations in tubes (de Duve *et al.*, 1959). It becomes a serious practical limitation in long tubes. I have observed, for example, that in the centrifugation of microalgae in 12-cm tubes (Section 9.1.1), that the portions of particle zones near the walls could become concentrated to the point of aggregation, whereas those in the center remain dilute.

The theoretical implications of density gradient centrifugation in tubes only occasionally complicate what is normally an extremely useful method, but we shall simplify our discussion by turning to separations in sector-shaped rotors.

3.2.2   Rate Separations in Zonal or Sector-Shaped Rotors

Let us modify the lateral walls of a tube, as in an analytical cell, or extend it through 360°, as in a zonal rotor (Fig. 3.10). Once again, we load the rotor with a density gradient and a thin layer of particles.* As the particles sediment

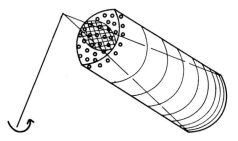

Fig. 3.9.   Scheme of rate separations in swinging buckets. A thin layer of particles is layered over a density gradient in a tube. Ideal sedimentation behavior is exhibited only by those particles in the cross-hatched zone that escape striking the wall.

* The mechanics of loading and unloading of gradients in zonal rotors is discussed in Section 6.3. It suffices here to note that fluids may be moved into or out of zonal rotors at the edge or at the center.

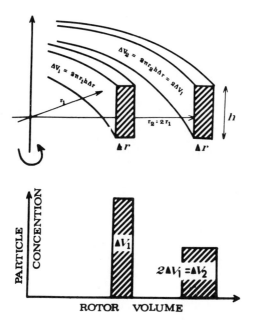

Fig. 3.10. Rate separation in a sector-shaped rotor. With lateral walls oriented along radial lines, wall effects are avoided, but particle zones are spread over a progressively longer circumference. The usual consequence is sectorial dilution. The lowered concentration will be evident if viewed directly within the rotor or recovered from the rotor.

outward the circumference of the particle zone becomes progressively longer (Fig. 3.10). The volume of the zone can be represented as

$$\Delta V = 2\pi r h \Delta r$$

Thus even if the thickness of the zone Δr remains constant, the volume in which the particles are contained must increase with increasing r, while the concentration of the particles proportionately decreases. This *radial* or *sectorial dilution** is a constant nuisance in rate separations. The extent of sectorial dilution is exactly proportional to the increase in the distance r from the axis of rotation. We can see mathematically by letting the concentration of particles as a function of radius $c(r)$ be equal to a constant amount of particles p divided by the zone volume ΔV in the equation

$$\frac{p}{\Delta V} = \frac{p}{2\pi h \Delta r} \cdot \frac{1}{r}$$

* A military analogy: a line of soldiers advances into a widening valley; as they march along, their numbers remain constant but the line becomes progressively thinner; that is, the concentration of the soldiers decreases.

This decrease in concentration is observed if one monitors the particles within the rotor or when recovering the gradient from the rotor (Fig. 3.10).

The actual sedimentation rate of the particles usually changes during passage through the gradient in a complicated way. Again referring to Eq. (3.10), the sedimentation rate will tend to increase as the particles move farther into the gradient because of the increasing value of r, but at the same time it will tend to decrease because of the decreasing difference in density between particles and medium $\rho_p - \rho_m(r)$ and also the increasing viscosity of the medium $\eta_m(r)$ in the denominator. The exact resultant, whether a deceleration, an acceleration, or constant velocity, depends on the shape of the gradient.

3.2.3 Gradient Shape

Isokinetic Gradients

We can control the properties of the sedimenting zone of particles to some extent by the choice of the gradient material and the *shape of the gradient*. (This latter phrase means the concentration of gradient material as a function of radius or volume.) As first shown by Harrison and Nixon (1959), de Duve et al. (1959), and later by Martin and Ames (1961), one can select a gradient shape to accomplish a specific purpose: to make the distance that a protein moves in a gradient proportional to the sedimentation coefficient of the protein, which is equivalent to making the sedimentation rates of any one protein constant throughout the gradient. Noll (1967) has called such gradients *isokinetic*.

An isokinetic gradient works on the principle, noted previously, that the sedimentation rate is the resultant of three opposing factors which must exactly cancel one another. Specifically, we ask that for each species of particle

$$dr/dt = \text{constant}$$

To achieve this we discard fixed elements from Eq. (3.10) and write

$$\frac{[\rho_p - \rho_m(r)]r}{\eta_m(r)} = K_r \qquad (3.15)$$

where K_r is the isokinetic gradient constant.

For each value of r in the rotor we choose a concentration of the gradient solute such that Eq. (3.15) holds. Since an indefinitely large number of gradient constants will satisfy Eq. (3.15), we can compute a large family of isokinetic gradients for each class of ρ_p. The shape of one such isokinetic gradient is shown in Fig. 3.11. The behavior of ribosomes in this gradient is

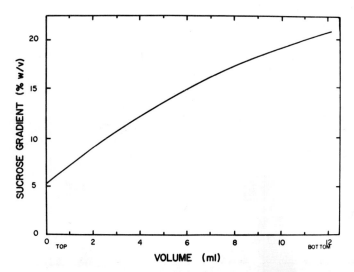

Fig. 3.11. Shape of an isokinetic gradient. This gradient was computed from Eq. (3.15) for the separation of particles of $\rho_p = 1.4$ gm/cm^3, such as ribosomes (R. A. Bowen, unpublished).

illustrated in Figs. 3.12 and 3.13. Tables for the construction of isokinetic gradients are presented in Appendices D1 and D2.

There are a number of advantages to the use of isokinetic gradients. Suppose we wish to predict the distance Δr that a particle will move in a certain time. If we start with the general sedimentation equation [Eq. (3.10)], we can solve for dr and integrate

$$\Delta r = \int dr = \frac{s^*\eta_w}{\rho_p - \rho_w} \int_0^{\Delta t} \frac{r\omega^2(\rho_p - \rho_m r)}{\eta_m r}\, dt \tag{3.16}$$

Equation (3.16) can be evaluated for any arbitrary gradient only as a finite series, preferably by computer. In the case of isokinetic gradients Eq. (3.16) reduces agreeably to

$$\Delta r = K_r s^* \int_0^{\Delta t} \omega^2 dt \tag{3.17a}$$

or, at constant rotor speed,

$$\Delta r = K_r s^* \omega^2 \Delta t \tag{3.17b}$$

Similarly, the calculation of the time required to sediment a particle a given distance in a gradient is simplified. For arbitrary gradients, the time required

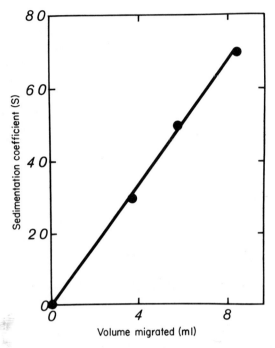

Fig. 3.12. Sedimentation rate of different sized particles in an isokinetic gradient. The distance sedimented by ribosomal particles of different sizes in the isokinetic gradient of Fig. 3.11 is proportional to the sedimentation coefficient of the particle (R. A. Bowen, unpublished).

to move a particle from r_1 to r_2 is

$$\Delta t = \frac{\rho_p - \rho_w}{s^* \eta_w} \int_{r_1}^{r_2} \frac{\eta_m(r)}{r\omega^2 (\rho_p - \rho_m(r))} \, dr \qquad (3.18a)$$

but for isokinetic gradients at constant rotor speed

$$\Delta t = \Delta r / K_r s^* \omega^2 \qquad (3.18b)$$

We should note here that, because of acceleration, deceleration, and fluctuation in speed, the proper measure of the amount of centrifugation required to move particles in any kind of rate separation is $\int \omega^2 dt$, rather than any simple product of speed^2 and time.

Another advantage of isokinetic gradients is in the estimation of sedimentation coefficients. Equation (3.17) says that the distance moved by a particle is proportional to its equivalent sedimentation coefficient. It becomes very simple therefore to interpolate sedimentation coefficients of unknown particles by the inclusion of two standard particles of the same density class in the gradient.

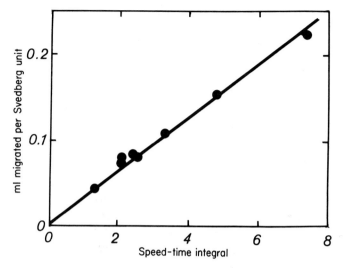

Fig. 3.13. Sedimentation in an isokinetic gradient as a function of the $\omega^2 dt$ for different particles (R. A. Bowen, unpublished). The distance migrated (measured here as volume of gradient) of ribosomal particles varies linearly with the $\omega^2 dt$ in isokinetic gradients. The gradient is the same as in Fig. 3.11. The units of the speed–time integral are in radians^2/sec $\times$ 10^{-11}.

Although isokinetic gradients have multiple advantages for density gradient centrifugation in tubes, we should note that their convenience in sector-shaped rotors is mitigated by sectorial dilution.

Acceleration Gradients

If a gradient shape can be manipulated to insure a constant rate of sedimentation, it follows that it can also be arranged to either decelerate or accelerate sedimentation rates. Kaempfer and Meselson (1971) designed an *acceleration gradient* in which homologous particles move at ever increasing rates the farther they are from the axis of rotation. With the usual density gradient materials the viscosity increases too rapidly with concentration to permit acceleration, but Kaempfer and Meselson found that the system of D_2O and CsCl at temperatures under $5°C$ shows strikingly anomalous behavior: viscosity decreases with concentration. The use of an acceleration gradient for the resolution of ribosomal subunits is shown in Fig. 3.14. The construction of the gradient is described in Appendix D7. Another strategy of designing an acceleration gradient is to impose an inverse gradient of a highly viscous material such as polyethylene glycol on a density gradient of another solute (Fig. 3.15).

Cowan and Trautman (1965) employed a similar strategy in devising a gradient that is nearly isokinetic by employing a gradient of KBr and an inverse gradient of $NaNO_3$. Although the two salts have similar densities,

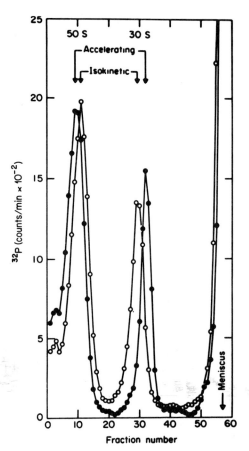

Fig. 3.14. Rate–zonal separation of ribosomal subunits in an acceleration gradient (Kaempfer and Meselson, 1971). The resolution of 30 S and 50 S subunits of *E. coli* ribosomal subunits, labeled with ^{32}P was compared in 0–12.6% CsCl/D$_2$0 acceleration gradients (Appendix D7) and 12.5–19.6% w/v sucrose isokinetic gradients (Appendix D1). In both cases 12.5 cm^3 of gradient containing 10 mM Tris–HCl pH 7.4, 10 mM magnesium acetate, and 0.1 mg gelatin/ml were centrifuged in an SB283 rotor at 41,000 rpm and 0°. The acceleration gradient (0) was spun for 3.9 hr and the isokinetic gradient (0) for 6.2 hr.

the viscosity of NaNO$_3$ is much greater than that of KBr. Thus, a negative viscosity gradient was imposed on a shallow density gradient.

Linear–Log Gradients

Isokinetic and acceleration gradients may have the disadvantage that the dynamic range is limited; that is, it would be difficult to obtain separate zones of particles of 50 S and 2000 S in the same gradient. To overcome this limitation Brakke and Van Pelt (1970) described a *linear–log gradient* in

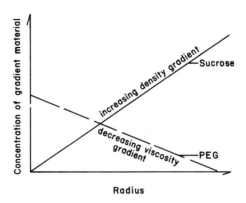

Fig. 3.15. Construction of an acceleration gradient by imposition of inverse viscosity gradient. An inverse gradient of polyethyleneglycol (PEG) on a regular gradient of sucrose could result in a sufficiently steep negative gradient of viscosity to counteract the effect of increasing buoyancy of sucrose and result in a progressive increase in sedimentation velocity as particles move into the gradient.

which the logarithm of the distance sedimented is proportional to the logarithm of the sedimentation coefficient. I think this should really be called a "log–log" gradient, but it again demonstrates the important principle that we can design gradient shapes to suit our needs. In general, gradients in which sedimentation rates are less than proportional to sedimentation coefficients will be steeper than isokinetic gradients.

Gradient-Induced Zone Narrowing

Let us return now to the problem of sectorial dilution as it affects zone width. Schumaker (1966) pointed out that not only the distance between zones but the shape and width of a sedimenting particle zone could be controlled by the shape of the gradient. We saw, as shown in Fig. 3.9, that zones of particles could sediment with constant zone widths but decreasing concentrations of particles in the zone. In isokinetic gradients, for example, we can expect that the particles in the leading edge of the zone will move as fast as those in the tail of the zone, thus, the radial width of the zone should remain constant. Now imagine a steeper gradient (Fig. 3.16); the particles in the leading edge will be decelerated with respect to those in the trailing edge by the increased viscosity and density of the medium. It is in fact possible to make the gradient sufficiently steep that the radial zone width shrinks. Schumaker calls this *gradient-induced zone narrowing*.

A simple use of gradient-induced zone narrowing is a *deceleration* or *collection gradient*, which can be achieved by imposing a sharp increase in slope at the foot of the gradient (Fig. 3.17). The effect of this is to crowd particle zones into a narrow region. It may be used effectively at the end of the

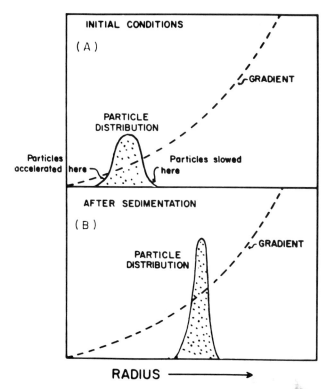

Fig. 3.16. Gradient-induced zone narrowing. If a gradient is sufficiently steep, the particles in the front of the zone will be accelerated less rapidly than those in the trailing edge (A). The result is a decrease in radial zone width (B).

gradient to concentrate faster moving particles after they have separated from slower moving ones.

Equivolumetric Gradients

Gradient-induced zone narrowing can also be employed to counteract or be coordinated with sectorial dilution. For example, we (Pollack and Price, 1971) designed an *equivolumetric gradient* in which gradient-induced zone narrowing exactly balances sectorial dilution. In this case a thin cylindrical zone of particles moves through units of volume (rather than radius) at a constant rate (Fig. 3.18).

$$dV/dt = \text{constant}$$

Since for a thin cylinder

$$dV = 2\pi rhdr$$

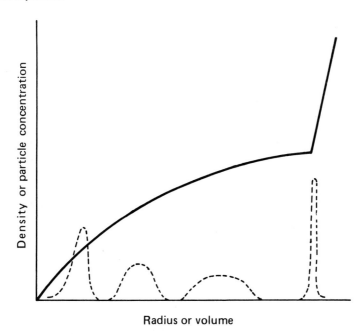

Fig. 3.17. Deceleration gradients. A steep region at the foot of a gradient can be used to compress strongly particle zones at the end of a rate separation.

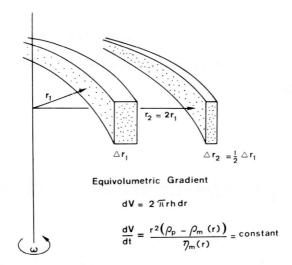

Equivolumetric Gradient

$$dV = 2\pi rh \, dr$$

$$\frac{dV}{dt} = \frac{r^2 \left(\rho_p - \rho_m(r) \right)}{\eta_m(r)} = constant$$

Fig. 3.18. Scheme of equivolumetric gradients. In contrast to the situation in Fig. 3.10, where the concentration of particles decreases progressively as the particle zone migrates into the rotor, we ask that zone width shrink to compensate for sectorial dilution.

the requirement for constant volumetric velocity translates to

$$dV/dt = 2\pi rh(dr/dt) = \text{constant} \qquad (3.19)$$

We can now combine Eqs. (3.10) and (3.19) and discard constant factors

$$\frac{r^2}{\eta_m(r)}\left[\rho_p - \rho_m(r)\right] = K_v \qquad (3.20)$$

where K_v is the equivolumetric gradient constant. The resulting equation describes equivolumetric gradients, which can be thought of as sectorial analogs of isokinetic gradients. The shape of one family of equivolumetric gradients is shown in Fig. 3.19.

In analogy with isokinetic gradients equivolumetric gradients greatly simplify the mathematics of rate separations. The time required for a particle to pass through a certain volume of gradient ΔV, which we call the *volumetric distance*, at constant rotor speed, is

$$\Delta t = \Delta V/K_v s^* \omega^2 \qquad (3.21)$$

Similarly, the volumetric distance traversed by a particle is

$$\Delta V = K_v s^* \int \omega^2 dt \qquad (3.22a)$$

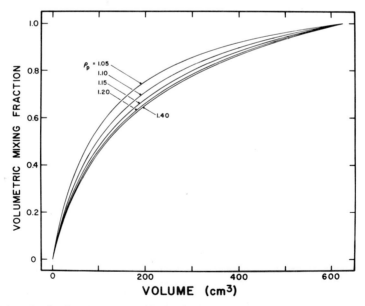

Fig. 3.19. Family of equivolumetric gradients for the B-XIV type of rotors (Eikenberry, 1973).

or, at constant rotor speed

$$\Delta V = K_v s^* \omega^2 \, \Delta t \qquad (3.22b)$$

Again, all particles of a given density class should sediment at volumetric rates that are proportional to their sedimentation coefficients. This is shown for polysomes in the inset of Fig. 3.20.

We also expect that zone widths should remain constant. This expectation is only partially realized; we find a slow, time-dependent zone enlargement (Fig. 3.21) which is independent of particle size and the distance migrated. For example, zones which are initially 5- to 10-cm³ wide are recovered 18 hr later in volumes of 15–20 cm³. This slow spreading of zones had been observed earlier by Spragg *et al.* (1969), who named it *anomalous zone broadening*.

The characteristic of all particle zones in equivolumetric gradients having substantially the same zone widths is advantageous in optimizing resolution (Section 3.2.5). In fact, the resolution of polysomes in equivolumetric gradients in zonal rotors is virtually the same as in isokinetic gradients in swinging buckets.

Exceptionally good resolution was also reported for ribosomal and messenger RNAs by Berns *et al.* (1971) (Fig. 3.22).

As in the case of isokinetic gradients, each equivolumetric gradient is specific to particles of a given density, but van der Zeijst and Bult (1972) and

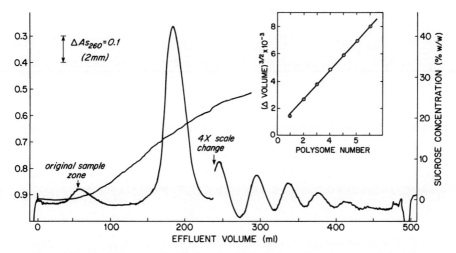

Fig. 3.20. Separation of polysomes in an equivolumetric gradient (Pollack and Price, 1971). Cytoplasmic ribosomes and polysomes were centrifuged in an equivolumetric gradient in a B-30 zonal rotor. The inset shows that the (volumetric distance migrated)$^{3/2}$ is a linear function of the polysome number, which is proportional to particle mass.

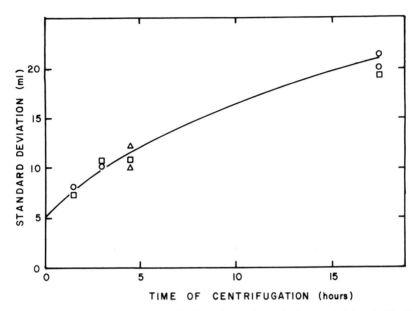

Fig. 3.21. Zone broadening in equivolumetric gradients (Pollack and Price, 1971). The gradual enlargement of particle zones in equivolumetric gradients is independent of the particle size or the distance migrated, but is dependent solely on time. The different symbols in the figure refer to ribosomal particles of different sizes and speeds of centrifugation. This phenomenon is called anomalous zone broadening.

Eikenberry (1973) have found that the gradient shape for $\rho = 1.2$ is a very close approximation for a wide range of particle densities (Fig. 3.19). The construction of equivolumetric gradients is detailed in Appendices D3 and D4.

Isometric Gradients

Gradient-induced zone narrowing was employed by Spragg *et al.* (1969) in their most elegant design of *isometric gradients*. These gradients were designed for the separation of the smallest possible particles in zonal rotors. The strategy was to start with the shallowest possible gradient to insure maximum sedimentation rates, and then steepen it progressively in order to compensate for sectorial dilution. The gradient shape is constructed with a Fortran program, and has the added refinement of specifying a gradient shape that is initially incorrect, but which will sediment and diffuse into the correct shape by the time the particles will have arrived at each location in the rotor. This modification of gradient shape by sedimentation and diffusion of the solute is not a trivial consideration in runs lasting many hours (McEwen, 1967).

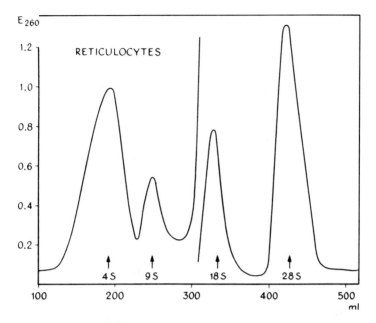

Fig. 3.22.   Separation of reticulocyte RNAs in an equivolumetric gradient (Berns *et al.*, 1971).

The isometric program also seeks to maintain constant zone widths, but the zones suffer from substantial anomalous zone broadening. A separation of serum globulins in an isometric gradient is shown in Fig. 9.21. Another application of gradient-induced zone narrowing is discussed in Section 3.2.4.

Step Gradients

An extreme but complex example of gradient-induced zone narrowing occurs during rate separations in another gradient shape called *step gradients*. A step gradient consists of segments of homogeneous solutions of increasing density (Fig. 3.23). We should note first that pure step gradients exist for only a few moments after they are formed. Diffusion of the solute serves to replace the sharp step with a steep but smooth ramp (dotted line in Fig. 3.23). The reason for this is instructive*: diffusion of a solute can be represented by

---

* I once squandered most of a summer learning respect for the significance of diffusion in density gradient centrifugation. I was trying to harvest algal cells into gradients of Ficoll. Although I knew that sucrose produced increases in density of the cells, which were fatal to the desired separations, I thought to use a layer of sucrose as a cushion under a Ficoll gradient in order to economize on this expensive polymer. Every experiment failed, since the cells ended not in the gradient, but at the edge of the rotor. After 6 weeks I finally realized that sufficient sucrose was diffusing several centimeters through the Ficoll to increase the density of the cells!

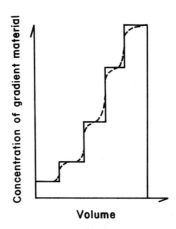

Fig. 3.23. Step gradients. Simple step gradients may be constructed by loading into the rotor discontinuous volumes of solution with stepped increases in solute concentration (solid lines). The sharp steps diffuse very quickly into rounded steps (dotted lines). Cline *et al.* (1970) have reported that step gradients lead to unusual resolution of particle mixtures.

the differential equation and Fig. 3.24.

$$\delta m/\delta t = -DA \, dc/dx \tag{3.23}$$

where $\delta m/\delta t$ is the time rate of diffusion of mass of the solute, D the diffusion coefficient; A the area across which diffusion occurs, and dc/dx the concentration gradient of the diffusing solute. The value of the diffusion coefficient varies widely in dependence on the weight of the particle or solute (cf. Appendix B1). In the case of a step, the value of dc/dx is initially infinite.

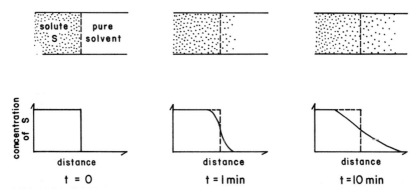

Fig. 3.24. Time course of diffusion. We imagine that at $t = 0$ a solution of sucrose forms a step gradient with water. At $t = 1$ min, the sucrose has already diffused some distance into the water. At $t = 10$ min the step has become well rounded.

Even though D may be very small, the product of a small but finite number with infinity is still infinity. Thus, there is initially an infinitely fast movement of solute across the step.

When a sedimenting zone encounters a partially smoothed but still steep step, three conflicting processes occur: (1) gradient-induced zone narrowing; (2) a widening of the zone as it passes to the top, shallow region of the step; and (3) a widening of the zone if overloading of the gradient occurs (see *capacity* immediately below). Cline *et al.* (1970) have reported that under appropriate conditions the net effect is increased resolution.

3.2.4   Zone Stability and Capacity

A gradient is *instantaneously stable* when no volume element of the gradient is less dense than an underlying element. Figure 3.25 shows the several simple configurations of particle zones in gradients, each of which is barely stable. Any addition of particles to such a zone would cause it to

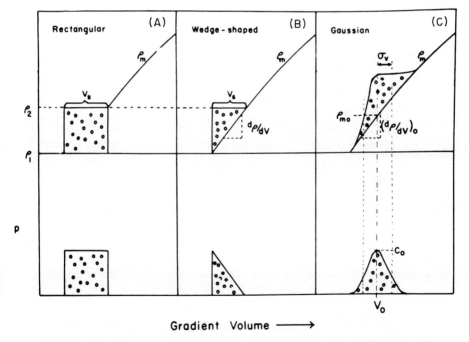

Gradient   Volume ⟶

Fig. 3.25.   Instantaneous static capacity of particle zones in three configurations. Rectangular zone (A), wedge-shaped zone or inverse sample gradient (B), and Gaussian zone (C) have each an instantaneous static capacity, which corresponds to the maximum amount of particles that can be introduced without producing a local density inversion.

become more dense than the underlying gradient. These maximum static capacities are the *instantaneous static capacity.*

We can compute this capacity for particle zones with the usual rectangular shape shown at the left of Fig. 3.25. The density of a solution containing particles is equal to the density of the medium plus the density increment due to the particles corrected for the volume of medium displaced by the particles.

$$\rho_t = \rho_m + C\bar{v}_p(\rho_p - \rho_m) \tag{3.24}$$

where ρ is the density of the total system (t), the medium (m), or the particle (p); C the concentration of the particles; and $\bar{v}$ the partial specific volume of the particles ($=1/\rho_p$). Note that ρ_t and ρ_m are at least potential variables in V_z, the volume of the particle zone measured from the top to the bottom or in sectorial coordinates from the inside to the outside.

The instantaneous static capacity of a rectangular zone is reached when the total density ρ_t just equals the density of the underlying gradient ρ_s. The mass of particles contained in such a zone of ΔV_z ml would be

$$m = V_z \frac{\rho_p(\rho_s - \rho_m)}{\rho_p - \rho_m} \tag{3.25}$$

where ρ_s is the density at the top of the gradient, ρ_m the density gradient of the solution in which the particles are suspended, and V_z the volume of the particle zone.

Although rectangular particle zones have the largest instantaneous static capacity of any particle distribution, numerous workers discovered to their vexation and puzzlement that gradients loaded beyond some critical level, which is substantially less than that predicted previously, are quite unstable (cf. Brakke, 1951; Anderson, 1956; Svensson *et al.*, 1957). After a few minutes, droplets, likened in appearance to intestinal villi, begin to descend from the particle zone and ultimately stream to the bottom of the gradient (Fig. 2.2). Many valuable samples have been lost or unintentionally diluted through this most peculiar phenomenon of *droplet sedimentation.*

The current interpretation of this phenomenon is as follows: the boundary between the particle zone and the gradient is initially sharp, which is to say that the gradients of solute and particles are both infinite at the boundary. This means that very rapid movements occur across the boundary in both directions, but the solute molecules that make up the gradient normally diffuse much more rapidly than the particles in the sample zone. The result is that solute molecules accumulate locally in the sample zone, raising the density in the regions immediately above the gradient, causing a density inversion (cf. Fig. 2.2). Small volume elements then begin to sink into the underlying gradient. Once an element begins to sink, the rate of movement of solute into the element is greatly accelerated. Finally the element breaks away from the sample zone and slowly drifts downward through the gradient as a discrete droplet or streamer.

Brakke (1955) observed that droplet sedimentation can be countered by gentle stirring of the sample zone. N. G. Anderson reports (personal communication) that one can in fact prevent droplet sedimentation by the simple expedient of placing the tube containing gradient and sample on the chassis of a centrifuge; the vibrations from the centrifuge are sufficient to stabilize the system. What happens in this case is that the sample zone slowly enlarges as locally dense regions mix with neighboring regions and are diluted.* Thus, droplet sedimentation is avoided without actually increasing the true capacity of a zone.

If this general model of droplet sedimentation is correct, one should be able to minimize the instability by either equalizing diffusion between sample zone and gradient or eliminating steep gradients in that region. The first possibility was tested by inserting a colored polymer ("Blue Dextran") between a lighter and denser solution and observing the widening of the colored zone (Schumaker and Halsall, 1970). When the lower zone was itself composed of a polymer, the colored zone was in fact much more stable than when it was composed of small molecules.

Since it appears that droplet sedimentation results not from a gross violation of the instantaneous stability criterion as illustrated in Fig. 3.25, but from the growth of locally dense perturbations, it follows that the system cannot be dealt with as a simple deterministic model. It is furthermore not surprising that two theoretical models have been put forward which make quite different predictions for the limiting conditions for stability (Svensson *et al.*, 1957; Sartory, 1969). The actual results in one study led to an empirical model, which is numerically about midway between the two (Halsall and Schumaker, 1971). That model [Eq. (3.26)] says that the stability of an upper zone containing particles p plus a solute s layered over a higher concentration of the solute alone is dependent on the ratios of two density increments $\Delta\rho_p$ and $\Delta\rho_s$, and that this ratio must be smaller than that of the diffusion coefficients of particle and solute

$$\frac{\Delta\rho_p}{\Delta\rho_s} = \frac{C_p(1 - \bar{v}\rho_s')}{\rho_s - \rho_s'} < \frac{D_p}{D_s} \tag{3.26}$$

where $\Delta\rho_p$ is the density increment due to the particles in the upper zone, $\Delta\rho_s$ the density increment due to the difference in concentration of solutes

---

* The object lesson for the practical centrifugationist is to commence centrifugation immediately after the sample has been layered over a gradient, or to select a laboratory over the boiler room.

in the two zones, C_p the mass concentration of the particle, $\bar{v}$ partial specific volume of the particle ($= 1/\rho_p$), ρ_s the density of the solute underneath the sample zone, and ρ_s' the density of the solute in the sample zone. D_p and D_s represent the diffusion constants of the particle and solute, respectively.

Equation (3.26) describes the *actual static capacity*, which is independent of time. The system, however, is not completely time independent, since diffusion gradually increases the volume of the particle zone and eliminates the concentration step between the zones.

Qualitatively it means that to optimize the stability of the sample zone, one should avoid large differences in concentration between the solute in the sample zone and that in the underlying gradient ($\Delta\rho_s$), that a gradient composed of a polymer with its small diffusion constant D_s should be more stable to droplet sedimentation than one composed of small molecules, and that larger particles with their smaller D_p will be more sensitive to this kind of instability than smaller ones.

Britten and Roberts (1960) proposed a means of eliminating steep gradients by continuing the underlying gradient through the sample zone (Fig. 3.26). What is actually done is to overlay the solute gradient with an *inverse sample gradient* or *wedge-shaped sample zone*. Such inverse gradients are prepared simply by constructing linear gradients of sample and the starting solution of the gradient (see Section 5.3). The use of wedge-shaped sample zones is practicable principally in the case of zonal rotors where the capacity of the gradient is challenged.

The instantaneous static capacity of an inverse sample gradient, as calculated by Eikenberry *et al.* (1970) is

$$m \cong \frac{1}{2}\left(\frac{\rho_p}{\rho_p - 1}\right)\left(\frac{d\rho}{dV_z}\right)\Delta V_z \tag{3.27a}$$

which is equivalent to

$$m \cong \frac{1}{2}\left(\frac{\rho_p}{\rho_p - 1}\right)(\rho_2 - \rho_1)\Delta V_z \tag{3.27b}$$

Although the concensus is that the actual static capacity of wedge-shaped particle zones is greater than of rectangular zones, the actual capacities are clearly less than the computed instantaneous capacities of Eq. (3.27). Brakke (1964) found actual capacities for tobacco mosaic virus in a variety of gradients to be between 0.74 and 2.15% of the instantaneous static capacity. Meuwissen (1973) has proposed a simple model based on the exclusion of solvent by particles-plus-solute. We shall develop the details of this model under the topic of *anomalous zone broadening*. Suffice it to say that Meuwissen's model predicts an actual static capacity of about 10% of the

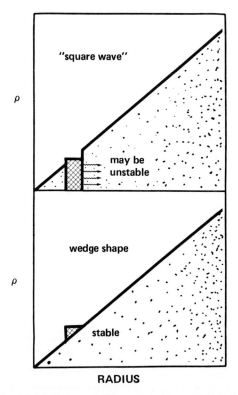

Fig. 3.26. Wedge-shaped sample zones (Britten and Roberts, 1960).

instantaneous static capacity. Meuwissen's own data (Fig. 3.27) show an actual capacity of 10–25% of the instantaneous static capacity. Given the complexity of these systems, the agreement is encouraging.

Narrow zones which are initially rectangular are often recovered as Gaussian distributions (Fig. 3.25). The equation for a Gaussian distribution of particles p about $V_z = 0$ is

$$C(V) = \bar{c}\epsilon \exp(-V_z^2/2\sigma_v^2) \tag{3.28}$$

where $\bar{c}$ is the concentration of particles at the center of the zone, V_z the volume measured from the center of the zone, and σ_v the first moment or standard deviation of the distribution. To compute the mass of particles in the zone, we integrate the concentration over the volume of the zone

$$m = \int_{-\infty}^{+\infty} c\, dV$$

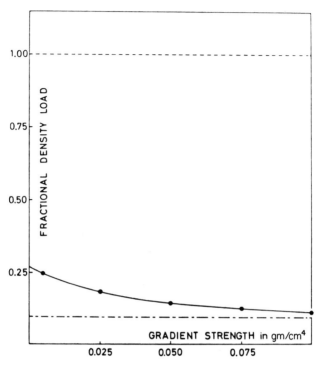

Fig. 3.27. Static capacity of triangular sample zones (Meuwissen, 1973). Serum albumin was loaded statically on sucrose gradients. The instantaneous static capacity (– – –) was calculated for the triangular shape in a manner similar to Eq. (3.27) and normalized to 1.00. The actual static capacity (0) was taken as the maximum amount before zone broadening occurred and is reported as the "fractional density load." The capacity estimated from Meuwissen's model of zero diffusional volume flow is shown as a horizontal line at about 0.1 (–·–).

For Gaussian distributions, this integral can be evaluated as

$$m = \sqrt{2\pi}\sigma_v\bar{c} \tag{3.29}$$

The static capacity of the zone occurs when the slope of density with respect to volume at the first moment reaches zero (cf. Fig. 3.26).

$$(d\rho/dV)_{v=\sigma_v} = 0 \tag{3.30}$$

Combining Eqs. (3.28), (3.29), and (3.30) the concentration of particles in the center of the zone is then

$$\bar{c}_{max} = [\sqrt{\epsilon}\sigma\rho_p(d\rho_m/dV_z)_0]/[\rho_p - \rho_{m,0} - 2\sigma(d\rho_m/dV_z)_0] \tag{3.31}$$

and the total mass of particles is (cf. Vinograd and Bruner, 1966)

$$m_{\max} = [\sqrt{2\pi\epsilon}\,\sigma^2 \rho_p (d\rho_m/dV_z)_0]/[\rho_p - \rho_{m,0} - 2\sigma(d\rho_m/dV_z)_0] \quad (3.32)$$

where the subscript 0 refers to the center of the particle zone.

Preliminary estimates of the dynamic capacities of Gaussian zones are near to 20% of instantaneous static capacity of Eq. (3.32) (Price, 1973), which is similar to the findings of Meuwissen (1973) for triangular zones.

As first pointed out by Berman (1966), the *dynamic capacity* of a gradient to support a zone may be different (and less) than its actual static capacity. The culprit in this case is gradient-induced zone narrowing, which was discussed under zone width. Berman observed* that a gradient which was initially stable could become unstable if gradient-induced zone narrowing were sufficiently severe to counteract the effects of both sectorial dilution and increased buoyancy. He suggested that a class of gradient shapes be considered, which have come to be called Berman gradients (see also Fig. 3.28):

$$\rho_m(r) = \rho_p - (k/r^n) \quad (3.33)$$

where k and n are arbitrary constants. Berman then imagined that the particles were initially loaded as inverse sample gradients to their instantaneous static capacities. He then computed the effects on the density profile of steepening the gradient through increasing the value of n. The results, shown in Fig. 3.28, led to the following generalizations: (1) $0 < n \le 1$ gradients will always be stable; (2) $1 < n \le 2$ gradients may become unstable; and (3) $2 < n$ gradients will become unstable as soon as the particle zone begins to sediment.

Gradients of $n = 1$ have a hyperbolic shape and would be the steepest Berman gradient that should be prudently used. Berman's predictions have been largely confirmed (Spragg and Rankin, 1967; Eikenberry *et al.*, 1970), such that up to 2 gm of ribosomes equivalent to 60% of the theoretical capacity have been separated in a single hyperbolic gradient (see Section 9.4.2). Larger loading resulted in a collapse of the gradient. The actual widths of zones, however, were found to increase substantially more than would have been predicted from Berman's relatively simple model. The finding that the gradient supported 60% of the instantaneous static capacity of the initial sample zone is not therefore necessarily in contradiction with Meuwissen's report of a limit of 20% of this capacity.

---

* Berman as a proper mathematician did not perform experiments; his observations were conducted on simulated centrifugations.

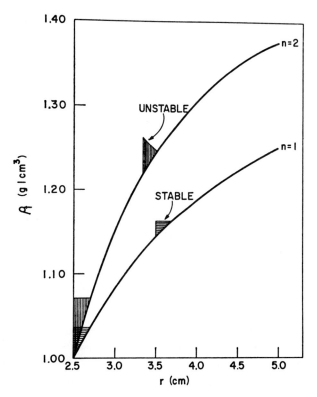

Fig. 3.28. Dynamic instabilities of particle zones (Berman, 1966). A zone initially stable may become unstable through gradient-induced zone narrowing. The values of n in the increasingly steeper gradients refer to the exponent in Eq. 3.33.

Anomalous Zone Broadening

The question of the widths of sedimenting zones is thorny and yet important both for capacity and for resolution to be discussed later. We learned previously that zones in equivolumetric and isometric gradients enlarge in a peculiar, time-dependent process called *anomalous zone broadening* (Spragg *et al.*, 1969). The models on which these gradient shapes are based predict constant zone width; the contradiction between expectations and observations is clear-cut in these cases, but zone spreading appears to be a general phenomenon in all kinds of gradients and rotors.

Spragg (1970) offered a model for anomalous zone broadening which points to the existence of a gradient of solvent (normally water) with direction opposite to that of the density gradient and whose magnitude increases sharply in the region of the particle zone. The gradient of water would result in a continuous diffusion of water into the particle zone, a kind of zonal edema.

In what is essentially an elaboration of Spragg's model, Meuwissen (1973) suggested that the diffusional flows of sucrose and water due to their oppositely disposed gradients normally balance one another, but that the presence of large concentrations of particles in a zone could exclude water and create a locally inverse gradient (Fig. 3.29). Diffusion of water would then not occur in direction or amounts to counterbalance the volume flow of sucrose. The result would be instability and local bulk flows of water with consequent enlargement of the particle zone.

We have compared zone broadening in equivolumetric gradients composed of sucrose and Ficoll (Table 3.1) (Price and Hsu, 1971). Although we expected that the shallower gradient of water in Ficoll should have decreased anomalous zone broadening, no such relief was observed. S. P. Spragg has

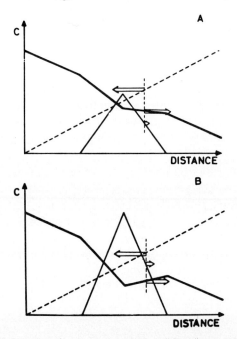

Fig. 3.29. Model for anomalous zone broadening (Meuwissen, 1973). One imagines a triangular zone of particles (——) loaded on a continuous gradient of sucrose (– – –). The presence of the particles will cause a local perturbation in what should be a continuous, oppositely disposed gradient of water (——). With low particle concentrations (A) the volume flows due to sucrose, water, and particles balance one another by simple diffusion and result in continuous enlargement of the zone. At high particle concentrations (B) the diffusion of water is insufficient in both direction and amount; so that the system becomes unstable.

Table 3.1.   Zone Broadening in Equivolumetric Gradients
of Sucrose and Ficoll[a,b]

Gradient material	Time of centrifugation (hr)	σ-value in cm³ for particle		
		30 S	50 S	70 S
Sucrose	4.6	13.6	10.8	9.4
Sucrose	19	17.9	17.5	16.0
Ficoll	4.6	19.0	13.4	12.7
Ficoll	19	20.4	18.3	18.5

[a] Price and Hsu, 1971.
[b] *Eschericia coli* ribosomes and subunits were centrifuged on equivolumetric gradients in the B-30 zonal rotor for 4.6 or 19 hr but to the same value of $\int \omega^2 dt = 4.8 \times 10^{11}$ rad²/sec. The sucrose and Ficoll gradients were each constructed with the same gradient constant.

countered (personal communication) that the activity of water in Ficoll does not lend itself to easy computation. Perhaps, as in the case of Meuwissen's model, the critical events concern the ternary system of particles, solute, and solvent.

Brakke (1964) pointed out a feature of anomalous zone broadening that is not accounted for in any of the quantitative models: for a given field–time integral, zone broadening is greater at low speed than at high speed. A complete understanding of this vexing phenomenon remains for the future.

3.2.5   Resolution

From time to time new procedures are said to improve resolution, which usually means that new zones of particles are revealed. Let us define resolution of sedimenting systems (i.e., *dynamic resolution*) more quantitatively in terms of pairs of specific particles. Borrowing from microscopy, we can define dynamic resolution Λ as the distance between two particle zones divided by the sum of the standard deviations of the particle distributions taken as Gaussian (cf. Fig. 3.30)

$$\Lambda \equiv \left| \frac{\bar{x}_1 - \bar{x}_2}{\sigma_1 + \sigma_2} \right| \tag{3.34}$$

We note that good separation of zone centers (Δx) and narrow zone widths (σ values) do not by themselves insure good resolution; both are required. The interaction of these factors is illustrated in Fig. 3.31. We can expect that resolution will be improved by increasing the distance that particles sediment, but this may be limited by increased zone widths.

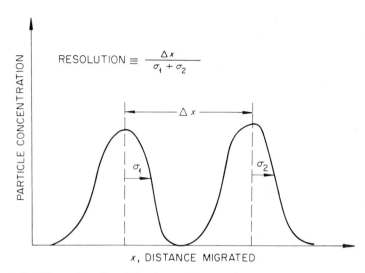

Fig. 3.30. The notion of resolution in particle separations (Price, 1971). The resolution of two Gaussian zones can be defined as the distance between the zones divided by the sums of their zone widths. "Distance" can be taken either as radial or as volumetric distance.

In measuring resolution, it is essential that we work with homogeneous particle populations. A broad band of mitochondria may mean not poor resolution, but rather good separation of size or density classes. Comparison of different methods should be done with the same quantity (preferably a negligible quantity) of particles, since anomalous zone broadening increases with the quantity of particles in a zone. Also one cannot compare the resolution of particle pairs that differ greatly in particle size, for anomalous zone

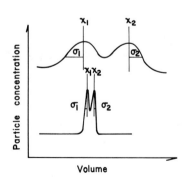

Fig. 3.31. Interaction of factors in resolution. Which profile shows better resolution? They may in fact be identical. The calculation of resolution must take into account both zone separations and zone width.

broadening is more likely with larger particles and particle diffusion more significant for smaller particles.

We have studied the resolution of ribosomes in equivolumetric gradients (Pollack and Price, 1971; Price and Hsu, 1971; Price, 1973) and found it superior to other zonal gradient shapes tested, and equal to that in isokinetic gradients in swinging buckets.

Hsu (1975) has deduced in an elegant mathematical anslysis that the optimal gradient profile for the separation of any pair of particles should have its density increase with $r^{2/3}$ and its viscosity increase with $r^{4/3}$. Hsu assumed that the dispersion of the particle zones would be negligible and that the particles would be optimally separated when the radial distance separating the centers of the two zones was maximal. This model may be appropriate for swinging bucket rotors, but certainly not for the cylindrically shaped zonal rotors (cf. Pollack and Price, 1971; Eikenberry, 1973).

Pretlow and Boone (1968) argue that better resolution may be obtained where the initial radius of the sample zone is as small as possible and have presented supporting data with a swinging-bucket rotor of very short arms. Their model predicts that the separation between the centers of particle zones will increase with decreasing initial radius and their data, obtained with two different size populations of latex beads, support the model. Since neither particle population was homogeneous, they could not determine the effect of shortening the rotor arms on zone width. They did report, however, that wall effects were more severe in the short-arm rotor.

In summary, we can seek to improve resolution by any tactic that will produce narrower particle zones without proportionately decreasing the relative rate of sedimentation. The principal factors will be the same as affect anomalous zone broadening (particle concentration and rotor speed) plus the shape of the gradient.

3.3   EQUILIBRIUM DENSITY, ISOPYCNIC SEPARATIONS, AND SEDIMENTATION EQUILIBRIUM

The principles of isopycnic separations may be disposed of in a small fraction of the space allotted to rate separations. It is not that they are less important, but that the situation is much simpler.

We note in Eq. (3.10) that the rate of sedimentation dr/dt is proportional to the reduced particle density.

$$dr/dt \; \alpha(\rho_p - \rho_m(r))$$

If the density gradient is sufficiently dense, dr/dt will decrease toward zero as ρ_p approaches $\rho_m(r)$ (Fig. 3.32). At infinite time the particle zone will be

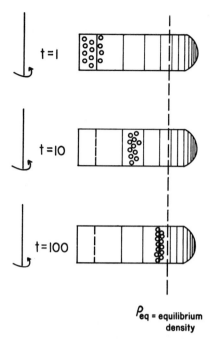

ρ_{eq} = equilibrium
density

Fig. 3.32.   Approach to equilibrium density. Particles move at progressively slower rates as they approach their equilibrium position in a density gradient.

centered on their equilibrium position. We define this as the *equilibrium density* ρ_{eq}.

$$\rho_p = \lim_{t \to \infty} \rho_m(r) \qquad (3.35)$$

In other words the particles migrate into the gradient at a progressively slower rate until they reach a level in the gradient where the densities of particles and medium are the same. Because high concentrations of gradient components will usually affect the density of the particle through changes in hydration, *inter alia*, the value of ρ_p at equilibrium will generally be different (probably greater) than the initial ρ_p under the usual conditions of preparation.

Since the equilibrium density is an equilibrium position, it may be approached by sedimentation from less dense regions of the gradient, from more dense regions (by *flotation*), or the particles may initially be dispersed throughout the gradient (Fig. 3.33). The final equilibrium position of the particles will be independent of the route, except in the case of particles sensitive to high concentrations of the gradient solute. For example, mitochondria, which may be irreversibly damaged by high osmotic pressures,

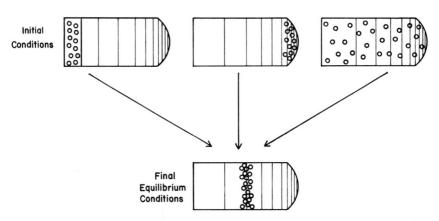

Fig. 3.33. All roads lead to Rome. Particles may sediment (left) or float (center) to their equilibrium position, or arrive there by a combination of the two; the final equilibrium position is normally the same.

could be expected to show a different equilibrium density if they were floated from the bottom of a gradient.

Observe that by isopycnic separation we denote the equilibrium position of the *particles; sedimentation equilibrium* refers to a condition where the distribution of all particles in the system is in true equilibrium between sedimentation and diffusion. Although we shall develop further the principle of sedimentation equilibrium (or *equilibrium sedimentation* or *isopycnic sedimentation equilibrium*) in Section 3.3.3 (cf. also Sections 4.3.8 and 7.11), two types of isopycnic centrifugation are distinguished here.

The term "isopycnic sedimentation" indicates that particles are centrifuged to a position in a gradient where their density is the same as that of the medium. However, the gradient itself is made of particles (the solute) dissolved in a solvent and the distribution of these solute particles is not necessarily in equilibrium with the centrifugal field. Thus the ternary system of sample particles, solute particles, and solvent may not be at a true equilibrium. We call the type of centrifugal separation, where relatively large sample particles are in equilibrium with a nonequilibrium gradient, a *pseudoequilibrium density separation*. However, we shall refer to it by the more general term *isopycnic sedimentation* (literally, equal density). The mean position of the large sample particles in the gradient may be called the equilibrium density, because the particles themselves are in a kind of secular equilibrium.

In *sedimentation equilibrium* we are to visualize that solute particles are sedimented toward the edge of the rotor, but diffuse back toward the center. Given a sufficiently long time, an equilibrium can be established

between sedimentation and diffusion. The resulting distribution of solute is a function *inter alia* of the speed of the rotor and the molecular weight of the solute. Indeed, the equilibrium distribution can be used as a measure of molecular weight.

The effect of centrifugation on the shape of a preformed gradient is commonly ignored (cf. isometric gradients, Section 3.2.3), but prolonged centrifugations at high speed can strongly alter the shape of a sucrose gradient (McEwen, 1967). The shapes of sedimentation–equilibrium gradients of sucrose and salt are shown in Appendix D9.

The distribution of solute also creates a density gradient. It becomes possible therefore to introduce a second set of particles, which will then seek a position of equilibrium density in the gradient. The presence of the sample particles will perturb the original gradient, but the final position of the particles will still represent a true equilibrium.

Thus particles may be centrifuged to their equilibrium density on either a preformed, nonequilibrium gradient or on a gradient generated by sedimentation equilibrium. The observed equilibrium density will be the same, but only in the latter case should we use the term "sedimentation equilibrium" (Table 3.2).

From Eq. (3.35), it is seen that particles reach their true equilibrium position only at infinite time. In practice isopycnic separations require much larger values (ca. $100 \times$) of $\int \omega^2 dt$ than corresponding rate separations. Experimenters often apply higher speeds or longer times than are required to give

Table 3.2. Two Kinds of Isopycnic Centrifugation

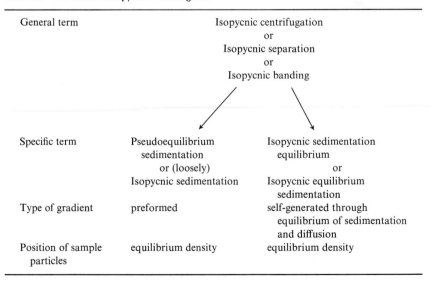

General term	Isopycnic centrifugation or Isopycnic separation or Isopycnic banding	
Specific term	Pseudoequilibrium sedimentation or (loosely) Isopycnic sedimentation	Isopycnic sedimentation equilibrium or Isopycnic equilibrium sedimentation
Type of gradient	preformed	self-generated through equilibrium of sedimentation and diffusion
Position of sample particles	equilibrium density	equilibrium density

identical results. For example, the distribution of mitochondria in a B-XIV rotor after centrifugation at 20,000 rpm for 30 min is indistinguishable from that at 35,000 rpm for 1 hr, which corresponds to a sixfold greater value of $\int \omega^2 dt$. Yet isopycnic sedimentation of mitochondria at maximum rotor speeds for 4–6 hr has been reported. In a somewhat different circumstance, solutions of CsCl require some 2 days at 40,000–60,000 rpm to reach sedimentation equilibrium, but DNA in such a gradient and speed will approach its equilibrium position in several hours. In a *preformed gradient* of CsCl the shorter time would clearly suffice for the banding of DNA.

3.3.1 Capacity

The capacity of gradients in isopycnic separations is essentially unlimited. I have seen particle zones so concentrated as to be semisolid. It follows that much smaller volumes of gradients are required for isopycnic separations than for rate separations. Indeed swinging buckets are usually adequate for all but the most massive preparations.

3.3.2 Resolution

Although homogeneous particle populations may have discrete values of equilibrium density the particles always range themselves on either side of this value in a Gaussian distribution. The particles cannot all occur at the same density because of diffusion. The equilibrium distribution represents an equilibrium between sedimentation or flotation on the one hand, which tend to concentrate the particles at their equilibrium density and diffusion on the other, which tends to move them away (cf. Fig. 3.34).

It follows from this qualitative model that the width of the particle zone at equilibrium is a function of the centrifugal field, the steepness of the gradient, and the particle size. Specifically Meselson *et al.* (1957) calculated that σ_r the standard deviation or first moment of the particle distribution with respect to radius is

$$\sigma_r = \left(\frac{RT\rho_0}{M^*(d\rho/dr)_0 \omega^2 r_0} \right)^{1/2} \tag{3.36}$$

where R is the universal gas constant, T absolute temperature, M^* particle mass in grams/mole, and subscript 0 center of particle zone.

In ordinary isopycnic sedimentation, steepness of the gradient, that is, the value of $d\rho/dr$, is fixed by the experimenter. In sedimentation equilibrium this value is a property of the gradient material in response to the centrifugal field $r\omega^2$. Tables of $(d\rho/dr)_0/r_0\omega^2$ are presented in Appendix C16a.

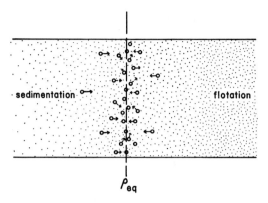

Fig. 3.34. Equilibrium between diffusion, sedimentation, and flotation at the equilibrium position. The sketch represents a portion of a gradient around the equilibrium density. Particles above their ρ_{eq} (left) are accelerated toward the equilibrium position in proportion to their distance from it (solid arrows). Similarly particles below their ρ_{eq} (right) tend to float upward in proportion to their distance from it (solid arrows). In addition, all particles, regardless of their position, have randomly distributed velocities due to diffusion (dotted arrows). At equilibrium all of these motions are in equilibrium.

Equation (3.36) shows that for preformed gradients in which the gradient shape is not affected by the centrifugal field, zone width is decreased and therefore resolution enhanced by high speeds. This relation also provides a test of the homogeneity of the particle population; if the observed r is greater than that computed from Eq. (3.36), one can expect additional variances are operating: from the measuring system, from heterogeneity among the particle, or from nonideality of the gradient system.

Where the gradient shape is controlled by rotor speed, as in gradients generated by sedimentation equilibrium, the changes in $d\rho/dr$ and ω^2 in Eq. (3.36) exactly cancel one another.

Equation (3.36) describes zone widths with respect to radius, which is appropriate for studies with the analytical ultracentrifuge, a topic developed more fully in Section 7.11. In preparative isopycnic separations, however, zone width and therefore resolution is significant with respect to its position in the gradient volume. We can compute a value of σ_v by transforming from radial to volume coordinates.* For small values of σ_r

$$\sigma_v \simeq 2\pi r_0 h \sigma_r$$

* If particles are in a Gaussian distribution with respect to radius, the distribution with respect to volume is

$$C = \bar{c}\epsilon \exp - \frac{\pi h(V_z - V_0)(r + r_0)^2}{\sigma_v^2}$$

which is not a Gaussian distribution. Nonetheless, for narrow zones σ_v is an approximate measure of zone width.

where r_0 is the center of the particle zone, and h the height of the rotor. The volumetric analog of Eq. (3.36) is then

$$\sigma_v = \left(\frac{2\pi h R T \rho_0}{M^*(d\rho/dV)_0 \omega^2} \right)^{1/2} \tag{3.37}$$

It follows from this that the zone width with respect to volume, while inversely related to the slope of the gradient and the square of the speed, is independent of the radial position within the rotor.

Resolution, as a function of zone separation as well as zone width, is strongly affected in opposite directions by the slope of the gradient. Substituting volume relations in Eq. (3.34) and discarding constants yields

$$\Lambda_v = k \left(\frac{M^* \omega^2}{\rho_0 (d\rho/dV)_0} \right)^{1/2} \tag{3.38}$$

where ΔV, the separation between zones, will be inversely related to the first power of $d\rho/dV$, while the σ_v values are inversely related to $\sqrt{d\rho/dV}$. It follows that the net effect of decreasing slope is to increase resolution.

This discussion constitutes only a barebones introduction to sedimentation theory: the companion Chapter 4 provides a more rigorous treatment of these same topics.

REFERENCES

Albertsson, P. A. (1972). "Partition of Cell Particles and Macromolecules," 2nd ed. Wiley, New York.

Anderson, N. G. (1956). Techniques for the mass isolation of cellular components. *Phys. Tech. Biol. Res.* **3**, 299–352.

Berman, A. S. (1966). Theory of centrifugation: Miscellaneous studies. *Natl. Cancer Inst. Monogr.* **21**, 41–76.

Berns, A. J. M., de Abreu, R. A., van Kraaikamp, M., Benedetti, E. L., and Bloemendal, H. (1971). Synthesis of lens protein in vitro. V. Isolation of messenger-like RNA from lens by high resolution zonal centrifugation. *FEBS Lett.* **18**, 159–163.

Brakke, M. K. (1951). Density gradient centrifugation: A new separation technique. *J. Am. Chem. Soc.* **73**, 1847–1848.

Brakke, M. K. (1955). Zone electrophocesis of dyes, proteins and viruses in density-gradient columns of sucrose solutions. *Arch. Biochem. Biophys.* **55**, 175–190.

Brakke, M. K. (1964). Nonideal sedimentation and the capacity of sucrose gradient columns for virus in density-gradient centrifugation. *Arch. Biochem. Biophys.* **107**, 388–403.

Brakke, M. K., and Van Pelt, N. (1970). Linear-log sucrose gradients for estimating sedimentation coefficients of plant viruses and nucleic acids. Anal. Biochem. **38**, 56–64.

Britten, R. J., and Roberts, B. B. (1960). High-resolution density gradient sedimentation analysis. *Science* **131**, 32–33.

Cline, G. B., Ryel, R. B., and Dagg, M. K. (1970). High-resolution separations in zonal centrifuge rotors. *In* "Microsymposium on Particle Separation from Plant Materials" (C. A.

Price, ed.), Oak Ridge Natl. Lab. CONF-700 11 9, pp. 58–65. Natl. Tech. Inf. Serv., Springfield, Virginia.

Cowan, K. M., and Trautman, R. (1965). Antibodies produced by guinea pigs infected with foot-and-mouth disease virus. *J. Immunol.* **94,** 858–867.

Day, E. D., Mcmillan, P. N., Mickey, D. D., and Appel, S. H. (1970). Zonal centrifuge profiles of rat brain homogenates. Instability in sucrose, stability in iso osmotic ficoll-sucrose. *Anal. Biochem.* **39,** 29–45.

de Duve, C., Berthet, J., and Beaufay, M. (1959). Gradient centrifugation of cell particles. Theory and applications. *Prog. Biophys. Biophys. Chem.* **9,** 325–369.

Doppler-Bernardi, F., and Duane, M. (1969). Interaction des ions metalliques avec le DNA. II. Adsorption préférentielle de l'ion césium par les acides nucléiques. *Biopolymers* **7,** 671–680.

Eikenberry, E. F. (1973). Generation of density gradients. Approximations to equivolumetric gradients for zonal rotors. *Anal. Biochem.* **55,** 338–357.

Eikenberry, E. F., Bickle, T. A., Traut, R. R., and Price, C. A. (1970). Separation of large quantities of ribosomal subunits by zonal ultracentrifugation. *Eur. J. Biochem.* **12,** 113–116.

Halsall, H. B., and Schumaker, V. N. (1971). A stability criterion for measurement of diffusion coefficients in the zonal ultracentrifuge. *Biochem. Biophys. Res. Commun.* **43,** 601–606.

Harrison, B. D., and Nixon, H. L. (1959). Separation and properties of particles of tobacco rattle virus (potato stem mottle virus) with different lengths. *J. Gen. Microbiol.* **21,** 569–581.

Hsu, H. W. (1975). Transport phenomena in zonal rotors. X. Optimal gradient solution for velocity sedimentation. *Math. Biosci.* **23,** 179–189.

Kaempfer, R., and Meselson, M. (1971). Sedimentation velocity analysis in accelerating gradients. *In* "Methods in Enzymology" (K. Moldave and L. Grossman, eds.), Vol. 20, Part C, pp. 521–528. Academic Press, New York.

Laties, G. G., and Treffry, T. (1969). Reversible changes in conformation of mitochondria of constant volume. *Tissue Cell* **1,** 575–592.

McEwen, C. R. (1967). Computation of density distributions in solution at sedimentation equilibrium. *Anal. Biochem.* **19,** 23–39.

Martin, R. G., and Ames, B. N. (1961). A method for determining the sedimentation behavior of enzymes: Application to protein mixtures. *J. Biol. Chem.* **236,** 1372–1379.

Meselson, M., Stahl, F. W., and Vinograd, J. (1957). Equilibrium sedimentation of macromolecules in density gradieuts. *Proc. Natl. Acad. Sci. U.S.A.* **43,** 581–588.

Meuwissen, J. A. T. P. (1973). Hydrodynamic instability: An explanation of anomalous zone spreading in density gradient methodology. *Spectra 2000* **4,** 21–31.

Noll, H. (1967). Characterization of macromolecules by constant velocity sedimentation. *Nature (London)* **215,** 360–363.

Novikoff, A. B. (1957). Biochemical heterogeneity of the cytoplasmic particles of liver. *Symp. Soc. Expl. Biol.* **10,** 92–109.

Pertoft, H. (1966). Gradient centrifugation in colloidal silica-polysaccharide media. *Biochim. Biophys. Acta* **126,** 194–596.

Pollack, M. S., and Price, C. A. (1971). Equivolumetric gradients for zonal rotors; separation of ribosomes. *Anal. Biochem.* **42,** 38–47.

Pretlow, T. G., and Boone, C. W. (1968). Centrifugation of mammalian cells on gradients in a new rotor. *Science* **161,** 911–913.

Price, C. A. (1971). Zonal centrifugation. *In* "Manometric Techniques" (W. W. Umbreit, R. H. Burris, and J. H. Staufer, eds.), 5th ed. pp. 213–234. Burgess Pub. Co., Minneapolis, Minn.

Price, C. A. (1973). Equivolumetric gradients: Apparent limits on resolution and capacity imposed by gradient-induced zone narrowing. *Spectra 2000* **4,** 71–81.

Price, C. A., and Hsu, T. S. (1971). The capacity of equivolumetric gradients in zonal rotors in the separation of ribosomes. *Vierteljahrsschl. Naturforsch. Ges. Zuerich* **116,** 367–375.

Sartory, W. K. (1969). Instability in diffusing fluid layers. *Biopolymers* **7,** 251–263.

Schumaker, V. N. (1966). Limiting law for boundary spreading in zone centrifugation. *Sep. Sci.* **1,** 409–411.

Schumaker, V. N., and Halsall, H. B. (1970). Zone diffusion. *In* "Microsymposium on Particle Separation from Plant Materials" (C. A. Price, ed.), Oak Ridge Natl. Lab. CONF-700119, pp. 69–80. Natl. Tech. Inf. Serv., Springfield, Virginia.

Spragg, S. P. (1970). Resolution in zonal rotors. *In* "Microsymposium on Particle Separation from Plant Materials" (C. A. Price, ed.), Oak Ridge Natl. Lab. CONF-700119, pp. 81–88.

Spragg, S. P., and Rankin, C. T., Jr. (1967). The capacity of zones in density-gradient centrifugation. *Biochim. Biophys. Acta* **141,** 164–173.

Spragg, S. P., Morrod, R. S., and Rankin, C. T., Jr. (1969). The optimization of density gradients for zonal centrifugation. *Sep. Sci.* **4,** 467–481.

Steck, T. L., Straus, J. H., and Wallach, D. F. H. (1970). A model for the behavior of vesicles in density gradients: Implications for fractionation. *Biochim. Biophys. Acta* **203,** 385–393.

Svensson, H., Hagadahl, L., and Lerner, K. D. (1957). Large-scale density gradient electrophoresis. Part I. The mathematics of a gradient mixing device with two series-coupled mixing chambers. *Sci. Tools* **4,** 37–41.

Tedeschi, H., and Harris, D. L. (1955). The osmotic behavior and permeability to nonelectrolytes of mitochondria. *Arch. Biochem. Biophys.* **58,** 52–67.

van der Zeijst, B. A. M., and Bult, H. (1972). Equivolumetric glycerol and sucrose gradients for the B-XIV and B-XV zonal rotors. *Eur. J. Biochem.* **28,** 463–474.

Van Holde, K. (1971). "Physical Biochemistry." Prentice-Hall, Englewood Cliffs, New Jersey.

Vinograd, J., and Bruner, R. (1966). Band centrifugation of macromolecules in self-generating density gradients. II. Sedimentation and diffusion of macromolecules in bands. *Biopolymers* **4,** 131–156.

4

Sedimentation Theory: A More Rigorous Approach (by Eric F. Eikenberry)

4.1 PHYSICAL DESCRIPTION

Samples subjected to centrifugation consist of one or more classes of particles (often referred to as species) dispersed in a liquid medium. We use the word "particle" to emphasize the independent mechanistic aspect of the dispersed entities. In cases where continuous solution properties are more important, the terms solute, solute particles, or solute molecules are more appropriate. Physically, there is no distinction among these designations.

The dispersion is spun in a centrifuge rotor for a specified interval to effect the desired analysis. Under the influence of the centrifugal field, the particles will tend toward one of three actions: (1) they will sediment (move outward from the center of the rotor) if they are more dense than the surrounding fluid; (2) they will float (move toward the center) if they are less dense than the surrounding fluid; or (3) they will remain stationary with respect to the rotor if they are isopycnic with respect to the surrounding fluid. The speed of the particles depends on (1) the configuration and angular speed of the rotor, (2) the size, shape, and buoyant density of the particles, (3) the nature of any interactions among the particles, and (4) the physicochemical properties of the dispersing medium.

It is assumed throughout the following discussion that there is no circulation in the fluid column containing the particles and, hence, that convection does not influence the particles' motions. Experimental realization of this usually requires that a gradient of solution density be present in the fluid column to stabilize it.

4.2 EQUATION OF MOTION OF A SINGLE PARTICLE IN A CENTRIFUGAL FIELD

4.2.1 Transformation of Newton's Second Law to a Rotating Coordinate System

Consider a particle of fixed mass m located at position r in a coordinate system at rest with respect to a fixed observer. This particle is immersed in a fluid medium contained in a rotor which turns with angular velocity ω, the magnitude of which is equal to the angular speed of the rotor. The direction of the vector ω is along the axis of rotation of the rotor in the direction given by the right-hand rule. There is no loss of generality if the fixed coordinate system is chosen so that its positive z axis is coincident with ω.

The basis for the equation of motion is Newton's second law, $\mathbf{F} = m\mathbf{a}$, in which $\mathbf{F}$ is the total force acting on the particle and $\mathbf{a}$ is the acceleration to which the particle is subjected. If the earth's gravitational field is neglected, the acceleration is given by the second derivative of the position vector with respect to time

$$\mathbf{a} = d/dt(\mathbf{dr}/dt)$$

It is convenient to transform the equation for $\mathbf{a}$ to a coordinate system fixed with respect to the rotor. If the angular velocity ω is constant, this transformation requires only that the differential operator be rewritten as (Symon, 1954)

$$d/dt = (d^*/dt + \omega \times)$$

where * indicates measurements made with respect to the rotating coordinate system. Newton's law then becomes

$$\mathbf{F} = m\left(\frac{d^*}{dt} + \omega \times\right)\left(\frac{d^*\mathbf{r}}{dt} + \omega \times \mathbf{r}\right)$$

which, upon performing the algebra, becomes

$$\mathbf{F} = m[\mathbf{a}^* + 2\omega \times \mathbf{v}^* + \omega \times (\omega \times \mathbf{r})] \tag{4.1}$$

where $\mathbf{a}^*$ is the acceleration and $\mathbf{v}^*$ the velocity of the particle.

4.2.2 Evaluation of the Components of the Acceleration

The first term on the right-hand side of Eq. 4.1 is the acceleration of the particle with respect to the rotor, the second term is the Coriolis acceleration, and the third term is the centripetal acceleration, commonly referred to as the centrifugal acceleration* or "centrifugal force." The magnitudes of these respective terms have been compared in the range encountered in centrifugation (Berman, 1966). The acceleration of the particle was found to be negligible in all circumstances in liquid media because of the viscous damping. The Coriolis acceleration is always small and almost always negligible. Its effect may be visualized by considering a particle that moves from an initial radius r_1 to a larger radius r_2 in the rotor. At the new larger radius the particle will necessarily be moving with a larger tangential speed, ωr^2 than it had previously. For the fluid in the rotor to impart this increase of speed to the particle, the particle will have to slip sideways with respect to the fluid in a direction opposite to the rotation and hence will follow a curved trajectory in the rotor, rather than moving exactly radially. This effect is significant only when the radial motion of the particles is extremely rapid; hence the Coriolis term may be safely neglected in the usual experimental circumstances of centrifugation.† Equation 4.1 may now be simplified by eliminating these two terms together with vector notation to obtain

$$F = -m\omega^2 r \qquad (4.2)$$

where the negative sign indicates that the force is directed toward the center of the rotor. The significance of the negative sign is that for a particle to move in a circular path it must be constrained by the presence of a force directed toward the axis of rotation, otherwise the particle would move away in a straight line. This constraining force is provided by the supporting fluid in centrifugation. The assumption has been made that gravity is negligible, which may not be adequate for centrifugation at a very low speed (e.g., <800 rpm.)

4.2.3 Sources of the Force, F

The force F, which acts on a particle to constrain its path to the very nearly circular trajectory found in centrifugation, is derived from three sources: (1)

---

* The acceleration component $\omega \times (\omega \times r)$ is directed toward the axis of rotation and hence is properly termed a centripetal acceleration.

† I have often observed the effect of the Coriolis acceleration while centrifuging an unclarified brei from plant cells in a density gradient in a zonal rotor. A heavy green pellet would form at the outer wall of the rotor and on one side only of the septum near the outer wall. The other side of the septum and the adjacent portion of the outer wall would be nearly free of sediment. This one-sided accumulation is precisely what would be predicted by the effect of the Coriolis acceleration.

the pressure acting on the surface of the particle which gives rise to the Archimedean buoyancy, (2) the viscous drag imparted by the fluid medium as the particle moves through it, and (3) a component from the thermal agitation in the surrounding fluid. The latter component results in no predictable motion of a particle considered individually, but it is the mechanical basis of diffusion which is considered below.

Pressure at a Point in the Fluid

Equation (4.2) applies also to every element of volume of the fluid itself and in that case is exact, since $a^* = v^* = 0$ in the absence of circulation. If dV is an element of fluid volume, the force per unit volume or body force acting on each such element in the liquid is

$$dF/dV = -\rho\omega^2 r \qquad (4.3)$$

where ρ is the density of the solution. In the case of an isolated particle, this density is the same as that of the pure solvent, but the presence of other particles, which must also be supported by the liquid, modifies the pressure distribution in a way that may be expressed by using the total solution density rather than the solvent density. This point is unambiguous in a thermodynamic derivation (see Fujita, 1962; cf. Section 4.2.5).

In a column of fluid at hydrostatic equilibrium, the pressure difference between two points is given by a line integral of the body force between those points. In our simple case this reduces to

$$P_r = \int_{r_m}^{r} \rho\omega^2 r \, dr + P_m$$

where P_r is the pressure at radius r, r_m the radius to the meniscus of the fluid column; and P_m the pressure at the meniscus. If ρ is independent of r, and if $P_m \cong 1$ atm is ignored, this equation may be integrated to give:

$$P_r \cong \rho(r^2 - r_m^2)/2 \qquad (4.4)$$

Archimedean Buoyancy

The Archimedean buoyant force, F_b, is the resultant of the pressure acting across each element of surface, dA, of a particle. This force may be expressed as an integral over the surface S of the particle

$$F_b = -\iint_S P(r) \, dA$$

where dA is the outward directed normal vector at the surface of the particle with magnitude dA. This is transformed by Green's Theorem to an integral over the volume of the particle V_p

$$F_b = - \iiint_{V_p} (\nabla P) dV$$

The gradient of the pressure, ∇P, is assumed to be approximately constant over the very small volume of the particle so that this equation may be approximated to give

$$F_b \cong -(\nabla P) \iiint_{V_p} dV = -(\nabla P) V_p$$

The gradient of the pressure is the negative of the expression in Eq. (4.3), so that F_b is directed along a radius. If we drop the vector notation the buoyant force becomes

$$F_b = -\rho \omega^2 V_p \tag{4.5}$$

where the negative sign indicates that this force is directed toward the rotor axis.

Viscous Force

If a spherical particle passes with velocity $\mathbf{v}$ through a perfect Navier–Stokes fluid, the viscous force $\mathbf{F}_v$, acting on the particle is given by Stokes' law

$$\mathbf{F}_v = -3\pi\eta d\mathbf{v} \tag{4.6}$$

where d is the diameter of the spherical particle, and η the viscosity of the medium. For nonspherical particles, this relation is generalized by the introduction of a frictional coefficient, f, such that

$$\mathbf{F}_v = -f\mathbf{v} \tag{4.7}$$

which may be simplified by dropping the vector notation since in this case the motion is directed radially. The frictional coefficient f_0 for a sphere is thus

$$f_0 = 3\pi\eta d$$

The frictional ratio, $\theta = f/f_0$, has been derived theoretically for several simple geometrical shapes, including long rods and ellipsoids of revolution (cf. Tanford, 1961, and Appendix A). Such simple shapes are the only ones that permit exact solution of the hydrodynamic equations describing the motion of a particle through a fluid medium (Happel and Brenner, 1973, Kuntz and Kauzmann, 1974). Frictional coefficients for bodies of more complex shape, such as bacterial viruses, have been obtained by numerical methods using collections of nonidentical spheres to represent approximately the shape of the body (Garcia de la Torre, 1977a,b, Teller *et al.* 1979).

4.2.4 Sedimentation Equation

If we neglect for the moment the effects of diffusion, Eqs. (4.2), (4.5), and (4.7) may be combined to give the equation of motion for a particle in a liquid medium in a centrifuge rotor

$$-fv - \rho\omega^2 r V_p = -m\omega^2 r \tag{4.8}$$

which may be rearranged to give

$$v = dr/dt = s\omega^2 r \tag{4.9}$$

where $s = (m - \rho V_p/f)$. This is the well-known sedimentation equation in which s is the sedimentation coefficient, defined here for a single particle. The sedimentation coefficient has dimensions of time and is usually reported in Svedbergs.

The sedimentation coefficient s may be transformed to a more useful form by several substitutions. The molar mass M of a substance,* usually called the molecular weight, is related to the mass of an individual particle of the substance by

$$M = N_0 m$$

where N_0 is Avogadro's number. That is, M is the mass of N_0 particles and as such is well defined even where the particle is not strictly a molecule.

Let ρ_p be the average density of the particle

$$\rho_p = m/V_p = M/N_0 V_p$$

Thermodynamic derivations of the sedimentation equation usually are expressed in terms of the partial specific $\bar{v}$ of the particles under investigation, where for practical purposes $\bar{v} = 1/\rho_p$, the reciprocal of the buoyant density

---

* M is reported on a scale of grams (gram-moles) or kilograms (kilogram-moles), respectively, in the cgs and mks systems. The particle mass or molecular mass m is measured on the scale of the unified atomic mass unit u defined as one-twelfth of the mass of an atom of the neutral ^{12}C nuclide. Thus $1\ u = 1.6605655 \times 10^{-24}$ gm. Masses of single particles are also reported in daltons, which are not SI units and of which there are two kinds: 1 dalton (chemical) = 1.66024×10^{-24} gm; 1 dalton (physical) = 1.65979×10^{-24} gm. The Avogadro constant is the number of atoms in exactly 12.0 gm of pure ^{12}C and is 6.022045×10^{23} mole^{-1}.

of the particles. Hence s may be expressed as either

$$s = \frac{M(1 - \rho/\rho_p)}{N_0 f}$$

or   (4.10)

$$s = \frac{M(1 - \bar{v}\rho)}{N_0 f}$$

4.2.5 Partial Specific Volume and Its Relation to Buoyant Density

The partial specific volume always occurs together with M; hence if M is to be measured $\bar{v}$ must also be known or measured.

The partial specific volume $\bar{v}_i$ of substance i is defined by (Tanford, 1961)

$$\bar{v}_i = (\partial V/\partial g_i)_{T,P,g_j}, \qquad (j \neq i)$$

where V is the total solution volume, g_i the mass of substance i and T, P, g_j refer to constant temperature, pressure, and mass of all other components of the solution. Conceptually the partial specific volume may be measured as follows. First, take a large volume of the solution to be used under specified conditions of composition, pressure, and temperature. Then, add to this a very small, known mass of the particles under investigation. Finally, measure the volume displaced by the particles and divide by their combined mass to obtain the partial specific volume. Hence, the partial specific volume is by definition the ratio of volume displaced to the mass of a particle and is thus the reciprocal of the buoyant density.

This simplistic definition masks several formidable problems: (1) how should the solution to be used be defined; (2) how should the test particle be treated before being introduced to the solution; and (3) how could such a measurement actually be made in a laboratory. Apparently, as defined previously, the partial specific volume is not just a property of the particle under investigation, but depends also on the solution environment (temperature, pressure, the presence of other components) and on the concentration of the particles themselves. Many authors, however, prefer a definition of $\bar{v}$ which, to the greatest extent possible, is a property only of the substance itself, not of its environment. For this definition the solution must be pure water (or, more realistically, very dilute buffer) and the test particles must be thoroughly washed in water and dried. When a partial specific volume is reported without qualification, it is assumed that these are the conditions implied: very dilute aqueous solution at 20°C and 1 atm pressure.

These ideal conditions are difficult to realize in many experimental systems. It is preferable to define partial specific volume as described previously under conditions closely related to those of an actual experiment. In this circumstance $\bar{v}$ varies according to solution composition. Using again the conceptual method of measuring $\bar{v}$, the test particles would be taken from a solution of the same composition as the large test volume, thoroughly shaken off to remove from them all adhering fluid, weighed, and placed into the test volume for the displacement measurement.

Casassa and Eisenberg (1964) have formalized this facetious approach and made precise the conditions under which meaningful results can be obtained. They showed that a consistent and workable definition of all thermodynamic parameters needed in this work could be obtained if one first exhaustively dialyzed the solution of particles against an appropriate solvent and then used the outer dialyzate as the reference solvent for all measurements. Under these conditions, M and $\bar{v}$ refer to that substance which did not redistribute across the dialysis membrane. Apparent specific volume ϕ is determined by measuring the density of the solution ρ and using the equation

$$\phi = [1 - (\rho - \rho_s)/c]/\rho_s$$

where ρ_s is the density of the outer dialysate in which the concentration of the species under investigation is zero. The concentration c of particles in the inner dialysate is expressed in gm/cm^3. The partial specific volume may be gotten from several measurements of ϕ at different concentrations using graphical or numerical methods and the equation

$$\bar{v} = \phi + w(d\phi/dw)$$

where w is the weight concentration of particles in grams per gram of principal solvent, usually water. Hence, at low concentrations of particles, the value of ϕ corresponds closely to $\bar{v}$; this is especially true of biological particles in aqueous solvents which generally show a very low dependence of apparent specific volume on concentration. In that case the distinction between the c and w scales of concentration measurement could be ignored for extrapolation to zero concentration.

Casassa and Eisenberg further point out that it is not $\bar{v}$ per se which is generally of interest but rather the density increment

$$d\rho/dc = 1 - \bar{v}\rho_s$$

which is needed for computation. This increment is precisely the quantity $(\rho - \rho_s)/c$ measured as described to find ϕ except here the density measurements must be made of a series of concentrations to define a true differential. The equality sign represents an approximation in that strictly it would hold for centrifugation only under conditions of constant chemical potential and for solutions infinitely dilute with respect to the particle species of interest. The density increment is more closely related to s measurements than is the derived quantity $\bar{v}$ and is more nearly independent of concentration than is $\bar{v}$. Hence measured density increments can be used directly without the necessity of calculating $\bar{v}$. Solution density measurements can be made easily on small volumes with excellent accuracy using a digital density meter (Elder, 1979).

This method is still not free of experimental hazards. One must make an absolute concentration measurement c in gm/cm^3 of solution. One approach is to dry and weigh known volumes of the solution and the reference solvent and substract the latter from the former to obtain the net weight of material of interest. Another approach is to measure concentration by some independent means (e.g., nitrogen analysis or optical absorbance). These methods give different results depending on the composition of the solutions due to the effects of "binding" of components. The differences will be slight for dilute solutions, but may be highly significant in the presence of concentrated salts. This point is discussed lucidly by Casassa and Eisenberg (1964). Finally the preceding discussion largely neglects the effects of pressure, which may be a real problem in ultracentrifugation, but which one usually hopes may be ignored. With these limitations in mind, the partial specific volumes referred to in subsequent discussions will be taken to mean under the conditions of the experiment and in the case of isopycnic centrifugation may be taken to be the reciprocal of the particle's buoyant density.

4.2.6   Transformation of *s* to Standard Conditions

The sedimentation coefficient s depends both on the nature of the particle and on the medium in which it is immersed. Experimental determinations of s are customarily corrected to standard conditions of solvent viscosity and density according to the formula

$$s_{20,w} = s_{T,m} \frac{\eta_{T,m}}{\eta_{20,w}} \frac{(\rho_p - \rho_{20,w})}{(\rho_p - \rho_{T,m})} \tag{4.11}$$

where the subscripts T and m denote properties at temperature T in the experimental medium, while the subscripts 20 and w refer to water at $20°C$. The assumption that we are dealing with an isolated particle here permits the use of the density and viscosity of the pure solvent rather than those of the solution. In actual practice, it is often required that experimental values of $s_{20,w}$ be extrapolated to infinite dilution to remove concentration effects and to justify the use of pure solvent parameters in calculations. The extrapolated quantity is designated $s_{20,w}^{\circ}$ (cf. Section 4.4.4). Eq. (4.11) is not exact in that solvation of the particles under investigation has not been taken into account. This results in an underestimation of the sedimentation coefficient that may become significant in a high gradient density (Nieuwenhuysen, 1979). An empirical relation of molecular weight to sedimentation coefficient for a wide range of proteins has provided evidence that the degree of solvation of proteins is large (0.5 g of H_2O per g of protein) and highly variable from one protein to another (Squire and Himmel, 1979).

4.2.7 Integrated Forms of the Sedimentation Equation

Equation (4.9) may be integrated to give implicitly the radial position of a particle as a function of time

$$\int_{r_0}^{r} \frac{d(\ln r)}{s(r)} = \int_{t_0}^{t} [\omega(t)]^2 dt \tag{4.12}$$

where r_0 is the position of the particle at time t_0. The right-hand side of this equation is called the speed–time integral. Frequently $\omega(t)$ can be regarded as a constant during an experiment so that the speed–time integral evaluates to $\omega^2 t$ if t_0 is chosen to be equal to zero. If s is not a function of r, that is, if the particle dispersion is dilute and uniform throughout, then the left-hand side of Eq. (4.11) may also be integrated to give

$$\ln(r/r_0) = s\omega^2 t \tag{4.13}$$

This equation is applicable to pelleting material from a uniform initial suspension, to differential centrifugation, and to boundary sedimentation in analytical centrifugation.

In the presence of a density gradient, $s(r)$ will generally have a complicated dependence on r because of the variations in viscosity and density. These variations may be expressed explicitly in the following form of Eq. (4.12)

$$\int_{r_0}^{r} \frac{\eta_{T,m}(r)d(\ln r)}{[\rho_p - \rho_{T,m}(r)]} = \frac{s_{20,w}\eta_{20,w}}{(\rho_p - \rho_{20,w})}\omega^2 t \tag{4.14}$$

This equation may be evaluated numerically if adequate data are available concerning the density and viscosity of the liquid medium as functions of temperature and concentration. The required density and viscosity data often may be estimated to adequate precision from published data on pure solutions. The approximation required is that any effects of dissolved salts, buffers and other low-molecular-weight solutes on the desired parameters be negligible.

The design of arbitrary density gradients for particular applications may be aided by a procedure based on Eq. (4.12), given by Eikenberry (1973). An approach to the problem of making numerical calculations with Eq. (4.14) has been presented by Hsu (1970).

4.3 MOTION OF DILUTE COLLECTIONS OF PARTICLES IN A CENTRIFUGAL FIELD

4.3.1 Diffusion

Fick's First Law and the Diffusion Coefficient

The thermal agitation, or Brownian motion, present in any body of liquid causes particles suspended in the liquid to be transported in a direction opposite to the gradient of concentration of the particles. This mass transport process is called diffusion. The rate of diffusional mass transport across any infinitesimal area in a solution is given by Fick's first law

$$\mathbf{J}_{\text{diff}}(\mathbf{r}, t) = -D\nabla c(\mathbf{r}, t) \tag{4.15}$$

where $\mathbf{J}_{\text{diff}}(\mathbf{r}, t)$ is the time-dependent vector field representing mass transported by diffusion across unit area per unit time, $c(\mathbf{r}, t)$ the scalar field representing concentration, and D is the coefficient of diffusion. In centrifugation a representation in cylindrical coordinates is appropriate and it is assumed that both c and $\mathbf{J}$ are constant along both the azimuthal and z coordinates. The remaining radial component of Fick's first law may be written

$$J_{\text{diff}}(r, t) = -D\left[\partial c(r, t)/\partial r\right] \tag{4.16}$$

The diffusion coefficient D of solute particles depends, as does the sedimentation coefficient, on the viscosity and density of the solvent and on the concentration of the solute particles themselves.

Relation of the Diffusion Coefficient to the Frictional
Coefficient in a Two-Component System

The form of Eq. (4.15) may be derived in several ways. Fick's original formulation was empirically based (cf. Jost, 1960). Einstein (1905) has given a derivation based on statistical mechanics (reviewed also by Tanford, 1961). A derivation based on the thermodynamics of irreversible processes using the phenomenological equations has the advantage of giving the form of the first order corrections for nonidealities, even though some of the parameters involved are not subject to experimental determination. This derivation is reviewed by Tanford (1961) and presented in detail by de Groot and Mazur (1969). The phenomenological equations postulate that the flow of matter in a system should be proportional to the gradient of total potential (chemical plus mechanical plus other forms if required) associated with that flow. For a simple two component system in which one dilute solute is present in a great excess of solvent, the phenomenological equation may be written as

$$J_2(r) = -L(\partial \mu_2 / \partial r)_t$$

where L is the phenomenological coefficient, μ the total potential of the solute, and the subscript t denotes evaluation at a particular time. The subscript 2 refers to the dilute component of primary interest in the system, the subscript 1 being reserved for the solvent.* The theory of irreversible processes identifies the coefficient L to be the ratio of the concentration to the molar frictional coefficient so that this equation becomes

$$J_2 = -c_2 / N_0 f (\partial \mu_2 / \partial r)_t \tag{4.17}$$

where c_2 is the concentration. If c_2 is on a scale of gm/cm^3 of solution, then J_2 has units of $gm/(cm^2 \ sec)$. In the absence of any nonchemical contribution, the total potential may be written as

$$\mu_2 = \mu_2{}^0 + RT \ln a_2 \tag{4.18}$$

where $\mu_2{}^0$ is the standard chemical potential for the solute, and a_2 the activity of the solute. The activity a_2 may be expressed in terms of the concentration and an activity coefficient y_2 by

$$a_2 = c_2 y_2$$

The quantity $(\partial \mu_2 / \partial r)_t$ may then be evaluated to give

$$\left(\frac{\partial \mu_2}{\partial r}\right)_t = \frac{RT}{c_2}\left[1 + \left(\frac{\partial \ln y_2}{\partial \ln c_2}\right)_{T,P}\right]\left(\frac{\partial c_2}{\partial r}\right)_t$$

where the subscript T,P indicates a derivative made at constant temperature and pressure. Upon combining this with Eq. (4.17) and comparing it with Eq. (4.16) we obtain the relation between the diffusion coefficient and the frictional coefficient in a two-component system

$$D_2 = \frac{RT}{N_0 f}\left[1 + \left(\frac{\partial \ln y_2}{\partial \ln c_2}\right)_{T,P}\right] \tag{4.19}$$

For a two-component system, the quantity in brackets approaches a limit of unity as the concentration is reduced to zero. Thus, experimental measurements of the diffusion coefficient may be extrapolated to zero concentration

---

* The solvent, component 1, is generally considered to include low-molecular-weight compounds (e.g., buffers, dilute salts) which are sufficiently dilute to have negligible effects on the thermodynamic properties of the solvent. Component 2 refers to the macromolecular solute under investigation; however, it is not implicit that it be of high molecular weight. Component 3 will be a low-molecular-weight solute which is present in high concentrations and must be treated apart from the solvent.

to yield the quantity denoted as $D_2{}^0$, which is related to the frictional co-efficient by

$$D_2{}^0 = RT/N_0 f = kT/f \tag{4.20}$$

where k is Boltzmann's constant.

4.3.2 Mass Transport Due to Combined Sedimentation and Diffusion

Consider a unit element of area oriented perpendicularly to a radius in a rotor. We obtain the rate of mass transport by sedimentation through each such element of area J_{sed}, by multiplying $s\omega^2 r$ in Eq. (4.9) by the concentration

$$J_{\text{sed},2}(r) = s_2 \omega^2 r c_2(r)$$

Thus, at a given time, the combined rate of mass transport per unit area due to sedimentation and diffusion is given by

$$J_{\text{total},2} = s_2 \omega^2 r c_2(r) - D_2 \left(\frac{\partial c_2(r)}{\partial r} \right)_t \tag{4.21}$$

4.3.3 Conservation of Mass

Conservation of mass in any system requires that the divergence of the mass transport rate vector $\mathbf{J}$ equal the negative of the time rate of change of mass concentration at every point. For a two-component system in which a single dilute solute is present in a great excess of solvent, the transport of solvent can be ignored to a good approximation and conservation of mass then requires that

$$\frac{\partial c_2(\mathbf{r}, t)}{\partial t} = -\nabla \cdot \mathbf{J}_2(\mathbf{r}, t) \tag{4.22}$$

If we make the familiar assumption that no variations take place along the azimuthal and z coordinates of a cylindrical coordinate system, then the radial component of this equation becomes

$$\frac{\partial c_2(r, t)}{\partial t} = -\frac{1}{r} \frac{\partial}{\partial r} [r J_2(r, t)] \tag{4.23}$$

4.3.4 Fick's Second Law

An equation known as Fick's second law, or as the diffusion equation, may be obtained by applying the equation describing conservation of mass,

Eq. (4.22), to the equation of Fick's first law, Eq. (4.15). If it is assumed that D_2 does not depend on position over small regions of the fluid, the general result is

$$\frac{\partial c_2(\mathbf{r}, t)}{\partial t} = D_2 \nabla^2 [c_2(\mathbf{r}, t)] \qquad (4.24)$$

or, in cylindrical coordinates in which variations in concentration occur only as a function radius, one obtains

$$\frac{\partial c_2(r, t)}{\partial t} = \frac{D_2}{r} \frac{\partial}{\partial r} \left[r \frac{\partial c_2(r, t)}{\partial r} \right] \qquad (4.25)$$

This equation describes radial diffusion in cylindrical coordinates in the absence of sedimentation. In centrifugation in preformed density gradients of low-molecular-weight solutes, the effect of sedimentation on the gradient-forming solute frequently may be ignored, and, in that case, Eq. (4.25) accurately describes the diffusion of the gradient. However, the concentrations of the gradient-forming solute generally are not small and thus D_2 will vary with position. Numerous useful forms of solutions to this equation are given by Jost (1960).

4.3.5 Lamm Equation

If the equation expressing conservation of mass in a centrifuge rotor, Eq. (4.23) is combined with Eq. (4.21), which expresses the mass transport rate under the influence of both sedimentation and diffusion, one obtains

$$\frac{\partial c_2(r, t)}{\partial t} = -\frac{1}{r} \frac{\partial}{\partial r} \left\{ r \left[s_2 \omega^2 r c_2(r, t) - D_2 \frac{\partial c_2(r, t)}{\partial r} \right] \right\} \qquad (4.26)$$

This is known as the Lamm equation and is the general equation of motion of dilute ideal diffusing particles in a centrifugal field.

A general solution of this equation is not possible, but a number of approximate solutions, valid under particular boundary conditions, have been published. Among these are the Faxén solutions, which are widely applicable to the determination of sedimentation coefficients of diffusing solutes, and the Archibald solution, which is used for molecular weight determination in the method of approach to equilibrium (see Tanford (1961) or Fujita (1962) for more information on these solutions).

In density gradient centrifugation, both s and D depend on radial position because of the changes in the viscosity and density of the medium. The differences in s and D between the top and the bottom of a density gradient may be quite large, frequently more than an order of magnitude, and the form of their dependence on radius is usually quite complicated. Thus, only numerical solutions of the Lamm equation are generally applicable to density gradient centrifugation.

4.3.6 Svedberg Equation

The sedimentation coefficient s and the diffusion coefficient D are related through their common dependence on the frictional coefficient f. Equation (4.9), the definition of the sedimentation coefficient, may be combined with Eq. (4.19) to give

$$\frac{s_2{}^0}{D_2{}^0} = \frac{M_2(1 - \bar{v}_2\rho)}{RT} \tag{4.27}$$

This is known as the Svedberg equation.

This equation provides the basis of a widely used method for the determination of molecular weight based on independent measurements of $s_2{}^0$ and $D_2{}^0$. Although the Svedberg equation is strictly valid only for an ideal solute, the condition of ideality may be satisfactorily approximated in practice by the use of a very dilute solute in a dilute buffered solvent. A technique for measuring extremely small diffusion coefficients in density gradients has allowed this approach to be used for determining molecular weights in the range of 2×10^6 gm, where molecular weight measurements are very difficult (Halsall and Schumaker, 1972).

4.3.7 Sedimentation-Diffusion Equilibrium
in a Two-Component System

If a centrifugation experiment is sufficiently prolonged, the processes of sedimentation and diffusion will eventually come into equilibrium. For a single ideal solute, the equilibrium distribution of solute may be obtained from the Lamm equation (4.26) by noting that at equilibrium the left-hand side of the equation is zero

$$\frac{\partial c_2(r, t)}{\partial t} = 0 = -\frac{1}{r}\frac{\partial}{\partial r}\left\{r\left[s_2\omega^2 r c_2(r, t) - D_2\frac{\partial c_2(r, t)}{\partial t}\right]\right\}$$

The subsidiary condition is imposed that, if $\omega = 0$, then the solute concentration at equilibrium should be uniform throughout the rotor

$$\frac{dc_2(r)}{dr} = 0$$

Because there is no time dependence at equilibrium the total derivative has been used in place of the partial derivative. Using this with the Svedberg equation (4.27), we obtain

$$\frac{1}{rc_2(r)} \frac{dc_2(r)}{dr} = \frac{M_2(1 - \bar{v}_2\rho)\omega^2}{RT} \tag{4.28}$$

This equation is the basis for the widely used method of molecular weight determination by sedimentation equilibrium in the analytical centrifuge. The advantages of this approach are that M_2 is obtained without reference to any other unknown except $\bar{v}_2$, and that the method has very good accuracy. The range of molecular weights which may be determined by this method extends from less than 10^3 gm to more than 2×10^6 gm. Detailed accounts of the application of this method may be found in Tanford (1961), Van Holde (1971), Yphantis (1964), and Hill et al. (1969).

Definition of Components

Equation (4.28), which gives the concentration distribution of an ideal solute at sedimentation–diffusion equilibrium, contains a term in ρ, the solution density, which is difficult to evaluate. This may be circumvented by an appropriate choice of the definition of components in the system. Casassa and Eisenberg (1964) demonstrated that if the solution containing the macromolecular component was dialyzed to equilibrium against the pure solvent then it was appropriate to use the outer dialysis fluid as the reference solvent and the dialyzed solution as the sample solution for all measurements. If this procedure is followed, the Eq. (4.28) holds with ρ equal to the density of the reference solvent, providing that the measurement of the apparent $\bar{v}_2$ is also carried out with the same two solutions. The molecular weight M_2 measured in this case is that of the unsolvated macromolecule: that is, of the nondialyzable entity if it may be assumed that bound material has the same density as the bulk solvent (see Section 4.2.5).

Time to Equilibrium

True sedimentation–diffusion equilibrium for a two-component system has no application in preparative centrifugation because the time required to establish equilibrium with a high-molecular-weight solute is prohibitive for fluid columns longer than a few millimeters. The time required for the solute concentration to be within 0.1% of its equilibrium value at every point in the fluid column is given approximately by

$$t_{0.1\%} \cong 0.7h^2/D_2 \tag{4.29}$$

where h is the column height in centimeters. In the analytical centrifuge, h is typically 3 mm and the time required for a solute of $M_2 = 10^4$ gm to reach equilibrium is about 24 hr.

4.3.8 Sedimentation–Diffusion Equilibrium in a Density Gradient

In this technique, a density gradient of a low-molecular-weight solute (e.g., CsCl) is formed at sedimentation–diffusion equilibrium. If a small amount of high-molecular-weight polymer is present, it will move to its isopycnic position in the density gradient. Theoretical treatment of this situation is complicated by the presence of high concentrations of the low-molecular-weight solute, which requires corrections for nonideality, and by the effects of solvation on the polymer.

Physical Density Gradient

In the absence of the macromolecular component, we will have a two-component nonideal system. The concentration as a function of radius is obtained from the assertion that at equilibrium the total potential, chemical plus mechanical, must be constant throughout the system. The potential of the low-molecular-weight solute, which will be designated as component 3, is given by

$$\mu_3 = \mu_3^0 + RT \ln a_3 - (M_3\omega^2 r^2/2)$$

The last term represents the centrifugal potential. If μ_3 is constant throughout the fluid column, one may evaluate the solute distribution by setting

$$0 = \frac{d\mu_3}{dr} = \left(\frac{\partial\mu_3}{\partial c}\right)_T \frac{\partial c_3}{\partial r} + \left(\frac{\partial\mu_3}{\partial P}\right)_{T,c_3} \frac{\partial P}{\partial r} - \frac{\partial\mu_3}{\partial r}$$

The second term on the right is related to the partial specific volume $\bar{v}_3$ by

$$(\partial\mu_3/\partial P)_{T,c_3} = M_3\bar{v}_3$$

Using this and Eqs. (4.3) and (4.18) we obtain

$$\frac{d(\ln a_3)}{dr} = \frac{M_3(1 - \bar{v}_3\rho)\omega^2 r}{RT} \tag{4.30}$$

This is the same as Eq. (4.28) except that the concentration has been replaced by the activity; we define $\beta(\rho)$ to be

$$\beta(\rho) = \frac{d(\ln a_3)}{d\rho} \frac{RT}{M_3(1 - \bar{v}_3\rho)}$$

which allows us to write Eq. (4.30) as

$$d\rho/dr = \omega^2 r/\beta(\rho) \tag{4.31}$$

At atmospheric pressure the quantity $\beta(\rho)$, designated $\beta^0(\rho)$, is a function only of the composition and temperature of the gradient. This quantity may be evaluated graphically from published data, and tables of $\beta^0(\rho)$ for several solutes have been published by Ifft *et al.* (1961), Vinograd and Hearst (1962), and Hu *et al.* (1962) (cf. Appendix C). An improved method for calculating β^0 and its application to certain salts has been presented by Sharp and Ifft (1979). It is important to note that the gradient achieved depends very much on the salt selected.

The physical density gradient present in the rotor has two components, the composition density gradient and the compression density gradient. The dependence of $\beta(\rho)$ on pressure is sufficiently small that the variation may be neglected, but compression does increase the physical density significantly in high-speed centrifugation. The physical density gradient is given by the expression (Vinograd and Hearst, 1962)

$$d\rho/dr = [1/\beta^0(\rho^0) + \chi(\rho^0)^2]\omega^2 r \qquad (4.32)$$

where χ is the isothermal compressibility of the solution, and ρ^0 the density of the solution at radius r evaluated at atmospheric pressure.

For preparative centrifugation, the composition gradient can be estimated directly from measurements made on collected fractions. For analytical centrifugation, evaluation of the composition gradient depends on knowing the density at one point in the fluid column, or, equivalently, knowing at which radius the density of the gradient is equal to the average density of the original solution. The location of this radius is dependent on the geometry of the fluid column, and thus sector-shaped cells require a different formula than cylindrical tubes. Ifft *et al.* (1961) have presented several methods for evaluation of the composition gradient. The physical gradient may be estimated using the method of Vinograd and Hearst (1962).

The published buoyant densities of particles are normally derived from the density ρ^0 of that part of the gradient where the particles were found to be located. It is evident from the foregoing discussion that these densities may differ somewhat from the physical buoyant densities of the particles. Further, estimates of buoyant densities can be expected to vary if they are based on different experiments in which one macromolecular species is brought to equilibrium at different depths in the fluid column.

Macromolecular Components in Density Gradients at Equilibrium

The presence of a dilute macromolecular component in a density gradient leads to certain theoretical problems if all of the possible interactions are considered. The composition of the surrounding fluid will modify the solvation of the macromolecules and the presence of the macromolecule zone will modify the physical density gradient in the rotor. It may be assumed in many cases that there is no thermodynamic interaction between the macromolecule (designated as component 2) and the gradient-forming solute (component 3).

Fujita (1962) shows that this requires that

$$\lim_{m_2 \to 0} (\partial \ln \gamma_2/\partial m_3)_{P,m_2} = 0$$

where γ_i is the activity coefficient of component i, and m_i the concentration of component i, and where both quantities are expressed on a molal scale. If this holds, then the sedimenting force on component 2 vanishes when

$$\rho(r)\bar{v}_2 = 1$$

where $\rho(r)$ is the physical density of the gradient at radius r. Casassa and Eisenberg (1964) show that if this condition does not hold precisely, then the position of the band is slightly displaced from the radius at which the solution density equals the reciprocal of the partial specific volume of the particles. This is caused by the fact that the presence of the particles slightly modifies the density gradient.

Given the assumption of no thermodynamic interaction between the macromolecules and the gradient-forming solute, the concentration profile of the zone of macromolecules may be derived. The assumption is made that the zone is centered at r_0 and that it is very narrow, so that the total density in the fluid column may be approximated by the first term in a Taylor series

$$\rho(r) \simeq 1/\bar{v}_1 + (r - r_0)d\rho/dr$$

We assume further that $d\rho/dr$ is approximately a constant over the width of the zone. Let

$$x = r - r_0$$

and

$$\sigma^2 = (RT/\omega^2 M_2 \bar{v}_2 r_0)(d\rho/dr)_{r_0}^{-1} \qquad (4.33)$$

If we substitute these relations into Eq. (4.28), and neglect x in comparison to r_0 we obtain

$$d \ln c_2/dx \cong -x/\sigma^2$$

and upon integration

$$c_2(x) \cong c_2(0) \exp(-x^2/2\sigma^2)$$

which is the equation of a Gaussian centered at r_0.

Thus, a macromolecular species at equilibrium in a density gradient is expected to have a Gaussian concentration profile, the width of which is inversely proportional to the square root of the molecular weight. In principle this could be used to measure the molecular weight of a macromolecular species, but in practice it is quite difficult to do so for two reasons. First, the zones are very narrow for high-molecular-weight substances and the width is not a very sensitive function of molecular weight. Second, the zone profile is very sensitive to heterogeneity in either M_2 or $\bar{v}_2$. Experimental difficulties notwithstanding, Schmid and Hearst (1969) have used this method to measure molecular weights of phage DNA in the range of 20 to 100×10^6 gm, a range that is difficult to work in by any other method. This method is also very useful in separating macromolecular species which possess small differences in buoyant density (cf. Section 8.3). The bands of proteins at sedimentation equilibrium in density gradients are wider than those formed by high-molecular-weight nucleic acids; therefore, the approximations leading to Eq. (4.33) may not hold for proteins. Measurement of protein molecular weight by this method is discussed by Lundh (1977).

The separation or resolution expected between two species of particles may be easily derived from the foregoing if we make some reasonable assumptions. If two types of particles have respective apparent buoyant densities of ρ_1 and ρ_2, then their radial separation at equilibrium will be given by

$$\rho_2 - \rho_1 = (r_2 - r_1)d\rho/dr$$

If one defines resolution to be

$$\lambda = \left| \frac{r_2 - r_1}{\sigma_1 + \sigma_2} \right|$$

and if we further assume that the two particle types are very similar in molecular weight, then, using Eqs. (4.31) and (4.33), one may predict that

$$\lambda \cong (\rho_2 - \rho_1)(\beta M/RT\rho_0)^{1/2}/2 \qquad (4.34)$$

where ρ_0 is a density midway between the two densities ρ_2 and ρ_1. Hence, the expected resolution does not depend at all on the speed of centrifugation but only on β and the density difference between the two particle types.

It is worth noting that in preparative sedimentation equilibrium in density gradients, the time required to reach equilibrium can be greatly reduced by using a preformed density gradient. This is due to two factors. First, if the preformed gradient approximates the equilibrium distribution, then only a small amount of physical transport is required to reach equilibrium, and this takes place quickly. Second, in a preformed gradient, the macromolecular component can immediately begin to move toward its equilibrium position without waiting for the formation of the density gradient to take place. Further, a preformed density gradient may produce the desired separation without the necessity of attaining true equilibrium. Brunk and Leich (1969) report time reductions of more than 50% using simple preformed step gradients.

Anet and Strayer (1969) have described another approach for reducing the time required to perform isopycnic separations (cf. Section 4.4). In their procedure a steep density gradient is initially formed using a high rotor speed, after which the speed is reduced. The macromolecular zones become resolved during the period at reduced speed. Even though the system does not arrive at true equilibrium, they claim that preparative amounts of macromolecules are resolved as well as in a comparable equilibrium experiment requiring more than twice the time.

4.3.9 Quasiequilibrium Sedimentation in a Density Gradient

A useful variation of the above equilibrium techniques is obtained by using a preformed density gradient which does not come to true sedimentation–diffusion equilibrium during the course of the experiment. A sample of macromolecular particles layered on top of such a gradient can sediment rapidly to the particles respective isopycnic positions in the density gradient and form zones of particles with concentration profiles given by Eq. (4.26). This technique, which does not arrive at true equilibrium, is referred to as isopycnic centrifugation or *isopycnic separation*. It is widely used in preparative work.

The radial position of the center of a zone in isopycnic centrifugation is determined by the same criteria that determine the zone position at true equilibrium, namely that $\rho \bar{v}_2 = 1$. In order for Eq. (4.23) to be used to predict the width of the zone, however, it is necessary that the zone itself be at true equilibrium in the gradient. Since the density gradient is continuously diffusing, this condition is difficult to fulfill. Thus, using zone width to estimate molecular weight is more hazardous than in the equilibrium case.

4.4 MOTION OF BOUNDARIES AND ZONES

4.4.1 Formation of Boundaries and Zones

If a uniform suspension of particles is subjected to a centrifugal field, the sedimentation eqation (4.9) indicates that every particle should begin to move outward along radii with velocities which are a function only of r. Thus, after a period of time, those particles which were initially at the meniscus will have moved to a larger radius r_1 and a region of solvent depleted of particles will have appeared between the meniscus and the particle-containing region of the fluid. The interface between the particle-depleted region and the particle-containing region is called a *boundary*. The boundary is formed at the meniscus and, in the absence of diffusion, should be perfectly sharp; that is, the particle concentration for $r < r_1$ is zero, while for $r > r_1$ the concentration is uniformly equal to the plateau concentration. In the presence of diffusion, the boundary will not be perfectly sharp, but, if the sedimentation has not proceeded too far, there should nonetheless be a plateau region radially distal to the boundary in which the concentration is constant with respect to radius at a given time.

If there is more than one species of particle in the suspension, it would be expected that a separate boundary should form for each species so long as they do not interact. In the limit of a continuous distribution of sedimentation coefficients among the particles, it would be expected that a continuous distribution of boundaries should be formed.

A zone is the name given to a distribution of particles which does not extend to both radial limits of the fluid column. The formation of a narrow zone of macromolecules at sedimentation–diffusion equilibrium was discussed previously. In zone sedimentation a small volume of a suspension of particles is layered on top of a density gradient, after which the centrifugal field causes the particles to move through the gradient. If there is no circulation within the zone, then at every time subsequent to the beginning of sedimentation, the zone should consist of an image of the original zone as modified by diffusion and sedimentation. We can see that the motion of boundaries and the motion of zones should be closely related if there are no interactions among the particles.

In general, we will confine our attention to relatively narrow zones (for any given species of particle). A narrow zone is a distribution in which the particle concentration is significantly different from zero only over a radial distance which is short in comparison to the total height of the fluid column.

4.4.2 Motion of Nondiffusing Boundaries and Zones

Sedimentation Velocity of Ideal Boundaries

In the absence of diffusion the sedimentation equation (4.9) holds for every particle in a system and, in particular, for particles in the region of a boundary. Thus, a perfect boundary moves at the same speed as the speed of sedimentation of the particles which mark the boundary.

Radial Dilution

The concentration of particles in the plateau region radially distal to a boundary decreases as a function time due to radial dilution or sectorial dilution. The expression for this may be readily obtained. Let r_p represent the radius to a position in the plateau region. In the plateau region $\partial c_2/\partial r = 0$ and the Lamm equation (4.26) becomes

$$dc_2(r_p)/dt = -2s_2\omega^2 c_2(r_p)$$

Let $\hat{r}$ be the position of the boundary as a function of time: $\hat{r} < r_p$. Using Eq. (4.10) and assuming that s_2 is not a function of r, we obtain

$$d[\ln c_2(r_p)]/dt = -2[d(\ln \hat{r})/dt]$$

At the start of the experiment, $c = c_0$ everywhere and $\hat{r} = r_m$, the radius to the meniscus. Thus, upon integration, we obtain

$$c_2(r_p) = c_0(r_m/\hat{r})^2 \tag{4.35}$$

Therefore, at a particular radius in the plateau region distal to a perfect boundary, the concentration of particles decreases as the square of the radial position of the boundary.

The expression for the radial dilution of a zone takes a different form because we do not make observations at a fixed radius. It is readily visualized that in the absence of wall effects a zone of constant radial width should occupy progressively larger solution volumes as its distance from the center of the rotor increases. The absence of wall effects implies the consideration of a sector-shaped solution compartment or of the central portion of a swinging-bucket tube. For a zone of constant radial width, the volume occupied by the zone increases in inverse proportion to its radius, so that the expression for radial dilution in this case is apparently

$$c_2(r) = c_0(r_0/r)$$

where $c_2(r)$ is the average concentration of the zone as a function of radius r, and c_0 initial average concentration of the zone at radius r_0.

Width of Sedimenting, Nondiffusing Zones

The width of an ideal thin zone should be inversely proportional to its velocity. This may be shown as follows. Consider a particle which marks the leading edge of the zone and a second particle which marks the trailing edge. If the gradient is invariant with time, the velocities of the particles will depend on position only. This implies that the trajectory of both particles will be identical except for a displacement in time Δt. If the path of the leading particle as a function of time is $r_1(t)$, then the path of the trailing particle is given by

$$r_t(t) = r_1(t - \Delta t)$$

If the zone is sufficiently thin that its width may be approximated by the first-order term of a Taylor series with respect to t, we obtain

$$\text{width} = r_1 - r_t \cong (dr_1/dt)\Delta t$$

If dr_1/dt is identified as the velocity of the zone, assuming that the velocity variation across the width of the zone is negligible, we obtain

$$\text{zone width/zone velocity} = \Delta t = \text{constant} \tag{4.36}$$

This result, which is true for any gradient profile, is implicit in the derivation by Berman (1966). He worked directly with the integral form of the sedimentation equation (4.12) and also made the thin zone approximation. The Lamm equation (4.26) with $D_2 = 0$ may be solved to give a representation of the development with time of an ideal thick band, but this will ultimately require numerical evaluation; hence, it seems to be more useful to include the effects of diffusion in that case.

Gradient-Induced Zone Sharpening

Equation (4.36) suggests that the width of a zone may be manipulated during an experiment by controlling the velocity of sedimentation in a density gradient. In particular, one may seek to reduce the width of a zone by reducing its velocity. The increased time required may, however, aggravate problems caused by diffusion. It may be noted that the markers used in deriving Eq. (4.36) could equally have marked the space between two zones. Thus, gradient-induced zone narrowing will also generally reduce the separation between zones. A practical application of gradient-induced zone narrowing has been presented by Spragg *et al.* (1969).

4.4.3 Motion of Diffusing Boundaries and Zones

Boundaries

In the presence of diffusion, the exact position of a boundary is no longer well defined, and may become difficult to evaluate. An unambiguous determination of the position of a boundary may be obtained in the following way. Consider a point r_p located in the plateau region distal to a sedimenting boundary. In that region, $\partial c/\partial r$ is zero if there is no appreciable gradient of particle velocity (e.g., caused by a density gradient) and Eq. (4.21) and (4.26) take on the following forms, respectively

$$J(r_p) = s(r_p)\omega^2 r_p c(r_p) \tag{4.37}$$

$$dc(r_p)/dt = -2s(r_p)\omega^2 c(r_p) \tag{4.38}$$

in which we have omitted the subscript 2 for clarity and substituted the total derivative with respect to time because there is no variation of c with radius at r_p.

The rate of mass transport through unit area of the cylindrical surface at r_p must be equal to the rate of decrease in the total mass of material which lies between the meniscus and r_p in the same cylindrical sector

$$r_p J(r_p) = -\frac{\partial}{\partial t} \int_{r_m}^{r_p} rc(r)dr \tag{4.39}$$

We now define the radius of an equivalent ideal boundary to be $\hat{r}$. This radius will be such that if the region from $\hat{r}$ to r_p were filled with solute at concentration $c(r_p)$, the mass of solute would equal the mass actually contained between r_m and r_p, the region which contains the diffuse boundary: viz

$$\int_{\hat{r}}^{r_p} rc(r_p)dr = \int_{r_m}^{r_p} rc(r)dr$$

The left-hand side of the equation is readily evaluated and we obtain:

$$\hat{r} = \left[r_p^2 - \frac{2}{c(r_p)} \int_{r_m}^{r_p} rc(r)dr \right]^{1/2} \tag{4.40}$$

The equation of motion of $\hat{r}$ is

$$d\hat{r}/dt = s(r_p)\omega^2 \hat{r} \tag{4.41}$$

as may be verified by differentiation of Eq. (4.40) and substitution of Eqs. (4.37), (4.38), and (4.39). Thus, $\hat{r}$ moves with the same sedimentation coefficient as that of the individual particles in the plateau region. The equivalent boundary position $\hat{r}$ is readily evaluated from data giving $c(r)$ at a given time.

This derivation was adapted from Tanford (1961), who also gives an alternative formulation for use when $(\partial c/\partial r)_t$ is given rather than $c(r)_t$. These relations demonstrate two important points. The first is that the equivalent position of a diffuse boundary is not readily related to any easily measured parameter, such as the inflection point of the concentration distribution. The second is that the sedimentation coefficient of the particles in a boundary may be inferred from the motion of such a boundary if the appropriate computations are made. These equations may be of use in evaluating the behavior of the trailing boundary of a thick zone.

It may be noted that the derivation of Eq. (4.35), the expression for radial dilution, is valid in the presence of diffusion so long as a plateau region continues to exist.

Zones

An equation analogous to Eq. (4.41) may be obtained for the motion of diffusing zones. As in Eq. (4.39), one should note that the mass transport through unit area of the cylindrical surface at r must equal the rate of decrease of mass in the region above r in the same cylindrical sector

$$rJ(r) = -\frac{\partial}{\partial t}\int_{r_m}^{r} rc(r)dr$$

Using Eq. (4.21), we obtain

$$-\frac{\partial}{\partial t}\int_{r_m}^{r} rc(r)dr = s(r)\omega^2 r^2 c(r) - rD(r)\frac{\partial c(r)}{\partial r}$$

If we assume that s and D are independent of r, we may multiply both sides of this equation by $1/r$ and integrate from the meniscus of the fluid column r_m to the base r_b to obtain

$$-\frac{\partial}{\partial t}\int_{r_m}^{r_b} d(\ln r)\int_{r_m}^{r} rc(r)dr = s\omega^2\int_{r_m}^{r_b} rc(r)dr - D\int_{r_m}^{r_b}\frac{\partial c(r)}{\partial r}dr \quad (4.42)$$

in which $\partial/\partial t$ may be placed outside the integration because none of the factors introduced depends on time. The second term on the right-hand side of Eq. (4.42) is the integral of a perfect differential and evaluates to zero if the zone is not present at either r_m or r_b. The left-hand side may be integrated by parts to give

$$-\frac{\partial}{\partial t}\int_{r_m}^{r_b} d(\ln r)\int_{r_m}^{r} rc(r)dr$$
$$= -\frac{\partial}{\partial t}\left[\ln r\int_{r_m}^{r} rc(r)dr\right]_{r=r_m}^{r=r_b} + \frac{\partial}{\partial t}\int_{r_m}^{r_b} rc(r)\ln r\,dr \quad (4.43)$$

The first term on the right is a constant with respect to time, so that its time derivative is zero. We may define the position $\hat{r}$ of an equivalent ideal zone in the following way:

$$\ln\hat{r} = \int_{r_m}^{r_b} rc(r)\ln r\,dr \Big/ \int_{r_m}^{r_b} rc(r)dr \quad (4.44)$$

We thus obtain the following expression from Eqs. (4.42) and (4.43)

$$d(\ln\hat{r})/dt = s\omega^2$$

The apparent zone position $\hat{r}$ thus moves with the same sedimentation velocity as the particles in the zone. In cylindrical coordinates, the volume element

dV is given by

$$dV = \theta h r dr$$

where θ is the sector angle, and h the height of the volume element. An element of mass of solute dm is then given by $c(r)dV$, and Eq. (4.44) may be written as:

$$\ln \hat{r} = \int_{r_m}^{r_b} (\ln r)dm \bigg/ \int_{r_m}^{r_b} dm \qquad (4.45)$$

Thus, $\ln(\hat{r})$ is a mass-averaged value of $\ln(r)$ over the entire contents of the fluid column.

The above derivation is due to Schumaker (1967). He also gives similar derivations for sedimentation in a gravitational field, and in a swinging-bucket rotor. The latter is of restricted value due to the neglect of wall effects. Further, Schumaker gives expressions for the sedimentation and diffusion of zones in the presence of gradients of density and viscosity. These expressions are somewhat complex and require numerical integration for their evaluation.

4.4.4 Concentration-Dependent Sedimentation

As the concentrations of sedimenting particles are increased, it is generally observed that the sedimentation coefficients of the particles decrease, sometimes dramatically. This may be caused in part by electrostatic interactions or mechanical interactions such as the tangling of long, rod-shaped molecules. No general theory exists to predict the degree of this dependence of s on concentration for real solutions.

Measured sedimentation coefficients are usually extrapolated to the conventional standard condition of infinite dilution. Two formulas which have been found to be useful in representing first-order variations in s as a function of concentration are

$$s = s^0(1 - k_1 c) \qquad (4.46)$$

$$s = s^0/(1 + k_2 c) \qquad (4.47)$$

where s^0 is the sedimentation coefficient at infinite dilution, and k_1, k_2 are constants. Equation (4.46) is useful for compact, globular particles while Eq. (4.47) is preferred for rod-shaped molecules such as nucleic acids or synthetic polymers (Tanford, 1961). Deviations of order higher than first are frequently observed at higher concentrations.

Dishon et al. (1969) have presented a series of numerical calculations of the sedimenting behavior of thin zones for a wide range of s and the coefficient k in Eqs. (4.46) and (4.47). These show that the presence of concentration-dependent sedimentation can lead, under some circumstances, to the production of highly skewed zones after short distances of migration.

Theoretical investigations of the hydrodynamic behavior of relatively large spherical particles sedimenting from suspensions in the earth's gravitational field have been presented (Famularo and Happel, 1965; Phillips and Smith, 1969; Happel and Brenner, 1973). Their results take the form of a correction to the terminal velocity derived from Stokes's law for spheres [Eq. (4.6)], and thus should be applicable to centrifugation. However, the calculations are quite complicated and numerous assumptions are made to allow the problem to be solved. Perhaps as a consequence of this, the agreement of their results with experimental determinations is not good. The correction to Stokes' law was given in the form

$$v/v_0 = 1/(1 + k_3 \phi^{1/3})$$

where v/v_0 is the ratio of particle settling velocity to the velocity of a free particle, ϕ the volume fraction occupied by the particles, and k_3 a constant. The value of k_3 for randomly arranged spheres was predicted to be 1.30 while other postulated distributions of the particles gave values in the range $1.30 \leq k_3 \leq 2.1$. Famularo and Happel (1965) also stated that, as the particle concentration increased, they found a tendency for the particles to form sedimenting dimers, and eventually clumps of particles, which sedimented more rapidly than the unaggregated particles. Thus, at high concentrations, the sedimenting particles were no longer mechanically independent entities. The assumption of mechanical independence was implicit in the derivation of the equations of motion given above.

4.4.5   Stability in Fluid Columns

Hydrostatic Stability

Hydrostatic stability in a fluid column subjected to an external force field, such as gravity or a centrifugal field, requires that the density throughout the fluid be a nondecreasing function of position in the direction of the gradient of potential of the external field. Stated simply, this means that one may not have a stable density inversion in which a more dense fluid overlays a less dense fluid.* This would imply that a column of fluid of uniform density should also be stable, but in practice perturbations arising from vibration or small differences in temperature within the fluid cause circulation. Thus, in centrifugation, it is required under nearly all circumstances that there be a

* Density inversions may be produced in capillary tubes and occur frequently in the atmosphere and in the oceans. They are not, however, stable.

gradient of fluid density, no matter how slight, in the fluid column in order to ensure stability. This must be a compositional density gradient, because a compressional density gradient offers no stability against convection.

In boundary sedimentation, in which the solute fills the entire fluid column except for a clear region near the meniscus, the required gradient is provided by the solute itself. The concentration gradient is quite strong near the boundary, and this, coupled with concentration-dependent sedimentation velocity, normally serves to stabilize the boundary. In the plateau region, there may be no density gradient and, indeed, convection is often observed in this region of the fluid column during analytical centrifugation experiments.

The density gradient may also be formed by the redistribution in the centrifugal field of a low-molecular-weight solute. The case of sedimentation–diffusion equilibrium has been discussed. In the case of band sedimentation in the analytical centrifuge, the stabilizing gradient results from the rapid diffusion of a low-molecular-weight solute from the sedimentation solvent into the sample zone, and from the rapid redistribution of the low-molecular-weight solute in the centrifugal field (cf. Section 8.2.3).

These gradients arise naturally during the course of the respective experiments. The other important class of density gradients is the preformed density gradients which serve the dual role of providing stability and aiding in the separation of various particle species (cf. Chapter 3).

Stability and Small Molecule Diffusion

If a solution of macromolecules (i.e., slowly diffusing molecules) is layered over (with respect to an external force field) a solution of small molecules, a stable situation results if the lower solution has a higher density than the upper solution. But, with the passage of time, the small molecules will diffuse into the region occupied by the macromolecules thus increasing the local density by an amount that may not be compensated by the diffusion of the macromolecules in the opposite direction. A density inversion can result and the macromolecules are then transported by convection. This leads to the formation of streamers, or droplet sedimentation, which has been described in detail by Nason *et al.* (1969). The same mechanism is involved in thermohaline convection, or the formation of salt fingers, and in this form has been studied extensively (Baines and Gill, 1969).

An expression relating the initial solution densities and molecular diffusion coefficients to the production of instability was obtained by Svensson *et al.* (1957). Their model was the infinite fluid column with an external force field directed along the negative x axis. The total solution density is given by

$$\rho = \rho_1 + c_2(1 - \bar{v}_2\rho_1) + c_3(1 - \bar{v}_3\rho_1) \tag{4.48}$$

where ρ_1 is the density of the pure solvent, and where the subscript 2 refers to the slower diffusing high-molecular-weight component and subscript 3 refers to the rapidly diffusing component. We make the following substitution:

$$\rho_2 = c_2(1 - \bar{v}_2\rho_1), \qquad \rho_3 = c_3(1 - \bar{v}_3\rho_1)$$

using as initial conditions

$$\left. \begin{array}{l} \rho_3(x, 0) = \begin{cases} \bar{\rho}_3, & x < 0 \\ 0, & x > 0 \end{cases} \\[2mm] \rho_2(x, 0) = \begin{cases} 0, & x < 0 \\ \bar{\rho}_2, & x > 0 \end{cases} \end{array} \right\} \, t = 0$$

where the barred quantities are the initial concentrations and it is assumed that $\bar{\rho}_3 > \bar{\rho}_2$ in order that initial stability obtains. In this case the diffusion equation (4.24) has a particularly simple solution

$$\rho_3(x, t) = \frac{\bar{\rho}_3}{2}\left[1 - \mathrm{erf}\left(\frac{x}{2\sqrt{D_3 t}}\right)\right]$$

$$\rho_2(x, t) = \frac{\bar{\rho}_2}{2}\left[1 + \mathrm{erf}\left(\frac{x}{2\sqrt{D_2 t}}\right)\right]$$

where $\mathrm{erf}(x)$ is the error function and D_3 and D_2 are the respective diffusion coefficients. We make the following substitution in Eq. (4.47):

$$y = \frac{x}{\sqrt{t}}$$

which gives

$$\rho(y) = \rho_0 + \bar{\rho}_3[1 - \mathrm{erf}(y/\sqrt{D_3})]/2 + \bar{\rho}_2[1 + \mathrm{erf}(y/\sqrt{D_2})]/2$$

If we set $d\rho/dy = 0$, we obtain

$$\frac{\bar{\rho}_3}{\bar{\rho}_2}\left(\frac{D_2}{D_3}\right)^{1/2} - \exp\left[y_{max}^2\left(\frac{1}{D_3} - \frac{1}{D_2}\right)\right]$$

where y_{max} is the value of y for the location of the extremum in space and time Since $D_3 > D_2$ by our initial assumption, y_{max} will have a real value only if

$$\bar{\rho}_3/\bar{\rho}_2 > (D_3/D_2)^n \qquad (4.49)$$

where $n = \frac{1}{2}$. The extremum will be a maximum in this case and, since any local maximum in density will constitute a density inversion, Eq. (4.49) gives a condition which guarantees that instability will eventually develop.

Several other analyses of density inversions caused by small molecule diffusion have been presented. Generally they take the form of Eq. (4.49) except that the exponent n is not agreed upon. Sartory (1969) used perturbation analysis to determine under which conditions a perturbation in a boundary layer would grow or decay with time. He found $n = \frac{3}{2}$ for the case of the infinitely thick sample zone discussed previously, and $n = \frac{5}{2}$ for a thin zone of slowly diffusing solute. An experimentally determined value of $n \cong 1$ was reported by Halsall and Schumaker (1971) based on measurements made in a zonal rotor in the presence of a solvent overlay.

It should be noted that the theoretical models discussed above are bounded at the top by an impenetrable barrier, the meniscus, and hence do not apply to a zone which has migrated into a density gradient: such a zone has solvent both above it and below it. In fact, a zone which has successfully penetrated a density gradient without becoming unstable should be relatively unaffected by small molecule diffusion. This may be appreciated in a qualitative way by noting that in rectangular coordinates (which were used for all the analyses mentioned above) an infinite linear density gradient does not change with time, so that if a given zone configuration were stable at one time, it should be stable at all times. This does not hold in cylindrical coordinates, but it is valid to say that diffusion-related changes take place very slowly in the central region of a density gradient so long as there are no "discontinuities" in the gradient. The result of Halsall and Schumaker (1971) referred to above may be explained by instability, which occurred before they were able to place the overlay.

4.4.6 Capacity of Zones

The material capacity of a zone is limited to that concentration which will not produce a density inversion. This was discussed by Svensson et al. (1957) and has come to be known as the Svensson criterion or Svensson limit. This limit as applied to centrifugation requires that

$$dp/dr \geqq 0$$

for all r. The maximum material load apparently coincides with the equality condition. We define the density increment due to the gradient-forming solute to be:

$$\rho_3 = c_3(1 - \bar{v}_3\rho_1)$$

and thus in the absence of a compressional gradient we may write the total solution density as

$$\rho(r) = \rho_1 + c_2(1 - \bar{v}_2\rho_1) + \rho_3$$

The Svensson limit is then given by

$$-\frac{dc_3}{dr} \leq \frac{1}{(1 - \bar{v}_2\rho_1)} \frac{d\rho_3}{dr}$$

Now, we define r_0 to coincide with the leading edge of a maximally loaded zone, so that $c_2(r_0) = 0$. The permissible solute concentration in this zone for any $r < r_0$ is given by

$$\int_r^{r_0} \left(-\frac{dc_2}{dr}\right) dr = c_2(r) = \frac{1}{(1 - \bar{v}_2\rho_1)} \int_r^{r_0} \left(\frac{d\rho_3}{dr}\right) dr$$

The maximum mass of solute m_2 which may be contained in a zone of thickness δ, the leading edge of which is at r_0, is given by

$$m_{2,\text{max}}(\delta) = \int_{r_0-\delta}^{r_0} c_2(r) dV$$

$$= \frac{1}{(1 - \bar{v}_2\rho)} \int_{r_0-\delta}^{r_0} dV \int_r^{r_0} \left(\frac{d\rho_3}{dr}\right) dr \qquad (4.50)$$

The evaluation of this depends on rotor geometry. It is often adequate to assume that the zone width δ is small compared to r_0 so that $d\rho_3/dr$ may be taken to be a constant across the width of the zone. If, for example, the rotor is a zonal rotor of internal height h, then Eq. 4.50 may readily be evaluated under the assumption of a thin zone to give

$$m_{2,\text{max}}(\delta) \cong \frac{2\pi h}{(1 - \bar{v}_2\rho_1)} \left(\frac{d\rho_3}{dr}\Big|_{r_0}\right) \int_{r_0-\delta}^{r_0} (r_0 - r) r\, dr$$

$$\cong \frac{\pi h \delta^2 r_0}{(1 - \bar{v}_2\rho_1)} \left(\frac{d\rho_3}{dr}\Big|_{r_0}\right) \qquad (4.51)$$

where terms of order δ^3 have been neglected.

In practice, achieving even a large fraction of the Svensson limit is difficult. If δ is initially very small, the zone profile is often altered by diffusion. If δ is taken to be somewhat larger, the indicated concentrations can become quite high, unless $d\rho_3/dr$ is small, and anomalous zone spreading is frequently the result (*vide infra*). Finally, if $d\rho_3/dr$ is too small, convective disturbances initiated by external perturbations may occur. The practical aspects of the application of the Svensson limit are discussed in Chapter 6.

4.4.7 Capacity Requirements in Density Gradients

A sedimenting zone of particles requires a certain amount of support from the density gradient if it is not to convect. It was found in the previous section that the maximum available capacity to support a collection of particles is proportional to the gradient of solution density $d\rho_3/dr$. Ideally, a density gradient should be designed to provide the needed particle support capacity at each radius. Several factors cause the requirement for capacity to decrease as a function of time. These are: (1) radial dilution of the sedimenting particles, (2) diffusion of the particle zone, and (3) the possible separation of different particle species, which allows the overall capacity requirement to be divided among various zones. One factor may cause the capacity requirement to increase; namely, gradient-induced zone narrowing. A fully optimized density gradient would strike a balance among these factors and would further seek to keep the time as short as practical by reducing the overall density change across the gradient to the minimum value compatible with an adequate stability margin everywhere. The diffusion and sedimentation of the gradient-forming solute must also be taken into account. An approach to this ideal has been made by Spragg et al. (1969), who, however, restricted themselves to very dilute samples on shallow, computer-optimized density gradients. A more general approach that would account for high concentrations of solute particles has not yet been presented.

4.4.8 Anomalous Motion of Zones

It is frequently observed that the width of a zone at the end of an experiment is greater than had been expected, even though Eq. (4.50) would have indicated that there should be no problem with hydrostatic instability. This has been referred to as anomalous zone broadening (Spragg, 1970). It should be apparent, in light of the preceeding discussion, that a variety of possible mechanisms is available to account for this phenomenon. In particular, concentration-dependent sedimentation velocity can lead to local convective motion in the zone which could give rise to observed broadening. Further, there may be factors outside of the theoretical treatment, such as mixing that occurs during the formation of the zone, which contribute to unexpected zone broadening. It should be noted that in the case of swinging bucket rotors, a large fraction of the sedimenting material will strike the wall of the tube during an experiment due simply to the geometry of the rotor. The region in which particles accumulate when they strike the wall can develop particle concentrations that exceed the limits of hydrostatic stability even though the concentration averaged over the entire section of the tube is below the predicted limit of stability.

REFERENCES

Anet, R., and Strayer, D. R. (1969). Density gradient relaxation: A method for preparative buoyant density separations of DNA. *Biochem. Biophys. Res. Commun.* **34,** 328–334.

Baines, P. G., and Gill, A. E. (1969). On thermohaline convection with linear gradients. *J. Fluid Mech.* **37,** 289–306.

Berman, A. S. (1966). Theory of centrifugation: Miscellaneous studies. *Natl. Cancer Inst. Monogr.* **21,** pp. 41–73.

Brunk, C. F., and Leich, V. (1969). Rapid equilibrium in isopycnic CsCl gradients. *Biochim. Biophys. Acta* **179,** 136–144.

Casassa, E. F., and Eisenberg, H. (1964). Thermodynamic analysis of multicomponent solutions. *Adv. Protein Chem.* **19,** 287–395.

de Groot, S. R., and Mazur, P. (1969). "Non-Equilibrium Thermodynamics," pp. 57–77, 267–270. North-Holland Publ., Amsterdam.

Dishon, M., Weiss, G. H., and Yphantis, D. (1969). Numerical solutions of the Lamm equation. V. Band centrifugation. *Ann. N. Y. Acad. Sci.* **164,** 33–51.

Eikenberry, E. F. (1973). Generation of density gradients: Approximations to equivolumetric gradients for zonal rotors. *Anal. Biochem.* **55,** 338–357.

Einstein, A. (1905). *In* "Investigations on the Theory of the Brownian Movement," pp. 1–18. Dover, New York, 1956.

Famularo, J., and Happel, J. (1965). Sedimentation of dilute suspensions in creeping motion. *AIChE J.* **11,** 981–988.

Fujita, H. (1962). "Mathematical Theory of Sedimentation Analysis," pp. 254–262. Academic Press, New York.

Garcia de la Torre, J. and Bloomfield, V. (1977). Hydrodynamic properties of macromolecular complexes. I. Translation. *Biopolymers* **16,** 1747–1763.

Garcia de la Torre, J. and Bloomfield, V. (1977b). Hydrodynamics of macromolecular complexes. III. Bacterial viruses. *Biopolymers* **16,** 1779–1793.

Halsall, H. B., and Schumaker, V. N. (1971). A stability criterion for the measurement of diffusion coefficients in the zonal centrifuge. *Biochem. Biophys. Res. Commun.* **43,** 601–606.

Halsall, H. B., and Schumaker, V. N. (1972). Zonal diffusion, a new technique. Application to the determination of the molecular weight of M13 viral deoxyribonucleic acid. *Biochemistry* **11,** 4692–4695.

Happel, J., and Brenner, H. (1973). "Low Reynolds Number Hydrodynamics," 2nd ed. Noordhoff Int., Gröningen, Leyden.

Hill, W. E., Rosetti, G. P., and Van Holde, K. E. (1969). Physical studies of ribosomes from *Escherichia coli. J. Mol. Biol.* **44,** 263–277.

Hsu, H. W. (1970). Theoretical approaches to sedimentation in gradient solutions. *In* "Microsymposium on Particle Separation from Plant Materials" (C. A. Price, ed.),Oak Ridge Natl. Lab. CONF-700119, pp. 89–96. Natl. Tech. Inf. Serv., Springfield, Virginia.

Hu, A. S. L., Bock, R. M., and Halvorson, H. O. (1962). Separation of labeled from unlabeled proteins by equilibrium density gradient sedimentation. *Anal. Biochem.* **4,** 489–504.

Ifft, J. B., Voet, D. H., and Vinograd, J. (1961). The determination of density distributions and density gradients in binary solutions at equilibrium in the ultracentrifuge. *J. Phys. Chem.* **65,** 1138–1145.

Jost, W. (1960). "Diffusion in Solids, Liquids, Gases," pp. 8–81. Academic Press, New York.

Kunz, I. D., Jr., and Kauzmann, W. (1974). Hydration of proteins and polypeptides. *Adv. Protein Chem.* **28,** 239–345.

Lundh, S. (1977). A new approach to analytical density gradient centrifugation. Simultaneous determination of molecular weight, specific volume, and preferential hydration of human transferrin. *J. Polymer Sci.* **15**, 733–748.

Nason, P., Schumaker, V. N., Halsall, H. B., and Schwedes, J. (1969). Formation of streaming convective disturbance which may occur at one gravity during preparation of samples for zone centrifugation. *Biopolymers* **7**, 241–249.

Nieuwenhuysen, P. (1979). Density-gradient-sedimentation velocity of solvated macromolecules: Theoretical considerations about the buoyancy factor. Biopolymers **18**, 277–284.

Phillips, C. R., and Smith, T. N. (1969). Random three-dimensional continuum models for two-species sedimentation. *Chem. Eng. Sci.* **24**, 1321–1335.

Sartory, W. K. (1969). Instability in diffusing fluid layers. *Biopolymers* **7**, 251–263.

Schmid, C. W., and Hearst, J. E. (1969). Molecular weights of homogeneous coliphage DNA's from density gradient sedimentation equilibrium. *J. Mol. Biol.* **44**, 143–160.

Schumaker, V. N. (1967). Zone centrifugation. *Adv. Biol. Med. Phys.* **11**, 245–339.

Sharp, D. S. and Ifft, J. B. (1979). Density gradient proportionality constants, density distributions, and pressure effects for three salt solutions. *Biopolymers* **18**, 3043–3065.

Spragg, S. P. (1970). Resolution in zonal rotors. *In* "Microsymposium on Particle Separation from Plant Materials." Oak Ridge Natl. Lab. CONF-700119, pp. 81–88. Natl. Tech. Inf. Serv., Springfield, Virginia.

Spragg, S. P., Morrod, R. S., and Rankin, C. T., Jr. (1969). The optimization of density gradients for zonal centrifugation. *Sep. Sci.* **4**, 467–481.

Squire, P. G. and Himmel, M. E. (1979). Hydrodynamics and protein hydration. *Arch. Biochem. Biophys.* **196**, 165–177.

Svensson, H., Hagdahl, L., and Lerner, K. D. (1957). Zonal electrophoresis in a density gradient. Stability considerations and separation of serum proteins. *Sci. Tools* **4**, 1–10.

Symon, K. R. (1954). "Mechanics," pp. 234–242. Addison-Wesley, Reading, Massachusetts.

Tanford, C. (1961). "Physical Chemistry of Macromolecules," pp. 317–390. Wiley, New York.

Teller, D. C., Swanson, E., and de Haen, C. (1979). The translational friction coefficient of proteins. *In* "Methods in Enzymology" (C. H. W. Hirs and S. N. Timasheff, eds.), Vol. 61, pp. 103–124, Academic Press, New York.

Van Holde, K. E. (1971). "Physical Biochemistry," pp. 79–121. Prentice-Hall, Englewood Cliffs, New Jersey.

Vinograd, J., and Hearst, J. E. (1962). Equilibrium sedimentation of macromolecules and viruses in a density gradient. *Fortschr. Chem. Org. Naturst.* **20**, 372–422.

Yphantis, D. (1964). Equilibrium ultracentrifugation of dilute solutions. *Biochemistry* **3**, 297–317.

5

Gradient Materials
and Construction of Gradients

5.1 CHOICE OF GRADIENT MATERIALS

Density gradients are usually prepared from solutions or sols of materials which are considerably denser than water: the density of most gradient solutions are greater than 1.0 gm/cm^3. Excluding nonaqueous gradients for the present, the properties of the ideal solute for gradients are simply stated: freely soluble in water, very dense, nonviscous, negligible osmotic pressure, physiologically and chemically inactive, transparent in visible and ultraviolet (UV) light, and cheap. Needless to say, this elixir has not yet been discovered, but combinations of these properties are available among a wide range of choices. The properties of a number of gradient materials in common and not-so-common use are listed in Table 5.1 and Appendix C.

5.1.1 Sucrose and Related Polymers

Sucrose

Common sugar, for all its faults, is easily the most widely used gradient material, dating from the pioneer work of Brakke (1951). In its favor are solubility, transparency, and cost. It is almost, but not completely, inactive physiologically: yeast cells can ferment and produce bubbles of CO_2 while sedimenting through it, and some membranes are damaged by concentrated sucrose solutions. The density of 65% w/w sucrose, which is about as concentrated as one can normally obtain, is 1.32 gm/cm^3. Although suitable for many purposes, this density is insufficient for the isopycnic separation of many viruses, glycogen, nucleic acids, etc. (cf. Fig. 1.6). The densities of

Table 5.1. Summary of Physical Properties of Some Gradient Materials[a]

Substance	Concentration	Stock solution[b] Density (gm/cm³) (°C)	Viscosity (centipoise)
CsCl	60% w/w	1.7900 (20°)	—
D₂O	100%	1.105 (20°)	—
Ficoll	46.5% w/w	1.1629 (4°)	1020
Glycerol	100%	1.2609 (20°)	1490 (20°)
Ludox AM[c]	30.1% w/w	1.206	16 (25°)
Metrizamide[d]	85% w/v	1.466 (5°)	246 (5°)
Sorbitol	60% w/w	1.2584 (4°)	102.9 (4°)
Sucrose	65% w/w	1.32600 (4°)	56.5 (20°)
Percoll	100%	1.13	10 (20°)

[a] Data compiled from various sources. Detailed information is tabulated in Appendix C.
[b] Stable at 4°C.
[c] The most widely used of the commercial silica sols.
[d] One of the iodinated benzoic acid derivatives.

sucrose solutions may be enhanced by the addition of sodium or potassium bromide, citrate, or tartrate.

Although sucrose gradients have been used more than any other for the separation of the membrane-bound organelles, they are almost certainly inferior to silica and Ficoll. The principal problem is the high osmotic potential of concentrated solutions of sucrose (Fig. 5.1).

Partly because of the largely deserved reputation of sucrose as a universal gradient material, excellent data are available on the physical properties of its solutions. Densities and viscosities for a range of temperatures and concentrations are tabulated in Appendix C. Investigators with direct access to computers may prefer to use the empirical formulas derived by Barber (1966) (cf. Appendix C2). Appendix C also contains tables of McEwen describing the sedimentation rates of particles through a variety of linear gradients of sucrose.

Although reagent grade sucrose is readily available, it usually contains some UV-absorbing material and ribonuclease activity. Some preparations contain a sedimentable contaminant. Grocery store sucrose is even cheaper than reagent-grade sucrose and may be purified sufficiently for most gradient work by passage through a column of activated charcoal. Solutions suitable for the most demanding gradient work can be easily prepared by passing a 65% w/w solution of sucrose through a mixed-bed ion-exchange column approximately 1 cm in diameter and 20 cm long (Fig. 5.2). Some

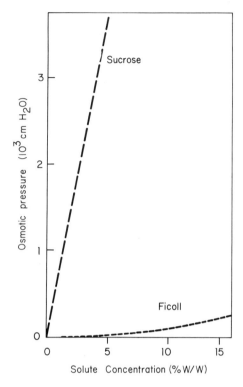

Fig. 5.1. Osmotic potential of different concentrations of sucrose compared to that of a sucrose polymer (Ficoll).

commercial grades may be used directly. Sucrose solutions prepared in this way are remarkably stable to microbial contamination.

In laboratories where density gradients are frequently used, it is convenient to prepare stock solutions of purified 65% w/w or 66% w/w sucrose and dispense aliquants for the preparation of specific gradients. Data for the dilution of the stock solutions appear in Appendix C4.

Sorbitol

Mannitol was greatly favored over sucrose by early physiologists as an osmoticum, presumably because it penetrated cell membranes less rapidly than sucrose. More recently mannitol has been recommended over sucrose in the isolation of mitochondria. However, mannitol crystallizes out from 15% w/v solutions; so that the densities obtainable are very slight. Sorbitol also appears to penetrate membranes slowly, but it is soluble up to about 50% w/w in water (Appendix C9). Avers *et al.* (1969) noted better preservation

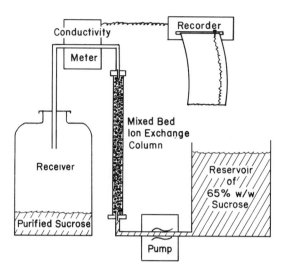

Fig. 5.2. Purification of sucrose by ion exchange. Flow of sucrose solution is upward because ion-exchange resins are less dense than 65% w/w sucrose. Conductivity will remain low until ion-exchange column becomes saturated.

of ultrastructure when yeast mitochondria were prepared in sorbitol as compared to sucrose.

The densities, viscosities, and refractive indices of sorbitol solutions have been determined by Curtis Suerth (unpublished; Appendix C9).

When preparing sorbitol solutions, note that commercial sorbitol comes in both anhydrous and monohydrate forms.

5.1.2 Carbohydrate Polymers

A number of polymers have been tried as gradient materials in order to eliminate adverse effects of osmotic potential.

It should be noted that the equilibrium densities of membrane-bound particles, including whole cells, are less (often dramatically so) in a non-osmotic or isosmotic gradient of a polymer than in sucrose. The reason, of course, is that water is drawn out of the particles and they become denser in gradients of high osmotic potential.

Glycogen

Glycogen is insufficiently soluble to be of much use. Moreover, glycogen, as normally obtained, is highly heterogeneous and varies among sources (cf. Barber *et al.*, 1966). Thus, its physical properties are difficult to quantitate.

Dextran

Dextrans obtained from *Micrococcus lysodeikticus* fermentations are commercially available (Pharmacia Fine Chemicals, Uppsala, Sweden) in defined fractions. The designations T-10, T-20, etc., refer to the mean molecular weights of the polymer. Dextran T-40, for example, has a weight-average molecular weight ($\overline{M}_w$) of 40,000. Dextrans are soluble to about 30% w/w, where they become extremely viscous. The lower weight fractions should in principle be more soluble, but are given to crystallizing out of solution. We find Dextran T-40 to be the easiest to use.

Mach and Lacko (1968) report dextran to be slightly superior to Ficoll for the separation of nuclei. Blue Dextran is a very high-molecular-weight dextran (ca. 200,000) to which methylene blue has been covalently bonded. It is most useful as an inert, nonsedimenting marker for sample zones in all but very high-speed separations.

Ficoll

Ficoll has become the most generally useful among polymeric gradient materials. It is a synthetic polymer of sucrose $\overline{M}_w$ 400,000 and is produced by Pharmacia Fine Chemicals (Uppsala, Sweden). It appears to be the gradient material of choice for the separation of lymphocytes (see Section 9.2.2).

Ficoll is soluble to about 50% w/w in water, but solutions more concentrated than 30% w/w can be pumped and stirred only with extreme difficulty. Some physical properties of Ficoll determined by Bell and Hsu (1974) are compiled in Appendix C.

Since dry Ficoll is very fluffy and dissolves rather slowly, it is convenient to prepare stock solutions by weighing the dry powder in a tared, wide-mouth, screw-cap bottle or flask which will fit on a shaker. We then add the desired amount of water, close the container tightly, and shake for several hours or overnight. Aliquants of the stock solution are measured by weight and the solution stored frozen.

Gorczynski *et al.* (1970), in their use of Ficoll gradients for the separation of antibody-producing cells, were concerned over the presence of salt (ca. 1%) in the commercial product. They deionized 500 gm of Ficoll in a 36% w/w solution with 100 gm of mixed-bed ion-exchange resin [AG-501-X8(D), Bio-Rad, Richmond, California]. "The solution was deionized twice, each time for 4 hr at 4°C with continuous stirring. Filtration of the deionized mixture through gauze removed the resin; subsequent filtration through Millipore filters sterilized the Ficoll solution allowing it to be stored for long periods at 4°" (Gorczynski *et al.*, 1970).

Pretlow *et al.* (1975) offer additional advice on problems encountered in preparing solutions of Ficoll. They warn that even sterile solutions increase osmolality and decrease viscosity when kept for many hours in the liquid state.

The high cost of Ficoll prompted us to investigate the feasibility of recycling. When a solution containing 15% w/w Ficoll in water was diluted three- to fivefold with 95% w/w ethanol and heated at 70°C for 1 hr, the Ficoll was largely precipitated. Ficoll is completely soluble in approximately 25% w/w ethanol.

5.1.3 Miscellaneous Polymers

Silica Sols—Ludox and Percoll

Small (ca. 150 Å diameter) particles of silica are stable as sols in mildly alkaline solutions. Silica sols, marketed as Ludox and Nalcoag, are available in several formulations (Appendix C11); one of them, Ludox AM, is partially substituted with Al^{3+}, which increases its stability to acid and salts. The preparations are colorless, have densities up to 1.29 gm/cm^3, are much less viscous than solutions of organic polymers, and are phenomenally inexpensive (ca. $1.00 per kilo in barrel quantities). The disadvantages of most silicas include a tendency to gel* at pH < 7 or in the presence of moderate concentrations of chloride or certain divalent cations. Ludox also contains toxic materials, which are apparently added to improve storage life.

Pertoft (1966 *et seq.*) has explored the use of silica sols as gradient materials and described procedures for the separation of particles ranging from whole cells (cf. Section 9.2.1) to viruses (cf. also Wolff, 1975). Lyttleton (1970) and this laboratory (Morgenthaler *et al.*, 1975; Price and Reardon, 1982) have used Ludox gradients successfully in the separation of chloroplasts (Section 9.3.2).

Pertoft has been much preoccupied with self-generating gradients (Section 5.3) for which Ludox is peculiarly suitable.

The addition of organic polymers, such as polyethylene glycol, Ficoll, and albumin, may be necessary to protect some cells from toxic effects of Ludox (cf. Pertoft, 1969, 1970; Morgenthaler *et al.*, 1975), but the addition of these polymers also affects the density of Ludox. The probable mechanism of this effect is solvent exclusion, a phenomenon described by Albertsson (1972). In a system of two polymers and water, one of the polymers will be more hydrophobic than the other. The presence of one polymer will affect the hydration of the other and therefore the density of the system. Beyond certain limiting concentrations the polymers will partition into two liquid, aqueous phases.

---

* Silica sols, valued commercially because of their controlled gelling properties, are used as surfacing agents.

The most important improvement in gradient materials within the last decade has been the invention of *Percoll* (Pertoft *et al.*, 1978; Pertoft and Laurent, 1977). As noted above, the toxicity shown by silica sols toward certain cells and membrane-bound organelles can be offset by the addition of various polymers, presumably through competition between the polymers and the membrane surface for active sites on the silica. Pertoft reasoned that the polymer could protect more efficiently if it were covalently bonded to the silica. Percoll is composed of a silica sol (Ludox HS) in which the particles of silica are coated with polyvinylpyrrolidone. Percoll has a density of 1.13 gm/cm^3, but gradients up to a density of 1.21 gm/cm^3 may be prepared by self-generation (cf. Section 5.3) or ultrafiltration (Section 9.1.1).

Because Percoll along with other silica sols is itself sedimentable, the complete removal of the gradient material from the separated particles may present problems. Dilution followed by sedimentation may be damaging to very sensitive particles. A more gentle procedure is gel filtration on columns of Sephacryl S-1000 (Pharmacia) (Hjort and Pertoft, 1982).

Percoll has a number of advantages. It is almost completely nontoxic, has low viscosity and low osmotic potential, is stable to low pH and high salt, and, unlike other silica sols, will not interfere with enzyme assays. Its disadvantages are that it absorbs in the UV and is expensive. It has, nonetheless, emerged as the gradient material of choice for the separation of membrane-bound particles.

Appendix C11 contains information on the physical properties of silica sols.

Thorium Oxide

De Duve *et al.* (1959) tested thorium oxide (Thorotrast) as a gradient material. It appears not to have been used subsequently.

Polyvinylpyrrolidone

Thomson and Klipfel (1958) employed gradients of polyvinylpyrrolidine (PVP). This synthetic polymer is not particularly dense and its solutions are rather viscous.

Albumin

Spleen and white blood cells have been separated by sedimentation in gradients of serum albumin (Vallee *et al.*, 1947; Haskill *et al.*, 1969; Leif *et al.*, 1972), but the solutions are extremely viscous and seem to have few advantages over Ficoll or dextrans. Indeed the presence of charged groups on the protein can produce serious artifacts, since a gradient of density will also be a gradient of counterions and osmotic potential.

Kneece and Leif (1971) describe procedures for the purification of albumin suitable for the separation of mammalian cells.

5.1.4   Iodinated Compounds

Holter *et al.* (1953) were the first to employ iodinated organic compounds as density gradient materials. The most readily available, water-soluble substances of this sort are radiological contrasting agents; thus, Holter *et al.* and Ottesen and Weber (1955) selected diiodon (compound VI in Fig. 5.3).

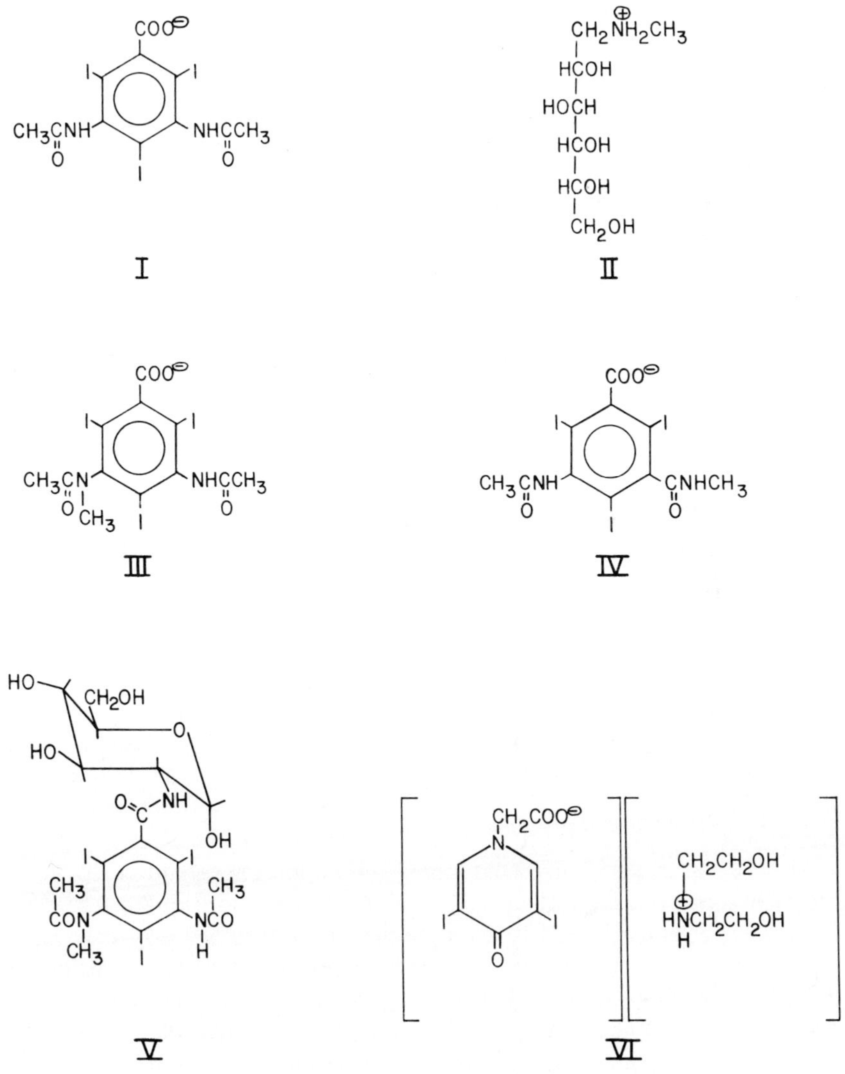

Fig. 5.3.   Structures of iodinated gradient materials.

Subsequently, Schatz *et al.* (1964) and Tamir and Gilvarg (1966) employed another opaqueing agent, Urografin (salts of diatrizoic acid; cf. Table 5.2 and Fig. 5.3), which, with a similar preparation, Renografin, became rather widely used. More recently, Metrizamide (Compound V in Fig. 5.3) was introduced with some significant advantages over the earlier materials.

Yet another radioopaque agent, "AG-6227," is claimed to be superior to Metrizamide and less expensive (Nordmann and Aunis, 1980).

All of these substances are extremely dense and have rather high molecular weights. The result is that dense solutions can be prepared with relatively low osmotic pressure and, as it turns out, low viscosity. Metrizamide has the additional advantage of being nonionic. Birnie *et al.* (1973) have shown that proteins, nucleic acids, ribosomes, and chromatin can be banded in gradients of Metrizamide without any apparent denaturation. In fact, nucleic acids exhibit extraordinarily low equilibrium densities (1.12–1.17 gm/cm^3) reflecting a fully hydrated state. Brain nuclei can also be banded (Mathias and Wynter, 1973).

The disadvantage of all of these materials stems from their original application: they are opaque not only to X rays, but throughout most of the UV range. The usual monitoring of gradients by absorption at 260 or 280 nm is therefore out of the question.

5.1.5   Salts

The greatest densities in aqueous systems can be achieved with solutions of salts. Cesium chloride is surely the most common, but cesium sulfate has somewhat greater density; rubidium salts are also employed (Appendix C6, C7, and C8).

Sodium bromide has been employed by itself and to augment the density of sucrose solutions (Wilcox and Heimberg, 1968). Potassium citrate and tartrate are also useful in increasing the densities of sucrose solutions marginally, but enough to permit isopycnic separation of several viruses (cf. Cline and Ryel, 1971).

Cesium and Rubidium Salts

Meselson *et al.* (1957) invented a new and important variant of isopycnic sedimentation; it is called density gradient sedimentation equilibrium (Sections 3.3, 5.3, and 8.3) and is distinguished from ordinary isopycnic separations in that both solute and particle are at equilibrium. They specifically described how DNA species with differing base ratios could be separated and detected with extraordinarily high resolution in equilibrium gradients of cesium chloride. The gradient in this case is established through the equilibrium of opposing processes of sedimentation and diffusion of the solute

Table 5.2. **Some Iodinated Compounds Suitable for Density Gradients**[a]

Name	Density (gm/cm^3) (°C)	Composition	Reference
Urografin	—	Mixture of sodium and II salts of I	Schatz et al., 1964
Renografin 76	1.412 (25°)	II Salt of I[b]	Tamir and Gilvarg, 1966
Hypaque	1.424 (25°)	II Salt of I	
Isopaque 440	1.479 (25°)	II Salt of III	
Cardiografin 400	1.462 (25°)	II Salt of I	
Angio-Conray	1.502 (25°)	Sodium salt of IV	
Conray 400	1.416 (25°)	II Salt of IV	
Diiodon		VI	Holter et al., 1953; Ottesen and Weber, 1955
Metrizamide	1.47 (5°–15°)	V	Birnie et al., 1973

[a] The roman numerals refer to the structure of the principal component as shown in Fig. 5.3. Metrizamide is available from Nygaard Inc.; the others are supplied by Winthrop Laboratories, with the exception of Urografin and Diidon. See also Appendix C.3.

[b] Some preparations of Renografin are mixtures of sodium and II salts of I.

itself. Equilibrium gradients are typically very shallow. The steepness and shape of the gradient described by Eq. (4.32) is dependent on the centrifugal field $r\omega^2$, the β-function, which depends on the choice of salt, and the geometry of the rotor (cf. Section 4.3.7). The β-functions for commonly used salts are tabulated in Appendix C8a. Cesium chloride and related salts were chosen for the high densities obtainable in principle, one can establish an equilibrium gradient with any solute, given sufficient time. One normally allows 24 to 48 hr for equilibrium within the space of the analytical cells of the Model E ultracentrifuge. In contrast, banding of macromolecules in these gradients is virtually at equilibrium within a few hours.

Clearly much longer (sometimes prohibitively long) intervals are required for true sedimentation equilibrium in angle or swinging-bucket rotors; with these it is preferable to employ preformed gradients (Brunk and Leich, 1969) or allow a gradient to form by diffusion across a step. Such gradients would not, of course, have the same shape as true equilibrium gradients.

Sedimentation equilibrium can be achieved much more rapidly in vertical rotors.

The shapes of equilibrium gradients and the densities obtainable are determined by the properties of individual salts (Appendix C6, C7, and C8), but the behavior of macromolecules is also determined by their ionic environment. For example, the densities of DNAs in CsCl are in the range of 1.7 gm/cm^3; in Cs_2SO_4 they are nearer 1.4 gm/cm^3. The choice of the salt is affected therefore by several considerations (cf. Chapter 7).

The buoyant density of DNA in gradients of alkali salts is controlled by the base composition of the DNA but is also affected in useful ways by substances that interact specifically with different kinds of DNA. Covalently closed circles, nicked circles, and linear DNA can be separated in gradients of CsCl containing ethidium bromide (Radloff et al., 1967). The rationale is that ethidium bromide intercalates into the double helices of DNA and the extent of intercalation is greater the more relaxed the molecule. Since ethidium bromide affects the buoyant density of the DNA, different conformers band at different densities in the gradient. The fluorescence of ethidium bromide also provides a sensitive means of detecting the bands of DNA.

CsCl–ethidium bromide gradients can also be used for rate separations of different size classes of DNA down to about 350 base pairs (El-Gewely and Helling, 1980) (cf. Section 9.5.3).

The resolution of eukaryotic DNAs can been achieved by the addition to gradients of Cs_2SO_4 of silver ion (Corneo et al., 1968) or 3,6-bis(acetatomercurimethyl)dioxane (Cortadas et al., 1977). The latter substance increases the buoyant density of DNA by binding preferentially to $(dA + dT)$ sequences.

The addition of $4M$ guanidium hydrochloride to CsCl gradients permits the isolation of glycoproteins which have been extracted with detergents (Sherblom et al., 1980).

The presence of covalently bound carbohydrate increases the ρ_{eq} of the protein. The guanidium ion apparently reverses the binding of detergents, such as sodium dodecyl sulfate or Triton X-100, which are required for the initial solubilization.

Cesium salts are very expensive. Lower grades may be purified in the laboratory with some savings (Szybalski, 1968). The absorbancy of saturated solutions should be less than 0.05 at 260 nm. An elaborate system for the recovery of large amounts of cesium chloride is described by Wright et al. (1966).

Alkali salts including cesium are extremely corrosive to aluminum alloys. Manufacturers universally warn against the use of cesium salts in aluminum rotors. This caveat also applies to the accidental leakage of salt solutions from plastic tubes in such rotors. The resulting pitting and hairline cracks can seriously weaken the metal, causing what Anderson sanguinely refers to as "catastrophic self-disassembly."

On the other hand, cesium salts may be used safely in titanium rotors. With all rotors an additional consideration is that the maximum speed must usually be lowered to allow for the high density and therefore mass of the load. Charts of such temporary derating are supplied by the manufacturer.

Cesium salts would have been at one time prohibitively expensive for zonal rotors because of the necessity of displacing the gradient with an equal volume of dense solution; edge-loading designs (cf. Section 6.3.9) now permit one to introduce a narrow gradient at the edge of the rotor and then to recover it by displacement with water.

5.1.6 Deuterium Oxide

Except for its expense and relatively low density, heavy water is an almost ideal gradient material. In sedimenting through a gradient of D_2O, particles "see" an invariant environment with respect to almost all parameters except density. However, since the water of hydration will be exchanged for D_2O of hydration, particle densities may be significantly greater in D_2O than in water.

Heavy water has been used for separations in swinging buckets (cf. de Duve et al., 1959) and a few heroic separations in zonal rotors (e.g., Corbett, 1967; Elrod and Anderson, 1967). De Duve et al. (1959) reported that mitochondria and lysosomes take up different amounts of D_2O and thus have distinctly different equilibrium densities in gradients of D_2O, whereas in sucrose they strongly overlap.

Millero et al. (1971) have determined the density and viscosity of D_2O solutions (Appendix C13). Solutions of D_2O–CsCl also have a special advantage for acceleration gradients (cf. Section 3.2.3) because the viscosity–concentration anomaly is more striking than in H_2O–CsCl solutions.

5.1.7 Other Gradient Materials

A large number of organic substances may lend themselves to density gradient centrifugation, although they seem to have received only limited attention (Parish and Hastings, 1966).

Nonaqueous Gradient Materials

Behrens (1938) used nonaqueous gradients in the earliest report on the use of density gradient centrifugation for the separation of particles. About the same time, Linderstrøm-Lang (1937) described a gradient of bromobenzene and kerosene for the estimation of the density of aqueous solutions. Centrifugation in nonaqueous gradients plays a minor role in current biological practice, but is of substantial importance in the analysis of clay and other minerals.

A list of the major classes of nonaqueous gradient materials is presented in Table 5.3 together with some of their properties.

Table 5.3.   Nonaqueous Gradient Materials

Name	Density (gm/cm³)	Reference	Comments
Kerosene	ca. 0.8	Linderstrøm-Lang, 1937	Flammable
Bromobenzene	1.495		Vapors of bromobenzene are toxic
Carbon tetrachloride	1.604	Behrens, 1938	Relatively nonvolatile pair
Benzene	0.879		
Ethyl ether	0.708	Behrens, 1938	
Chloroform	1.490		
Tetrabromoethane	2.96	Francis et al., 1970	Gradients prepared with miscible solvents, such as acetone and ethanol
Bromoform	2.89		

Gradient Additives

Just as buffers, salts, etc., are routinely added to gradients to maintain appropriate physiological conditions, salts and detergents may be incorporated in order to remove contaminating materials, or to achieve special effects. N-Dodecylsarcosinate* and lauryldimethylamine oxide† are detergents which remove lipids but leave many enzyme systems active (cf. Evans et al., 1973).

The sedimentation rates of RNAs in gradients of sucrose dissolved in formamide or dimethyl sulfoxide, unlike those in aqueous sucrose, are proportional to molecular weight, presumably because hydrogen bonds are broken and secondary structure cannot contribute to the frictional coefficient.

5.2   CONCENTRATION CONVENTIONS AND STOCK SOLUTIONS

We should remind ourselves of some rules governing the designation of concentrations which are particularly critical for the concentrated solutions used in preparing gradients. For even moderately dense solutions, the con-

---

* Ciba-Geigy offers this as Sarkosyl, the active ingredient of Gardol.

† The active ingredient of Joy; sold as Ammonyx LO by the Onyx Chemical Co., Jersey City, New Jersey. The commercial product contains a small amount of H_2O_2, which may be removed by successive treatment with catalase and heat sterilization (R. K. Clayton, personal communication).

centration expressed as percent weight by weight (% w/w) is numerically very different from that expressed as percent weight by volume (% w/v). For example, 65% w/w sucrose is at 0°C equal to about 86% w/v. *It is imperative therefore to specify the analytical base in reporting the composition of gradient solutions.* It is astonishing how many otherwise careful scientists overlook this point.

The relation between the two kinds of weight percentages is

$$C_{w/v} = \rho C_{w/w} \qquad (5.1a)$$

or

$$C_{w/w} = C_{w/v}\rho^{-1} \qquad (5.1b)$$

where $C_{w/v}$ is the concentration on a weight basis, $C_{w/w}$ the concentration on a volume basis, and ρ the density.

Physical chemists have traditionally favored the weight-by-weight basis in part because it is independent of temperature. One may find it convenient to measure out the components of concentrated stock solutions on this same basis, especially in the case of slowly soluble materials. Continuing with the same example, we prepare 65% w/w sucrose simply by mixing 65 gm of sucrose with 35 gm of water. If one were to prepare the same solution on a volume basis (=86% w/v), one should be obliged to weigh out 86 gm of sucrose, dissolve it in a minimum of water (how much?) and dilute to 100 cm^3 at 0°C, a formidable task!

On the other hand weight-by-weight solutions can become hopelessly complicated when two or more solutes are present. For example, how much dextran would one incorporate in a 20% w/w sucrose solution such that mitochondria would "see" the same concentration of dextran as in a solution containing 8% w/w sucrose and 10% w/w dextran? For such complex systems, we are much better off using weight-by-volume or, when appropriate, molar relations.

In all events we shall find it convenient to prepare concentrated stock solutions of gradient materials and dilute them to the desired concentrations. Suppose we wish to prepare 100 cm^3 of a 10% w/v solution of sucrose (at 0°C) from a stock solution of 65% w/w sucrose. The fundamental relation is that the amount of sucrose in the two solutions is the same

$$V_d C_d = V_s C_s$$

where the subscript d refers to the diluted solution and the subscript s refers to the stock solution.

$$100 \text{ cm}^3 \times 10\% \,(\text{w/v}) = V_s \times 65\% \,(\text{w/w}) \times \rho_s$$

The density of 65% w/w sucrose at 0°C is 1.3260 gm/cm^3 (cf. Appendix C1). Hence, the required volume of the stock solution is

$$V_s = 100 \text{ cm}^3 \frac{10\% \text{ (w/v)}}{65\% \text{ (w/w)} \, 1.3260}$$

$$V_s = 11.6 \text{ cm}^3$$

In general, for stock solutions specified on a w/w basis

$$V_s = V_d \frac{C_{d(w/v)}}{\rho_s C_{s(w/w)}} \tag{5.2a}$$

or

$$V_s = V_d \frac{\rho_d C_{d(w/w)}}{\rho_s C_{s(w/w)}} \tag{5.2b}$$

For stock solutions specified by volume w/v

$$V_s = V_d \frac{C_{d(w/v)}}{C_{s(w/v)}} \tag{5.3a}$$

$$V_s = V_d \frac{\rho C_{d(w/w)}}{C_{s(w/v)}} \tag{5.3b}$$

5.3 GRADIENT GENERATORS

As discussed elsewhere (cf. Section 3.2.3) the gradient shape is of crucial importance in optimizing resolution and capacity, particularly for rate separations. The ideal gradient generator, therefore, should be completely *programmable*; this means that it should be capable of generating a gradient of any desired shape. For zonal rotors the generator should also be capable of pumping up to several liters of quite viscous solutions, and be easy to clean and sterilize. For swinging buckets one needs gradient volumes ranging from $6 \times 3 = 18$ cm^3 to $6 \times 40 = 240$ cm^3.

Extremely simple and inexpensive devices can be fabricated in the laboratory for generating linear and exponential gradients (Fig. 5.4 and 5.6). These have proved quite practicable for swinging buckets and are generally useful whenever linear or exponential gradients suffice. Gradient engines suitable for zonal rotors must not only have a larger capacity, but be able to pump against a considerable back pressure. Some designs can be fabricated readily in the laboratory (Anderson and Rutenberg, 1967; Birnie and Harvey, 1968).

Linear gradient generators most commonly use two equal cylinders (Parr, 1954; Bock and Ling, 1954) (Fig. 5.4a) containing an *initial* or *starting* solution (right) and a *final* solution (left). The two cylinders communicate at or preferably under their base. The chamber on the right is mixed thoroughly. As solution is drawn off from the mixing chamber, final solution enters the

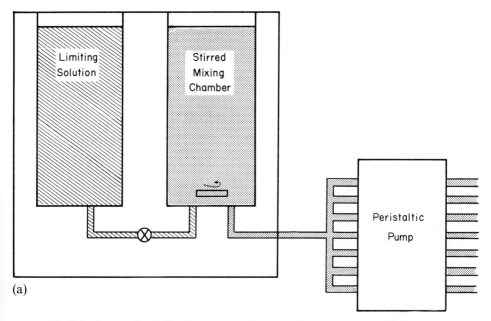

(a)

Fig. 5.4. Inexpensive devices for generating linear gradients. These can be easily fabricated in the laboratory shop. Any of the generators may be coupled to the stream splitter shown in a. (a) Two-cylinder system. Cylinders may be drilled out of block of Plexiglas or constructed of a Plexiglas cylinder cemented to a base. Valve connecting cylinders should be below the level of the cylinders to prevent tunneling. In this diagram a peristaltic or proportioning pump is arranged to split the output of the gradient engine into six identical streams. The Gilson Minipuls HP8 is particular suitable. (b) Proportioning pump system. A gradient stream is pulled from the mixing chamber at twice the velocity that limiting solution is drawn from a reservoir. To obtain the doubled velocity on the exit stream, one may either use two sections of the tubing marked "A" or select tubing with an internal diameter twice that of "A." (c) Twin-syringe pump (Moore, 1969) A motorized syringe pump, such as is used for infusions, drives two syringes. V1 empties into V2 which serves as the mixing chamber. The gradient is pumped from V2. Funkhouser found that disposable plastic syringes lend themselves easily to this system, especially since one can connect V1 to V2 with a hypodermic needle piercing the piston of V2. (d) A commercial two-cylinder gradient device (courtesy Pharmacia Fine Chemicals). The low-speed stirrer, valve connecting between the two cylinders, and a needle valve controlling the outflow are attractive features. (e) The B-XXI distributor rotor (Molecular Anatomy Program, Oak Ridge National Laboratories). A gradient stream is led into a groove near the center of an angle rotor, then split into each of the tubes. Equal distribution is assured by the centrifugal field. (See pp. 130–133.)

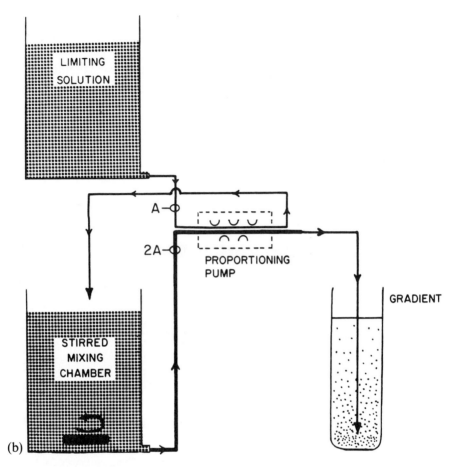

Fig. 5.4(b). *Continued*

mixing chamber so that the composition of the mixing chamber and of the gradient thus changes continuously.

In the simple versions of the two-cylinder generator gravity is relied on to maintain the levels in the two chambers approximately equal; in more sophisticated machines equal volumes are imposed by rigidly connected (Paris, 1970) or motor-driven (de Duve *et al.*, 1959) pistons. In all cases the concentration of the output changes linearly from the initial to the final solution (Fig. 5.5), provided only that the cross-sectional areas of the two cylinders are the same and that the volumes of fluid in the two chambers are always equal.* If the diameters of the two cylinders are unequal or if the

---

* This will not exactly obtain with two fluids of unequal density acted on by gravity alone.

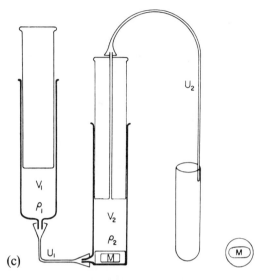

Fig. 5.4(c). *Continued*

pistons are driven unequally, a different gradient shape results. Moore (1969) has presented the following analysis of the generator shown in Fig. 5.4c in which the two cylinders have different cross-sectional areas. Let the final piston be represented by subscript F and the mixing piston by subscript M. The density of the effluent gradient is ρ_V. The mass of fluid in the mixing chamber is m. For equal incremental displacements of the two pistons, the increment of density in the mixing chamber is

$$d\rho_V = d(m/V)$$

$$= \frac{dm}{V_M} - \frac{mdV_M}{V_M{}^2}$$

The increment of mass dm must be the net of inflow and outflow

$$dm = \rho_V(A_F + A_M)dx - \rho_F A_F dx \qquad (5.4)$$

where A refers to the cross-sectional area of the pistons. Hence

$$d\rho_V = \frac{\rho_V(A_M + A_F)dx - \rho_F A_F dx}{A_M x} - \frac{\rho_V A_M{}^2 x dx}{(A_M x)^2}$$

$$= \frac{A_F}{A_M}(\rho_V - \rho_F)\frac{dx}{x}$$

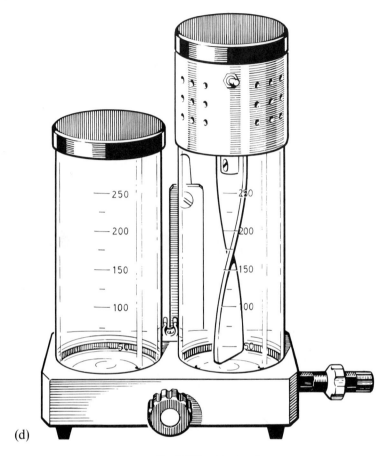

(d)

Fig. 5.4(d).   *Continued*

Integrating

$$\int_{\rho_M}^{\rho_V} \frac{d\rho_V}{\rho_V - \rho_F} = \frac{A_F}{A_M} \int_{x_0}^{x} \frac{dx}{x}$$

$$[\ln (\rho_V - \rho_F)]_{\rho_M}^{\rho_V} = \frac{A_F}{A_M} [\ln x]_{x_0}^{x} \tag{5.5}$$

$$\rho_V = \rho_F + (\rho_M - \rho_F) \left[\frac{x}{x_0} \right]^{\frac{A_F}{A_M}}$$

Plots of Eq. (5.5) for different ratios of A_F and A_M are shown in Fig. 5.5.
When the two cylinder cross sections are equal, the gradient is of course

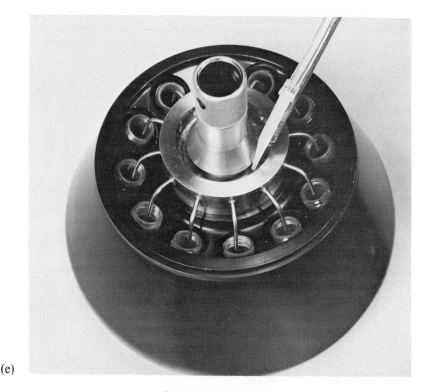

(e)

Fig. 5.4(e).   *Continued*

linear. If the mixing chamber is relatively thick, the gradient is concave; if thin, it is convex.

Several types of inexpensive linear gradient generators are shown in Fig. 5.4.

Exponential gradients can be made to approximate isokinetic and equivolumetric gradients and others with some fuss (Appendix D). We should look therefore at the mathematics of exponential and other nonlinear generators.

In the exponential generator (Fig. 5.6a), first described by Alm *et al.* (1952), let V_M be the volume of the mixing chamber, c_S the concentration of the *starting* solution in the mixing chamber, c_L that of the *limiting* solution in the reservoir, and c_V the concentration of the effluent ($=$ gradient) after V cm^3 has flowed from the system. The incremental increase in the amount of solute in the mixing chamber is

$$dc_V = (c_L - c_V)dV$$

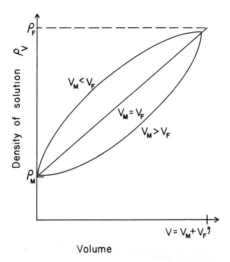

Fig. 5.5. Shapes of gradients from two-cylinder engines. The shape of the gradients depends on the diameters of the two cylinders. If they are equal, the gradient is linear; otherwise they may be concave or convex [cf. Eq. (5.5)].

(A)

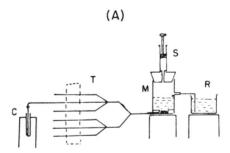

Fig. 5.6. Inexpensive exponential gradient engines. Most of these can be easily fabricated in the laboratory shop or with the aid of a glassblower. A stream splitter can be coupled to them, as in Fig. 5.4A. (A) The volume of fluid in the mixing chamber M can be adjusted with a syringe S (McCarty *et al.,* 1968). The volume of the reservoir can be used to gauge the total volume of the gradient. This generator is quite suitable for swinging buckets. (B) Zonal gradient engine of Anderson and Rutenberg (1967). The chamber is selected to approximate the volume of the rotor. A circulating pump maintains a vigorous vortex while gradient is drawn off from the lowest "T" on the stem of the chamber. Since it is a closed system, limiting solution from the reservoir is drawn in to replace the volume drawn off to the rotor.

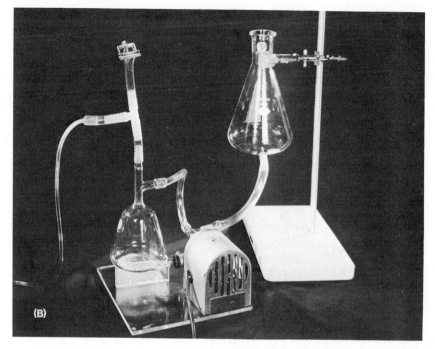

Fig. 5.6. *Continued*

Integrating between $V = 0$ and $V = V$

$$c_V = c_L - (c_L - c_S) \exp(-V/V_M) \qquad (5.6)$$

The range of gradient shapes possible with exponential generators is shown in Fig. 5.7.

Very handsomely designed mixing chambers suitable for swinging-bucket rotors are available in three sizes from Searle under the brand name Isograd. The chambers are components of a complete generator system which seems needlessly complicated.

An inexpensive exponential generator suitable for zonal rotors is shown in Fig. 5.6B. The principle of generating the gradient is the same as in other exponential generators, but the Anderson–Rutenberg machine is equipped with a circulating pump that insures adequate mixing for the volumes and viscosities encountered with zonal rotors.

Another type of gradient engine employs differential rates of flow through two channels followed by mixing. In one version of this, cylinders are discharged at different rates; for example, a linear gradient is formed if one piston displaces a starting solution at a steadily decreasing rate while another piston displaces a limiting solution at a steadily increasing rate. The Beckman

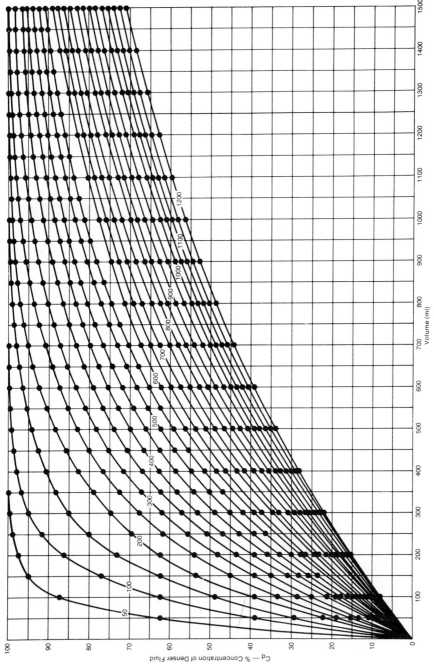

Fig. 5.7. Shapes of gradients from exponential generators (Courtesy of Damon/IEC Division). In all cases a limiting solution from a reservoir is drawn to a mixing chamber of constant volume. The rate of flow in and out of the mixing chamber is the same [cf. Fig. 5.6A and Eq. (5.4)].

Spinco 141 and ISCO generators (Figs. 5.8a and e) are commercial versions of these. The two pistons are programmed to discharge and fill repeatably at rates determined by the position of a cam (Spinco 141) or at selected control points (ISCO).

A few comments are in order about gradient generators.

(1) In the gradient generators discussed here we introduce two solutions, a starting and a final or limiting solution, which are mixed in continuously changing proportions. Note that mixing occurs by volume; so that volumetric factors occur throughout. In general we cannot assume that the concentration of solute in a mixture of equal volumes of two solutions will be the mean of the two concentrations. Therefore, we must compute the desired mixture at each point along the gradient. In the case of linear gradients in isopycnic separations one can safely interpolate the true equilibrium density of particles in a fraction from determined densities of adjacent fractions, so that the small departures from nonlinearity are usually insignificant.

(2) Multiple gradients can be formed by pulling the gradient stream through a manifold* with a peristaltic or proportioning pump (cf. also Wallach, 1970). Attempts to push a gradient into a manifold invariably result in unequal streams (cf. Fig. 5.4a).

Sheeler et al. (1978) describe an ingenious device for generating multiple gradients. A moveable, false bottom in each centrifuge tube is first placed at the top of the tube, and then drawn downward, pulling a portion of the gradient through a manifold. The system requires, however, specially constructed tubes equipped with special seals between the moveable bottom and the sides of the tube.

The B-XXI distributor head for angle rotors (Fig. 5.4e) is another means of splitting a gradient stream into multiple tubes. In this case the stream is led into a circular groove in an angle rotor and there split into separate streams leading into tubes in the rotor.

(3) Fittings should be selected with an idea to ready interchangeability; Luer and Swage-Lok connectors are suitable.

(4) The tunnel connecting the two cylinders of a two-cylinder generator may serve as a two-way channel for the uncontrolled mixing of the two solutions if it is too large or not placed below the bottom of the cylinder as shown in Fig. 5.4a. Generators available from Canadian Scientific, Buchler, BRL, Hoefer, and Pharmacia look particularly well designed in this respect.

(5) If channel or tubing connections are too small, the resulting pressure drops may interfere with hydrostatic equilibria; the two cylinders of a two-cylinder generator may empty unevenly, or air trapped in the exponential generator of Fig. 5.6a may expand and thus alter the mixing volume.

---

* Available from Small Parts, Inc.

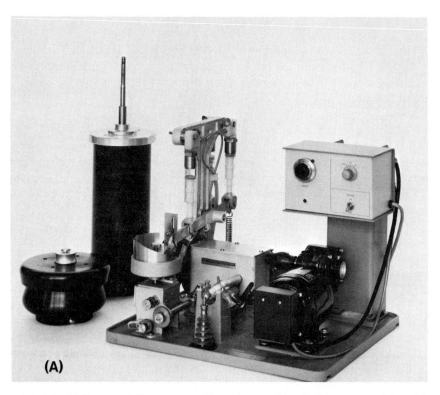

(A)

Fig. 5.8. Fully or partially programmable gradient engines. In these commercial models one may obtain linear or exponential gradients of different volumes or, in some cases, gradients of arbitrary shapes (cf. Table 5.5). (A) 141 Gradient Pump (Spinco Division, Beckman Instruments). The shape of the gradient is determined by a template, which may be cut to any desired shape. Starting solution is drawn from a reservoir to a measuring syringe (M) whose position is limited by the template. The volume of each stroke not taken by the measuring syringe is used to draw final solution from a second reservoir. A B-IV (tall) and Ti15 (short) zonal rotor are also shown. (B) Ultrograd (LKB). This system also uses a template for generating gradients of arbitrary shape (shown in the photograph as a sawtooth graph paper in the unit at the right). The machine in this case opens or closes power circuits over that fraction of a duty cycle determined by the height of the template. The power circuits are then used to open or close valves (stacked units at the center), which can connect any one of these solutions from Erlenmeyer flasks (at top) to a pump (at left). The system is shown connected to a chromatographic column, but the manufacturers report that it can be adapted to pump gradients to zonal rotors. (C) Two-cylinder gradient pump (Damon/IEC Division). This engine can deliver only linear or exponential gradients, but possesses a smooth and powerful drive suitable for viscous gradient materials and for pulseless displacement of rotor contents. The mixing chamber (right) is held at a fixed position for exponential gradients; both pistons are driven for linear gradients. (D) Two-cylinder gradient former (Du Pont/Sorvall). In this passive system fluid is drawn from the gradient generator by an external pump. The two pistons may be linked; so that the two cylinders empty at the same rate and a linear gradient is formed. Alternatively, the mixing chamber is fixed and the system forms an exponential gradient. (E) Dialagrad (ISCO). The contribution of two pumps (faces visible at right) are governed by settings of 12 dials. Smoothed arbitrary shapes of gradients can be obtained. (See pp. 139–142.)

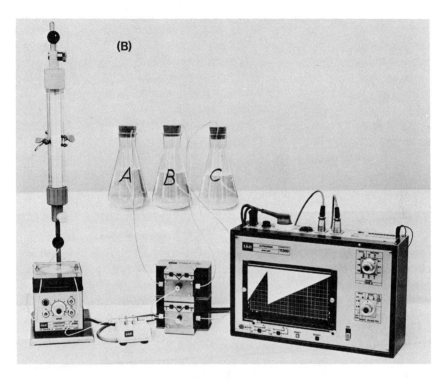

Fig. 5.8. *Continued*

(6) The closest attention must be given to ensure that mixing is efficient and uniform. Magnetic stirrers should be closely coupled, which requires that the magnet be close to the drive. Propellors and vibrators* may perturb liquid surfaces and thus upset the requirement that liquid levels in the two cylinders remain equal.

(7) The significance of volume becomes especially important with gradient generators for zonal rotors. In general we find that most gradient generators which were designed for swinging buckets or for the larger volumes of dilute solutions employed in column chromatography are beset by large coefficients of difficulty when asked to deliver 1 liter of 65% w/w sucrose.

Some commercially available gradient generators are shown in Fig. 5.8 and a comparison of their properties is presented in Table 5.5. Four gener-

* For example, Chemag, A. G. Männedorf/ZH, Switzerland.

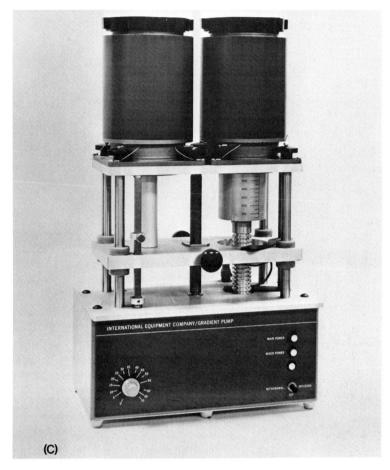

Fig. 5.8. *Continued*

ators (Isolab, MSE, Spinco, and LKB) achieve complete programmability by employing templates that may be cut or molded to any arbitrary shape. The Spinco template is rather imprecise and the Isolab even more so. Viscous solutions can be handled most securely with positive displacement pumps (ISCO, IEC, Spinco), but bubbles of air trapped in the partial vacuum of the Spinco 141 fluid system can destroy gradient shapes, especially in the case of extremely viscous solutions. Exponential generators have the marked disadvantage that, when the gradient is completed, the mixing chamber contains a substantial quantity of limiting solution, which may be very wasteful of expensive gradient materials.

E. F. Eikenberry (personal communication) has designed an omega-

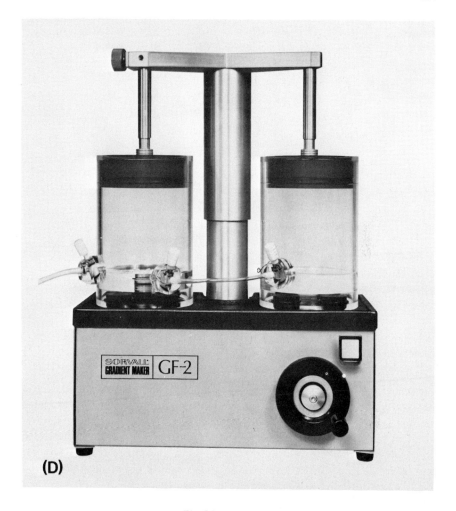

(D)

Fig. 5.8. *Continued*

gradient generator (Fig. 5.9) along similar lines; in this case the outputs of two metering pumps are controlled by a laboratory minicomputer which may be programmed to deliver completely arbitrary gradient shapes to any desired degree of precision. Although it would be difficult to justify the expense of a general purpose minicomputer simply to generate gradients, such a system could be implemented today with a microprocessor of quite modest cost.

Baxter-Gabbard (1972) recommends freezing and thawing as a means of generating any number of density gradients. Since solutes are excluded from

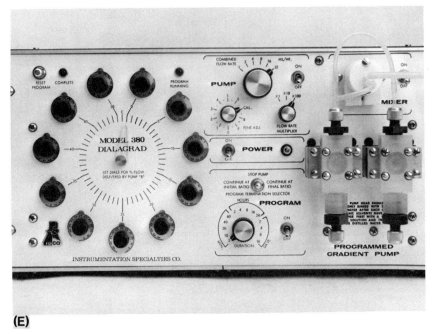

(E)

Fig. 5.8. *Continued*

the first part of a solution to freeze, the gradient material accumulates in the bottom of the tube. Upon thawing, a smooth, although arbitrary gradient results. It can be made more steep by repeated freezing and thawing. If gradient shape is not a serious consideration, the method is suitable for constructing gradients of single solutes; salts and other solutes will be subject to the same forces, however, and will result in unbalanced gradients.

Self-Generated Gradients

Density gradients may be generated through sedimentation of the gradient material in a centrifugal field. Such self-generated gradients are of two types, somewhat analogous to isopycnic and rate separations of sample particles. Equilibrium gradients are produced as a resultant of sedimentation and diffusion (cf. Sections 3.3.3 and 4.3.7–4.3.9). These gradients are usually made of alkali salts, notably cesium chloride, but not exclusively so. Spragg (1970) has also considered equilibrium gradients of sucrose, the idea being that such a gradient, once constructed, and maintained at a constant velocity, would be absolutely stable against diffusion. A distinct disadvantage is, however, that equilibrium gradients are disappointingly shallow and would be only marginally useful in rate separations.

Table 5.4.   Commercial Devices for Measuring Density

Name	Manufacturer	Principle	Comments
Abbé refractometer	Bausch & Lomb	Refractive index	Null instrument, batch only
		Refractive index	Direct reading, batch only
Refractometer	Waters Associates	Differential refractive index	Direct reading; continuous flow; corrected for light scattering
Refractometer	Pharmacia	Differential refractive index	Direct reading; continuous flow
Pycnometer	Various	Weight of precisely determined volume of liquid	Batch only; very slow
Density meter	Anton Paar	Natural frequency of tube containing the fluid	Direct reading, digital, continuous-flow, extremely precise
Density beads	Pharmacia	Color-coded beads of Sephadex ($1.017–1.142$ gm/cm^3)	Accuracy to 0.0005 gm/cm^3; sensitive to ionic strength and osmotic pressure.

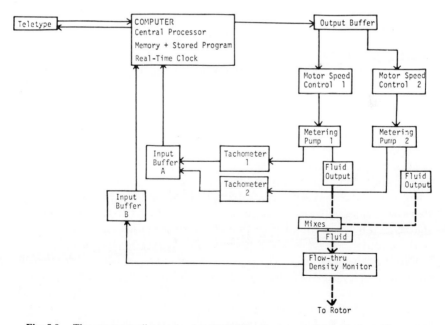

Fig. 5.9.   The omega gradient generator (E. F. Eikenberry, unpublished). A gradient pump could be controlled by a computer. The diagram shows one possible configuration for the flow of information (——) and fluids (– – –).

Pertoft (1966 *et seq.*) has advocated the use of a very different kind of self-generated gradient. One starts with a uniform colloidal sol of silica (cf. Appendix C11) to which has been added another polymer, such as dextran, and centrifuges the system at about 30,000 rpm for 30 min. Through a combination of simple sedimentation and solvent exclusion, one can obtain a nearly linear gradient of silica. We should note that the gradient obtained is based on a rate sedimentation of the silica; the particle size of the silica is such that continued centrifugation would result in the complete sedimentation of the silica particles. The gradient obtained is then used without transfer to another vessel for rate or isopycnic separation of much larger particles.

5.4   DENSITY MEASUREMENTS

An experiment may be judged successful merely if two or more kinds of particles have been separated; we then may not care to know the exact parameters of the gradient that brought about that happy juncture. If, however, we need to know the equilibrium densities of separated particles, or wish to compute a sedimentation coefficient, or perhaps wish to discover what failed in a separation, we shall certainly want to measure the densities of stock solutions and of fractions along the recovered gradient.

The most common method of measuring the density of gradient fractions is indirect: refractive index. Tables of refractive indices of different concentrations of a number of the common gradient materials are presented in Appendix C. The method is suitable for most materials except D_2O and Ludox, whose refractive indices do not differ appreciably from those of water.

The most widely used refractometer is the Abbé. The older version of this is completely manual: a drop of solution is placed on a prism, and a light "step" aligned manually with cross-hair. With a new version (Table 5.4) there is a direct optical read-out. After having read through several gradients, most workers will long for a fully automatic or continuous-flow refractometer. They exist but are expensive and have their limitations. One must be sure that the gradient stream is maintained at a constant temperature, and that the refractometer is insensitive to light absorption or light scattering by particle zones.

Direct determination of density by a pycnometer is in principle preferable to refractometry, since the determination of density is then direct rather than derived. Conventional pycnometers are inconveniently large for gradient work, but one can weigh micropipets to obtain densities of the contained fluid to within 0.001 gm/cm^3 (Vinograd and Hearst, 1962).

Considerably greater precision and accuracy may be obtained with a different pycnometric principle: a small sample of fluid is contained in or

Table 5.5. Characteristics of Commercially Available Gradient Generators

Manufacturers and designation	Kinds of gradients delivered			Maximum volume (cm³)	Maximum pumping rate (cm³/min)	Suitability with viscous materials	Ease of sterilization
	Linear	Exponential	Fully programmable				
Damon/IEC	+	+		2000	70	3+	2+
Damon/IEC	+	+		[a]	ca. 100	2+	3+
ISCO Dialagrad 380			[b]	∞	50	2+	-
ISCO Dialagrad 382			[b]	∞	10	2+	-
ISCO Dialagrad 570	+	+		50	16	3+	+
ISOLAB Gradipore			+	1500	[c]	-	-
LKB GM-1	+			500	[c]	+	
Ultragrad			+	∞	[d]	[d]	3+
MSE Fixed Profile	+	+		2000	ca. 150	2+	2+
MSE Automatic Variable			+	∞	ca. 120	2+	3+
Du Pont/Sorvall	+	+			[c]		
Beckman/Spinco 141			+	6000	66	-	-

[a] Depends on selection of mixing chamber. Commercial version of system shown in Fig. 1.3.
[b] Gradient determined by smoothed fit to nine specified points along gradient.
[c] Depends on gravity or choice of auxiliary pump.
[d] Pumps suitable for sucrose have not been fully described. A requirement is that the starting and final solutions be delivered to the mixing chamber at rates which are independent of their viscosities; some kind of positive displacement pump would seem to be necessary.

pumped through a vibrating, hollow tube. The natural frequency of the system is a sensitive function of the density of the fluid and can be recorded electronically. Vas Es and Bont (1974) have described such a device optimized for the flow rates and concentrations of sucrose normally encountered in zonal centrifugation. They report an accuracy of ± 0.001 gm/cm^3. This same principle has been incorporated into a commercial instrument, the Paar Digital Density Meter* (Persinger *et al.*, 1974).

Another instrumental approach to automatic pycnometry employs the absorption of β-rays, which is generally proportional to mass and hence density (Atherton *et al.*, 1973).

Density Markers

Still another means of calibrating a gradient is by means of visible particles whose densities are known. These include color-coded plastic or glass spheres covering a range of densities from 1 to 2 gm cm^3 or more. Plastic markers (Spinco Microspheres, etc.; cf. Appendix B3) are relatively inexpensive and also have fairly low precision. Glass floats (Techne) are available at considerably greater expense but with a claimed precision of 0.0002 gm/cm^3. Sets of color-coded Density Marker Beads are available from Pharmacia for calibrating gradients of silica. The exact banding densities are influenced by the ionic strength and osmotic pressure of the medium. Colored plastic chips from household items can be prepared with reasonably repeatable densities in the region of 1.05 gm/cm^3.

Richard *et al.* (1970) have described an organic liquid that can be used as a density marker in sedimentation–diffusion equilibrium of nucleic acids (cf. Section 8.3). The perfluorodated fluid FC-78 is available from Minnesota Mining and Manufacturing Co. Its density at atmospheric pressure is 1.705 gm/cm^3. Richard *et al.* provide the data to compute its density under conditions of ultracentrifugation.

REFERENCES

Albertsson, P.-A. (1972). "Partition of Cell Particles and Macromolecules," 2nd ed. Wiley, New York.
Alm, R. S., Williams, R. J. P., and Tisilius, A. (1952). Gradient elution analysis. I. A general treatment. *Acta Chem. Scand.* **6**, 826–836.
Anderson, N. G., and Rutenberg, E. (1967). Analytical techniques for cell fractions. VII. A simple gradient-forming apparatus. *Anal. Biochem.* **21**, 259–265.
Atherton, R. S., Boyce, I. S., Clayton, C. C., and Thomson, A. B. (1973). Flow-through density meter for zonal centrifugation and other procedures. *Prep. Biochem.* **3**, 237–267.

* Anton Paar, K. G.; Mettler Instrument Corporation in the U.S.A.

Avers, C. J., Szabo, A., and Price, C. A. (1969). Size-separation of yeast mitochondria in the zonal centrifuge. *J. Bacteriol.* **100,** 1044–1048.

Barber, A. A., Harris, W. W., and Anderson, N. G. (1966). Isolation of native glycogen by combined rate-zonal and isopycnic centrifugation. *Natl. Cancer Inst. Monog.* **21,** 285–302.

Barber, E. J. (1966). Calculation of density and viscosity of sucrose solutions as a function of concentration and temperature. *Natl. Cancer Inst. Monog.* **21,** 219–239.

Baxter-Gabbard, K. L. (1972). A simple method for the large scale preparation of sucrose gradients. *FEBS Lett.* **20,** 117–119.

Behrens, M. (1938). Zell- und Gewebetrennung. *In* "Handbuch der biologischen Arbeitsmethoden" (E. Abderhalden, ed.), Vol. V (10-II), pp. 1363–1392. Urban u. Schwarzenberg, Munich.

Bell, L. R., and Hsu, H. W. (1974). Transport phenomena in zonal centrifuge rotors. IX. Gradient properties of Ficoll and methylcellulose. *Separation Sci.* **9,** 401–410.

Birnie, G. D., and Harvey, D. R. (1968). A simple density-gradient engine for loading large-capacity zonal ultracentrifuge. *Anal. Biochem.* **22,** 171–174.

Birnie, G. D., Rickwood, D., and Hell, A. (1973). Buoyant densities and hydration of nucleic acids, proteins, and nucleoprotein complexes in Metrizamide. *Biochim. Biophys. Acta* **331,** 238–294.

Bock, R. M., and Ling, N.-S. (1954). Devices for gradient elution chromatography. *Anal. Chem.* **26,** 1543–1546.

Brakke, M. K. (1951). Density gradient centrifugation: A new separation technique. *J. Am. Chem. Soc.* **73,** 1847–1848.

Brunk, C. F., and Leich, V. (1969). Rapid equilibrium in isopycnic CsCl gradients. *Biochim. Biophys. Acta* **179,** 136–144.

Cline, G. B., and Ryel, R. B. (1971). Zonal centrifugation. *In* "Methods in Enzymology" (W. B. Jakoby, ed.), Vol. 22, pp. 168–204. Academic Press, New York.

Corbett, J. R. (1967). Purification of lysosomes by zonal centrifugation. *Biochem. J.* **102,** 43p.

Corneo, G., Ginelli, E., Soevo, C., and Bernardi, G. (1968). Isolation and characterization of mouse and guinea pig satellite deoxyribonucleic acids. *Biochemistry* **7,** 4373–4379.

Cortadas, J., Macaya, G., and Bernardi, G. (1977). An analysis of the bovine genome by density gradient centrifugation: Fractionation in ccsium sulfate-3,6-bis(acetatomercurimethyl)-dioxane density gradient. *Eur. J. Biochem.* **76,** 13–19.

de Duve, C., Berthet, J., and Beaufay, H. (1959). Gradient centrifugation of cell particles. Theory and applications. *Prog. Biophys. Biophys. Chem.* **9,** 325–369.

El-Geweley, M. R., and Helling, R. B. (1980). Preparative separation of DNA-ethidium bromide complexes by zonal density gradient centrifugation. *Anal. Biochem.* **102,** 423–428.

Elrod, L. H., and Anderson, N. G. (1967). A method for isolating nuclei using sucrose deuterium oxide gradients. *Oak Ridge Natl. Lab. [Spec.] ORNL-Spec. (U.S.) ORNL-***4171,** 86–88.

Evans, W. H., Hood, D. O., and Gurd, J. W. (1973). Purification and properties of a mouse liver plasma-membrane glycoprotein hydrolysing nucleotide pyrophosphate and phosphodiester bonds. *Biochem. J.* **135,** 819–826.

Francis, C. W., Tamura, T., and Bonner, W. P. (1970). Separation of clay minerals and soil clays using isopycnic zonal centrifugation. *Soil Sci. Soc. Am. Proc.* **34**(2), 351–353.

Gorczynski, R. M., Miller, R. G., and Phillips, R. A. (1970). Homogeneity of antibody producing cells as analyzed by their buoyant density in gradients of Ficoll. *Immunology* **19,** 817–829.

Haskill, J. S., Legge, P. G., and Shortman, K. (1969). Density distribution analysis of cells forming 19S hemolytic antibody in the rat. *J. Immunol.* **102,** 703–712.

Hjort, R., and Pertoft, H. (1982). Removal of Percoll from microsomal vesicles by gel filtration on Sephacryl S-1000 superfine. *Biochim. Biophys. Acta,* in press.

Holter, H., Ottesen, M., and Weber, R. (1953). Separation of cytoplasmic particles by centrifugation in a density gradient. *Experientia* **9,** 346–348.

Kneece, W. C., and Leif, R. C. (1971). The effect of pH, potassium, sodium, bicarbonate, and chloride ions and glucose on the buoyant density distribution of human erythrocytes in bovine serium albumin gradients. *J. Cell Physiol.* **78,** 185–200.

Leif, R. C., Neece, W. C., Jr., Warters, R. L., Grinvalsky, H., and Thomas, R. A. (1972). Density gradient system. III. Elimination of hydrodynamic, wall, and swirling artifacts in preformed isopycnic gradient centrifugation. *Anal. Biochem.* **45,** 357–373.

Linderstrøm-Lang, K. (1937). Dilatometric ultra-micro-estimation of peptidase activity. *Nature (London)* **139,** 713–714.

Lyttleton, J. W. (1970). Use of colloidal silica in density gradients to separate intact chloroplasts. *Anal. Biochem.* **38,** 277–281.

McCarty, D. S., Stafford, D., and Brown, O. (1968). Resolution and fractionation of macromolecules by isokinetic sucrose density gradient sedimentation. *Anal. Biochem.* **24,** 314–329.

Mach, O., and Lacko, L. (1968). Density gradient in a dextran medium. *Anal. Biochem.* **22**(3), 393–397.

Mathias, A. P., and Wynther, C. V. A. (1973). The use of Metrizamide in the fractionation of nuclei from brain and liver tissue by zonal centrifugation. *FEBS Lett.* **33,** 18–22.

Meselson, M., Stahl, F. W., and Vinograd, J. (1957). Equilibrium sedimentation of macromolecules in density gradients. *Proc. Natl. Acad. Sci. U.S.A.* **43,** 581–588.

Millero, F. J., Dexter, R., and Hoff, E. (1971). Density and viscosity of deuterium oxide solutions from 5-70°C *J. Chem. Eng. Data* **16,** 85–87.

Moore, D. H. (1969). Gradient centrifugation. *In* "Physical Techniques in Biological Research" (D. H.Moore, ed.), 2nd ed., Vol. 2, Part B, pp. 285–314. Academic Press, New York.

Morgenthaler, J.-J., Marsden, M. P. F., and Price, C. A. (1975). Factors affecting the separation of photosynthetically competent chloroplasts in gradients of silica sols. *Arch. Biochem. Biophys.* **168,** 289–301.

Nordmann, J.-J., and Aunis, D. (1980). Distribution of secretory granules from adrenal medulla and neurohypophysis on continuous isoosmotic density gradients formed with a new ioxaglic derivative AG-6227. *Anal. Biochem.* **109,** 94–101.

Ottesen, M., and Weber, R. (1955). Density-gradient centrifugation as a means of separating cytoplasmic particles. *C. R. Trav. Lab. Carlsberg* **29,** 417–434.

Paris, J. E. (1970). Preparation of large volumes of linear gradient solutions for zonal ultracentrifugation. *Experientia* **26,** 325–326.

Parish, J. H., and Hastings, J. R. B. (1966). Some alternatives to sucrose for density gradient centrifugation. *Biochim. Biophys. Acta* **123,** 202–204.

Parr, C. W. (1954). The separation of sugars and of sugar phosphates by gradient elution ion exchange columns. *Biochem. J.* **56,** 27P–28P.

Persinger, H. H., Lowen, J., and Tamplin, W. S. (1974). Evaluation of a density meter. *Am. Lab. (Fairfleld, Conn.)* Sept., 68–74.

Pertoft, H. (1966). Gradient centrifugation in colloidal silica-polysaccharide media. *Biochim. Biophys. Acta* **126,** 594–596.

Pertoft, H. (1969). The separation of rat liver cells in colloidal silica-polyethylene glycol gradients. *Exp. Cell Res.* **57,** 338–350.

Pertoft, H. (1970). Separation of cells from a mast cell tumor on density gradients of colloidal silica. *JNCl, J. Natl. Cancer Inst.* **44,** 1251–1256.

Pertoft, H., and Laurent, T. C. (1977). Isopycnic separation of cells and cell organelles by centrifugation in modified colloidal silica gradients. *In* "Methods of Cell Separation" Vol. 1, (N. Catsimpoolas, ed.), pp. 25–65. Plenum, New York.

Pertoft, H., Laurent, T. C., Låås, T., and Kågedal, L. (1978). Density gradients prepared from colloidal silica particles coated by polyvinylpyrrolidone (*Percoll.*) *Anal. Biochem.* **88**, 271–282.

Pretlow, T. G. II, Weir, E. E., and Zettergren, J. G. (1975). Problems connected with the separation of different kinds of cells. *Int. Rev. Exp. Pathol.* **14**, 91–191.

Price, C. A., and Reardon, E. M. (1982). Isolation of chloroplasts for protein synthesis from spinach and *Euglena gracilis* by centrifugation in silica sols. *In* "Methods in Chloroplast Molecular Biology" (M. Edelman, R. Hallick, and N.-H. Chua, eds.). Elsevier-North Holland, in press.

Richard, A. J., Glick, J., and Burk, R. (1970). An inert liquid marker for density gradient ultracentrifugation in CsCl. *Anal. Biochem.* **37**, 378–384.

Radloff, R., Bauer, W., and Vinograd, J. (1967). A dye-buoyant-density method for the detection and isolation of closed circular duplex DNA: the closed circular DNA in HeLa cells. *Proc. Natl. Acad. Sci., U.S.A.* **57**, 1514–1521.

St. Onge, J. M., and Price, C. A. (1975). Automatic sorting of ichthyoplankton: Factors controlling plankton density in gradients of silica. *Mar. Biol.* **29**, 187–194.

Schatz, G., Haslbrunner, E., and Tuppey, H. (1964). Deoxyribonucleic acid associated with yeast mitochondria. *Biochem. Biophys. Res. Commun.* **15**, 127–132.

Sherblom, A. P., Buck, R. L., and Carraway, K. L. (1980). Purification of the major sialoglycoproteins of 13762 MAT-B1 and MAT-C1 rat ascites mammary adenocarcinoma cells by density gradient centrifugation in cesium chloride and guanidine hydrochloride. *J. Biol. Chem.* **255**, 782–790.

Spragg, S. P. (1970). Resolution in zonal rotors. *In* "Microsymposium on Particle Separation from Plant Materials" (C. A. Price, ed.), Oak Ridge Natl. Lab. CONF-700119, pp. 81–88. Natl. Tech. Inf. Serv., Springfield, Virginia.

Szybalski, W. (1968). Use of cesium sulfate for equilibrium density gradient centrifugation. *In* "Methods in Enzymology" (S. P. Colowick and N. O. Kaplan, ed.), Vol. 12, Part B, pp. 330–360. Academic Press, New York.

Tamir, H., and Gilvarg, C. (1966). Density gradient centrigugation for the separation of sporulating forms of bacteria. *J. Biol. Chem.* **241**, 1085–1090.

Thomson, J. F., and Klipfel, F. J. (1958). Intracellular distribution of uricase and catalase in liver of tumor-bearing mice and mice given injections of aminotriazole. *Cancer Res.* **18**(2), 229–233.

Vallee, B. L., Hughes, W. L., and Gibson, J. G. (1947). A method for the separation of leukocytes from whole blood on serum albumin. *Blood* **1**, 82–87.

Van Es, W. L., and Bont, W. S. (1974). The simultaneous measurement of densities and absorbancies in sucrose gradients, applied to zonal centrifugation. *Anal. Biochem.* **58**, 139–145.

Vinograd, J. and Hearst, J. E. (1962). Equilibrium sedimentation of macromolecules and viruses in a density gradient. *Fortschr. Chem. Org. Naturst.* **20**, 372–422.

Wallach, D. F. H. (1970). Simple system for rapid generation of duplicate density gradients. *Anal. Biochem.* **37**, 138–141.

Wilcox, H. G., and Heimberg, M. (1968). The isolation of human serum lipoproteins by zonal ultracentrifugation. *Biochim. Biophys. Acta* **152**, 424–426.

Wolff, D. A. (1975). The separation of cells and subcellular particles by colloidal silica density gradient centrifugation. *Methods Cell Biol.* **10**, 85–104. Academic Press, New York.

Wright, R. R., Pappas, W. S., Carter, J. A., and Weber, C. W. (1966). Preparation and recovery of cesium compounds for density gradient solutions. *Natl. Cancer Inst. Monogr.* **21**, 241–249.

6

Techniques of Preparative Density Gradient Centrifugation

The upper end piece was positioned and pressed down, forcing the Lusteroid tube through the needle . . .

Martin and Ames, 1961

6.1 PLANNING A SEPARATION

6.1.1 Sample Characteristics and Choice of Rotor Types

Perhaps the most perplexing decision for novices in density gradient centrifugation is which rotor to use. There is no simple answer. We can start by asking, (1) how large are the particles that are to be separated? and then (2) is the separation based on rate or density?

Obviously, the smaller the particles, the faster (or longer) the particles must be sedimented. Figures 6.1 and 6.2 give the approximate centrifugal field required to separate particles of a given sedimentation coefficient and density in 8 hr. (The sedimentation coefficients of various subcellular particles are shown in Fig. 1.5.) I have constructed these approximations on the assumption that the particles are initially located over isokinetic or equivolumetric gradients and that the particles can be regarded as separated in a rate separation if they sediment an additional 1 cm or 100 cm^3 into the gradient. On the basis of experience, I assume the particles to be near their isopycnic position at about 100 times the minimum $\omega^2 \Delta t$ required to separate them according to rate. Obviously the estimates of the required speeds must be revised upward if the separation must be achieved in shorter times, if the selected gradients for rate separation are steeper, or if the

150

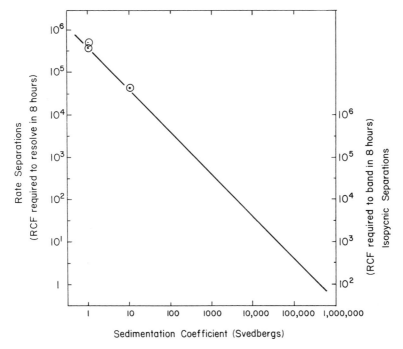

Fig. 6.1. Minimum centrifugal field required to achieve separations of particles in swinging-bucket rotors. The centrifugal field in g's is required to move particles 1 cm in 8 hr in shallow isokinetic gradients of sucrose (left ordinate). The curve was calculated for particles of 1.2 gm/cm^3, but differences for particles of 1.1 gm/cm^3 or 1.3 gm/cm^3 would be barely perceptible on this graph. To achieve an isopycnic separation in the same time interval one can arbitrarily assign a centrifugal field about 100 times greater (right ordinate). To select the swinging-bucket rotor capable of achieving a given separation, first locate the minimum centrifugal field on either ordinate corresponding to the particle density and sedimentation coefficient, then consult the column in Table 6.1 labeled g_{max}. Any rotor with at least this centrifugal field will suffice in most cases.

gradient material for isopycnic separations is more viscous than that of sucrose.

The performance and capacities of various swinging-bucket and zonal rotors are shown in Tables 6.1 and 6.2.

In general, I recommend that as a first step one try to estimate the isopycnic value of a particle by sedimenting the mixture in a swinging bucket using a step gradient with alternate steps tinted with about 0.2% Blue Dextran (Fig. 6.3). One may subsequently determine the ρ_{eq} more precisely and estimate the heterogeneity with respect to density by repeating the separation in a continuous gradient.

The choice of rotor depends principally on the quantity of the sample.

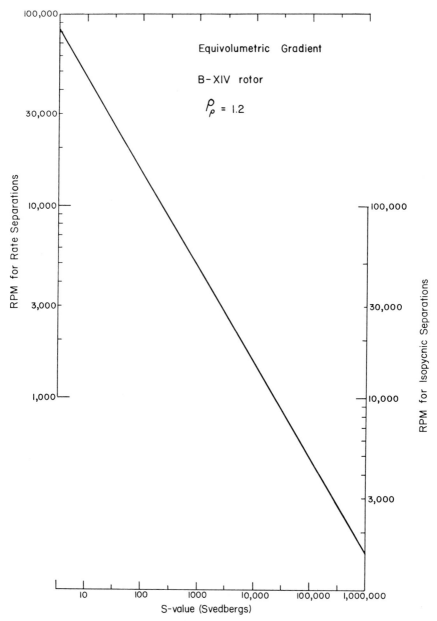

Fig. 6.2. Minimum rotor speed required to achieve separation of particles in a zonal rotor. The rotor speed in rpm required to move particles 100 cm^3 in 8 hr in an equivolumetric gradient (left ordinate) is illustrated. The curves were calculated for a particle density of 1.2 gm/cm^3 in the B-XIV rotor, but the curves for particles of 1.1–1.4 gm/cm^3 in other batch-type zonal rotors would be virtually indistinguishable on this scale. To achieve an isopycnic separation in the same interval one can arbitrarily assign a centrifugal field about 100 times greater (right ordinate). One can, of course, continue centrifugation for longer than 8 hr to achieve resolution at slower speeds.

Table 6.1. Characteristics of Some Swinging-Bucket Rotors Commonly Used for Density Gradient Centrifugation[a]

Manufacturer and type	Place × volume	Maximum speed rpm	Maximum speed rad²/sec²	g_{max}	r_{min} (cm)	r_{max} (cm)
Sorvall HL 8	8 × 100	3,700	1.50×10^5	3,720	14.5	24.5
	16 × 50	3,400	1.27×10^5	3,080	12.4	24.0
IEC 269	8 × 100	3,150	1.09×10^5	2,780	12.1	24.4
	8 × 50	4,100	1.84×10^5	3,720	10.5	19.8
IEC 253	12 × 50	3,000	1.27×10^5	2,400	13.4	22.7
	12 × 15	3,300	1.19×10^5	2,800	14.9	23.2
IEC SB-110	6 × 40	25,000	6.85×10^6	110,100	6.9	15.8
Sorvall AH-627	6 × 38.5	27,000	8.00×10^6	131,000	7.3	16.2
	6 × 17	27,000	8.00×10^6	135,000	6.5	16.7
Spinco SW 27	6 × 38.5	27,000	8.00×10^6	132,000	7.5	16.2
MSE 43127-106	3 × 70	23,500	6.06×10^6	100,000	6.4	16.2
Sorvall HB-4	4 × 50	13,000	1.85×10^6	27,500	4.7	14.6
Sorvall HS-4	4 × 50	7,000	5.30×10^5	9,343	6.1	16.5
Spinco DS-13	4 × 50	13,000	1.85×10^6	26,860	4	14.2
Spinco SW 25.2	3 × 60	25,000	6.85×10^6	106,900	6.7	15.4
IEC 940	4 × 40	12,000	1.58×10^6	20,800	4	12.9
Spinco 27.1	6 × 17	27,000	8.00×10^6	135,000	7.5	16.7
Spinco SW 25.1	3 × 34	25,000	6.85×10^6	90,000	5.6	13.0
MSE 43127-104	3 × 25	30,000	9.87×10^6	129,000	5.9	12.9
MSE 43127-501	6 × 16.5	25,000	6.85×10^6	110,000	6.1	15.8
MSE 43127-111	6 × 14	40,000	1.75×10^7	281,000	6.3	15.8
Spinco SW 40 Ti	6 × 14	40,000	1.75×10^7	285,000	6.7	16.0
Spinco SW 41 Ti	6 × 13	41,000	1.84×10^7	286,000	6.6	15.2
IEC SB-283	6 × 12	41,000	1.84×10^7	283,000	5.5	15.1
IEC SB:206	6 × 12	35,000	1.34×10^7	206,000	5.5	15.1
Spinco SW 36	4 × 13.5	36,000	1.42×10^7	193,000	5.8	13.4
Sorvall AH-650	6 × 5	50,000	2.74×10^7	300,000	5.7	10.8
Spinco SW 50.1	6 × 5	50,000	2.74×10^7	300,000	6	10.7
MSE 43127-115	6 × 5	56,000	3.44×10^7	404,000	5.6	11.6
IEC SB-405	6 × 4.2	60,000	3.95×10^7	405,900	??	10.1
Spinco SW 60 Ti	6 × 4.4	60,000	3.95×10^7	485,000	6.3	12.0
Spinco SW 56 Ti	6 × 4.4	56,000	3.44×10^7	408,000	6	11.7
MSE 43127-102	3 × 6.5	60,000	3.95×10^7	356,000	3.8	8.9
MSE 43127-103	3 × 5.5	40,000	1.75×10^7	178,000	4.8	9.9
Spinco SW 50L	3 × 5	50,000	2.74×10^7	274,000	4.8	9.9
Spinco SW 65 Ti	3 × 5	65,000	4.63×10^7	420,100	4.1	8.9
Spinco SW 65L Ti	3 × 5	65,000	4.63×10^7	420,000	3.8	8.9
MSE 43127-101	3 × 3	50,000	2.74×10^7	261,000	4.1	9.3

[a] Rotors stretch somewhat at high speed; Beckman–Spinco estimates that 0.58 mm is a reasonable approximation.

Table 6.2. Characteristics of Current, Batch-Type Zonal Rotors

Manufacturer and designation	Oak Ridge designation	Maximum speed rpm	Maximum speed ω^2	Core configuration	Gradient volume (cm^3)	Radius at edge (cm)	g_{max}	Special characteristics
IEC A-12	A-XII	4,600	2.32×10^5	center loading	1300	18	4,206	Transparent end caps, largest radius
MSE A	A-XII	5,000	2.74×10^5	center loading	1300	18	5,000	Transparent end caps, largest radius
IEC Z-8	—	8,000	7.02×10^5	center loading	1250	12	9,000	Transparent end caps, MACS option
				edge loading	1115	11	7,800	
MSE HS	—	10,000	1.10×10^6	center loading	695	10.3	11,400	Transparent end caps
Sorvall SZ-14	—	18,500	3.7×10^6	reorienting gradient	1373	9.5	36,424	Sample normally loaded while spinning, but unloaded at rest; gradient reorients slowly during deceleration
Spinco JCF-Z	—	20,000	4.39×10^6	center loading / reorienting gradient	1900 / 1700	8.9 / 8.9	40,000 / 40,000	Interchangeable cores
IEC B-29	B-XV	35,000	1.34×10^7	center loading	1670	8.9	121,100	MACS option
	B-XXIX	35,000	1.34×10^7	edge loading	1480	8.5	116,000	Sample may be loaded or unloaded at the center or the edge.
Christ B-XV	B-XV	30,000	9.87×10^6	center loading	1650	8.89	89,500	
MSE B-XV Ti	B-XV	35,000	1.34×10^7	center loading	1670	8.9	122,000	Dynamic seal remains in rotor
MSE B-XV A1	B-XV	25,000	6.85×10^6	center loading	1670	8.9	62,000	
MSE B-29	B-XXIX	25,000	6.85×10^6	edge loading	1430	7.6	52,800	
Spinco Ti 15	B-XV	32,000	1.12×10^7	center loading	1665	8.9	102,000	Interchangeable cores
	B-XXIX	32,000	1.12×10^7	edge loading	1350	8.4	95,600	Sample may be loaded or unloaded at the center or the edge

Spinco Al 15	B-XV	22,000	5.31×10^6	center loading	1675	8.9	48,100	Sample may be loaded or unloaded at the center or the edge
	B-XXIX	22,000	5.31×10^6	edge loading	1350	8.4	45,200	
Spinco B-4	B-IV	40,000	1.75×10^7	center loading	1750	4.9	86,000	Requires special L-4 drive unit MACS option
IEC B-30	B-XIV	50,000	2.74×10^7	center loading	659	6.7	186,500	
	—	50,000	2.74×10^7	edge loading	570	6.4	176,000	Sample may be loaded or unloaded at the center or the edge
Christ B-XIV	B-XIV	45,000	2.22×10^7	center loading	650	6.67	151,000	
MSE B-XIV Ti	B-XIV	47,000	2.42×10^7	center loading	650	6.7	165,000	Dynamic seal remains in rotor
MSE B-XIV Al	B-XIV	35,000	1.34×10^7	center loading	650	6.7	91,000	Interchangeable cores
Spinco Ti 14	B-XIV	48,000	2.53×10^7	center loading	665	6.7	172,000	
	—	48,000	2.53×10^7	edge loading	550	6.5	167,000	Sample may be loaded or unloaded at the center or the edge
Spinco Al 14	B-XIV	35,000	1.34×10^7	center loading	665	6.7	91,000	Sample may be loaded or unloaded at the center or the edge
	—	35,000	1.34×10^7	edge loading	544	6.4	87,000	
Spinco Z-60	—	60,000	3.95×10^7	center loading	330	6.35	256,000	Fastest zonal rotor
Electro-Nucleonics K-5	K-V	35,000	1.34×10^7	center loading	8390	6.6	90,000	Alternate core configuration of K-type continuous-flow centrifuge (see Table 6.4)
Electro-Nucleonics RK-5	—	35,000	1.34×10^7	center loading	4180	6.6	90,000	Alternate core configuration of RK-type continuous-flow centrifuge (see Table 6.4)

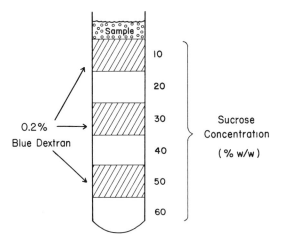

Fig. 6.3. Step gradients for locating approximate isopycnic values. A step gradient, in this case of sucrose, is prepared with alternate layers tinted with 0.2% w/v Blue Dextran. The positions of the various layers after centrifugation can be easily seen.

For rate separations one needs an absolute minimum of 1 cm³ of gradient per 1 mg of particles. Moreover, loads of this magnitude require special considerations and will fail under ordinary conditions (cf. Section 3.2.4); a safe load is 0.1 mg of particles per 1 cm³ of gradient.* We should remember that resolution usually decreases progressively with increasing loads starting at about 0.01 mg per 1 cm³ of gradient. On the other hand we should be wary of losing the particles in too vast a volume of gradient. For example, if 0.01 mg of ribosomes become spread homogeneously over 20 cm³ of gradient, the absorbance at 260 nm will be less than 0.01 and hence below the usual limit of detection. In general, for rate separations one should place the dividing line between swinging bucket and zonal rotors at about 20 mg.

The capacities of gradients in isopycnic separations is formally limited only by the physical displacement of the gradient by the particles (cf. Section 3.3.1), but such enormous quantities are normally recoverable only in continuous-flow with isopycnic banding methods, in which the initial particle suspensions are quite dilute. If initially dense suspensions are loaded into a swinging-bucket or zonal rotor, the resolution of isopycnic zones is often obscured by aggregation in one or more particle zones. Aggregation is particularly noticeable in swinging-bucket rotors because of the wall effect (q.v.). Nonetheless, one can load on the order of 10 mg of particles per 1 cm³ of gradient with some loss of resolution.

* Brakke (1964) reports that nonideal sedimentation limited the maximum concentration to 0.2 0.3 mg of plant viruses per 1 cm³.

I implied in the previous discussion that the choice between swinging-bucket and zonal rotors is simply a question of capacity; this is not completely true. Loading conventional zonal rotors involves passing the sample across a spinning seal. Special techniques are required to protect particles which are susceptible to shear, such as DNA (cf. Section 9.5.1), synaptosomes (cf. Section 9.3.4), and chloroplasts (cf. Section 9.3.2). These techniques include the use of extra-large channels in the seal or reorienting gradient methods (cf. Section 7.5). However, swinging buckets are especially sensitive to gradient overloading with its resultant droplet sedimentation. For this reason the resolution of micron-sized particles in rate separations in swinging buckets is noticeably inferior to that in zonal rotors (cf. the size resolution of cells, Section 9.2.3). Finally, vertical rotors have the advantage (and sometimes disadvantage) of a very short path length, combined with a relatively large volume.

The choice of continuous-flow rotors involves another set of questions, which are considered in a separate section (cf. Section 7.1). Suffice it to note here that continuous-flow or semibatch techniques may be advantageous for collecting particles from as little as 1 liter of sample.

6.1.2 Types of Separation: $s-\rho$ Methods

Few particles can be purified with a single slice through $s-\rho$ space (Fig. 1.7). The question is not whether s or ρ separations are preferable, but rather which should be done first.

If the sample is large and dilute, an isopycnic step should be employed first, because the particles can be concentrated in a small volume of the gradient. The partially purified particles can then be diluted (or diluted, sedimented, and resuspended) and recentrifuged in a rate separation. This sequence may be disadvantageous if the particles are sensitive to isopycnic sedimentation or to pelleting and resuspension.

The reverse sequence, with rate separation first is suitable enough if the sample is small (see Fig. 1.6), however, a crude cell brei is more likely to overload a gradient than an isopycnic "cut" of that brei. A distinct advantage of this sequence is that gradient fractions from a rate separation may be loaded directly over denser gradients for isopycnic separations.

If one is attempting a total subcellular fractionation, the $s-\rho$ sequence is preferable; the rate separation in a zonal rotor generates a large number of fractions, which then can be loaded onto isopycnic gradients in angle, vertical, or swinging-bucket rotors. Since, however, rate separations of larger particles are relatively unsuccessful in tubes, the reverse sequence requires multiple runs in zonal rotors, which would strain the logistics of the best organized of laboratories.

Another tactic in the purification of a single kind of particle is to employ continuous-flow harvest with isopycnic banding, which is in part an $s-\rho$ separation. If this is followed by a conventional rate separation, the overall purification strategy may be said to be $s-\rho-s$.

Brown *et al.* (1973) have proposed a sequential s system for total cell fractionation. A cell brei is loaded onto an equivolumetric gradient in an edge-loading zonal rotor and centrifuged for an $\int \omega^2 \, dt$ calculated to drive particles with a range of s^* values (say, 1,000,000–500,000 S) into a distal segment of the gradient. The rotor is slowed, the distal segment unloaded from the edge and replaced with a fresh segment of gradient. Centrifugation is continued for another interval to drive the next slower fraction of particles into the distal segment, the fraction unloaded, and the segment of gradient replaced as before. The process can be continued until the very slowest particles are driven clear of the sample zone and then the entire gradient unloaded. The advantage of Brown's procedure is that one can obtain fractions representing a very wide range of particle sizes in a single separation (cf. Section 9.3.3).

Even if different kinds of particles have overlapping ρ and s values, there is yet another card to play: *density perturbation* (Ryan and Headon, 1979). Many particles will specifically absorb certain materials in quantities sufficient to alter their densities. For example, the densities of lysosomes from rats fed Triton WR-1339 are substantially less than those from normal rats (Leighton *et al.*, 1968) and the density of mitochrondria incubated with the artificial electron acceptor, iodonitrotetrazolium, becomes greater from the accumulation of insoluble formazan (Headon *et al.*, 1978). A different type of density perturbation can occur in isopycnic sedimentation in silica sols (St. Onge and Price, 1975; Morgenthaler and Price, 1976). Addition of certain polymers to the sols causes the ρ_{eq} of a variety of particles to shift to either lower or higher densities. Although the cause of these density shifts is not known, they appear to involve interactions between the surface of the particle, the silica sol, and the polymer.

6.1.3   Choice of Gradient: Material and Shape

Chapter 5 was devoted to the characteristics of different gradient materials. Although sucrose is chosen more than nine times out of ten, we should be sure that it is in fact the best choice. Silica sols or one of the other polymers may be preferable over sucrose for the membrane-bound organelles. Buffer, salts, an osmoticum, and protective reagents if added, should be included throughout the gradient. Since gradients are commonly prepared by mixing a starting solution with a limiting solution, it is normally sufficient to test the integrity of the particles in these two extremes.

The choice of gradient shape depends on the kind of separation and the relative quantity of sample. Linear gradients are easily the simplest shapes for isopycnic separations and have no obvious disadvantages. The slope of the gradient will determine the resolution in part (Fig. 3.29).

Small quantities of particles (< 0.1 mg per 1 ml of gradient) can be safely managed on those gradient shapes designed for high resolution (cf. Section 3.2.3) (isokinetic and acceleration gradients in swinging-bucket rotors; equivolumetric and isometric in zonal rotors). Hyperbolic gradients in zonal rotors should be used for larger quantities (cf. Section 3.2.4). To my knowledge, no high-capacity gradient shape has been tested in the tube geometry of swinging-bucket rotors.

Although one can certainly imagine tailored gradients to resolve optimally specific mixtures of particles, I know of no specific advantage for other gradient shapes that have been tried in zonal rotors. Gradients that are linear with radius, however, have relatively good capacity and span a wide range of sedimentation rates. The use of step gradients (Cline and Ryel, 1971) remains experimental.

6.1.4 Size and Shape of Sample Zone

In the foregoing discussions, gradient capacity was mentioned in terms of the mass of particles per unit volume of gradient. Attention is now focused on the volume in which the sample should be contained, and where the particles should be with respect to the gradient.

In an isopycnic separation the sample volume may occupy 80% of the rotor volume or more (cf. Fig. 3.37); the final position of the particles within the gradient is usually quite indifferent to the route or distance they might have to travel. However, the practice of incorporating the sample throughout the gradient (i.e., using the entire rotor volume for gradient and sample) can be disadvantageous if there are contaminating small particles, such as soluble micromolecules of the cell, which would not move to their equilibrium positions during the course of centrifugation.

In continuous-flow (cf. Section 7.1) and semibatch operations (cf. Section 7.4) the sample volume may be indefinitely large.

In rate separations the sample volume is much more critical. Imagine two different volumes of sample in isokinetic gradients. The widths of the particle zones increase only slightly as the particles sediment into the gradient and remain approximately proportional to the initial widths of the sample zones. It follows that resolution, defined as the distance between the zones divided by the width of the zones, must decrease with the increasing volume of the sample zone.

The upper limiting volume of the sample zone is quite simply related to the poorest resolution that one is prepared to accept. The lower limit of sample volume is related to the static resolution and anomalous zone broadening of the system (cf. Section 3.2.4).

We (Price and Kovacs, 1969) determined the static resolution of a variety of zonal rotors and found that the lowest useful limit of sample volume is about 5 cm³. After centrifugation, particle zones can be recovered with dispersions (σ-values) of as little as 10 cm³.

I should emphasize that although these high levels of resolution may be obtained repeatedly, they are dependent on the system employed, including such variables as tubing diameter or laminar or plug flow. If resolution is an important consideration, one must pay fastidious attention to all of the elements in the gradient system.

It is not possible to concentrate particle concentration indefinitely in order to shrink sample volumes to the critical lower limit. As discussed in Section 3.2.4, instabilities occur at particle concentrations above some limit, which is a complex function of the size of the particles and the nature of the gradient material. In general inverse sample gradients should be used above about 5 mg/ml. The largest reported total load in a zonal rotor, achieved with an inverse sample gradient over a Berman gradient, corresponded to about 60% of the static capacity of the inverse sample gradient (Eikenberry *et al.*, 1970).

6.1.5 Length of Run: The Question of Speed

The time required to complete a rate separation can be computed directly from the sedimentation coefficient of the fastest moving particle and the properties of the gradient. From Eq. (3.18a) we can calculate the time required to move the distance from the sample zone (r_1) to the bottom of the gradient (r_2)

$$\Delta t = \frac{\rho_p - \rho_w}{s^* \eta_w} \int_{r_1}^{r_2} \frac{\eta_m(r)}{r\omega^2 [\rho_p - \rho_m(r)]} dr$$

For gradients of arbitrary shapes Eq. (3.18a) can be evaluated only numerically and preferably by computer. However, the repeatability of any given separation can be assured by centrifuging for a constant value of $\int \omega^2 dt$. For isokinetic and equivolumetric gradients, one obtains much simpler relations. The $\int \omega^2 dt$ required to move the fastest particle to the end of an isokinetic gradient is

$$\int \omega^2 dt = \Delta r/K_r s^* \tag{6.1}$$

where Δr is the length of the gradient, K_r the isokinetic gradient constant, and s^* the equivalent sedimentation coefficient. At constant angular velocity [Eq. (3.18b)]

$$\Delta t = \Delta r/K_r s^* \omega^2$$

In the case of equivolumetric gradients the corresponding equations are

$$\int \omega^2 dt = \Delta r/K_v s^* \tag{6.2}$$

or at constant angular velocity [Eq. (3.21)]

$$\Delta t = \Delta V/K_v s^* \omega^2$$

For long centrifugations we may choose to assume constant velocity. For short runs, where the times of acceleration t_a and deceleration t_d contribute significantly to the integral, we may approximate it by Eq. (6.3) (cf. Fig. 6.4).

$$\int \omega^2 dt \cong [\Delta t + (\Delta t_a + \Delta t_d)/2]\omega_{max}^2 \tag{6.3}$$

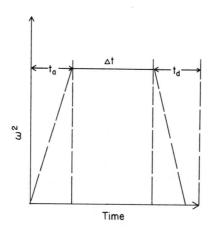

Fig. 6.4. Approximation of $\int \omega^2 dt$ in the absence of a direct means for recording the rotor speed during acceleration t_a and deceleration t_d, one may approximate the actual curve by assuming that ω^2 is linear with time during acceleration and deceleration. The value of $\int \omega^2 dt$ is then computed from Eq. 6.3.

A number of workers have noted that the speed of preparative centrifuges can vary substantially over a long run, resulting in much larger variations in the rpm^2 or ω^2. Even larger variations can occur when the speed control is set at supposedly identical values in successive runs.* Finally, analog speed indicators are inherently rather inaccurate. In order to obtain accurate values of the $\int \omega^2 \, dt$ and acceptable repeatability of rate separations, many investigators have turned to meters that compute and record the $\int \omega^2 \, dt$ from direct, digital measurements of the speed of the rotor.† Measurement of the $\int \omega^2 \, dt$ is also obtained as a dividend from the microprocessor-controlled systems of current centrifuges such as the Beckman L8.

In the case of isopycnic separations we are dealing with an *approach to equilibrium*. A rule of thumb is that the $\int \omega^2 \, dt$ for isopycnic separations should be 100 times greater than that for a comparable rate separation. This value should be compared with separations obtained at half and twice the $\int \omega^2 \, dt$ to ensure that the particles are in substantial equilibrium with the gradient.

All of the foregoing imply that the extent of sedimentation is determined by the $\int \omega^2 \, dt$, rather than time or speed. Thus 8000 rpm for 30 min yields the same $\int \omega^2 \, dt$ ($= 1.2628 \times 10^9$ radians^2/sec) as 2000 rpm for 8 hr (Appendix A). This implication is not always true. As a number of investigators have noted, certain particles are susceptible to high centrifugal fields. Wattiaux and Wattiaux-De Coninck (1970) found that mitochondrial fractions distribute themselves quite differently when banded at 50,000 rpm as compared to those banded at 39,000 rpm, and that the differences can be attributed to irreversible disruption of mitochondria by the higher hydrostatic pressure. Infante and Baierlein (1971) report analogous but reversible changes in the sedimentation behavior of ribosomes attributable to a dissociation into subunits under the influence of hydrostatic pressure. Simple prudence dictates that separations be compared at different speeds but constant $\int \omega^2 \, dt$.

The following section gives how-to-do-it accounts of swinging-bucket and zonal separations. Since successful procedures vary substantially from one laboratory to another, any specific protocol must be regarded as one among many equally valid alternatives.

6.2 SWINGING-BUCKET SEPARATIONS

6.2.1 Choice of Rotor

Since all commercial swinging-bucket rotors have substantially the same geometry, the principal consideration is one of volume and speed (cf. Table

6.1; Fig. 6.5 and 6.6). A few years ago there were real differences in path length and in the numbers of tubes per rotor (3–6) from manufacturer to manufacturer, but today the primary distinctions concern the ease of attachment and removal of the tubes from the rotors. Although advances in metallurgy and improved engineering design may produce yet another leap in the speeds of swinging buckets, the wise scientist will reserve judgment,

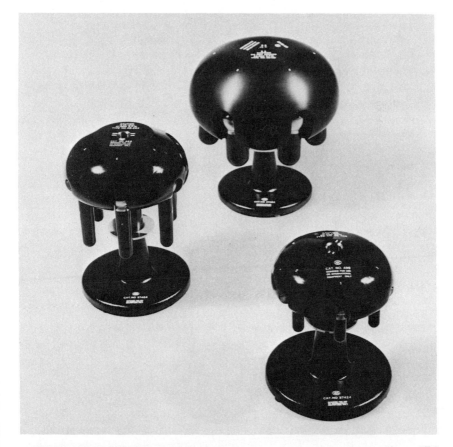

Fig. 6.5. Three principal sizes of swinging-bucket rotors used in ultracentrifuges (IEC Division/Damon Instruments). The SB-110 (top), SB-283 (left), and SB-405 (bottom right) are typical of the six equal place, swinging-bucket rotors covering the range from 25,000 to 60,000 rpm (cf. Table 6.1).

---

* It would be helpful if centrifuge manufacturers employed digital speed controls or rheostats with detentes at integral speeds.

† Such meters are available at considerable expense from centrifuge manufacturers.

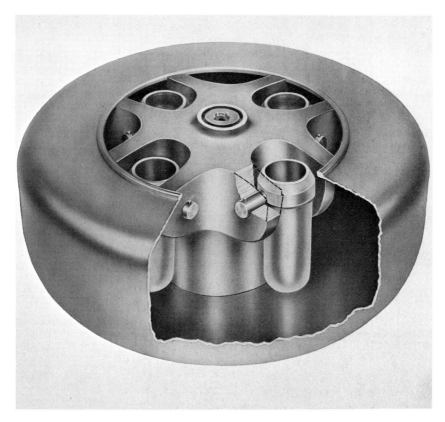

Fig. 6.6.   A wind-shielded, swinging-bucket rotor for use in air (DuPont Instruments/ Sorvall). The HB-4 rotor will spin four 50-cm^3 tubes at 13,000 rpm (cf. Table 6.1).

recalling that some earlier leaders in the "g-race" were permanently derated after a time when it was discovered that design speeds could not be maintained in practice.

If a small loss in resolution can be tolerated, the time required for separations may be greatly decreased by using only the bottom portion of the rotor tube (Griffith, 1978). For example, similar separations of serum proteins were obtained in a SW 65-Ti rotor in 5 hr using a 2.0-ml gradient and in 14 hr using the full volume of the tube.

6.2.2   Preparation of Loading of Gradients

Simple two-cylinder (Fig. 5.4) or exponential generators (Fig. 5.6) are usually quite suitable for the preparation of gradients for swinging-bucket tubes. It is usually advantageous to prepare six or more gradients simultaneously by splitting a larger gradient with a proportioning pump (Fig. 5.4a). The tubes may be cooled in an ice bath or cold room* and the gradients are stable for several hours.

It is especially important to prechill ultracentrifuge rotors and tube holders, since heat transfer is very slow in a vacuum.

6.2.3 Sample Preparation and Loading

Examine a drop of the sample under the microscope to ensure that the particles flow freely. The suspension should be free of clots and aggregates, or else the gradient will become contaminated with small molecules and other particles thrown off by rapidly sedimenting clumps so that the observed distribution of particles or activities will be misleading.

Observe the limits of particle concentration in the sample (cf. Sections 3.2.4 and 3.3.1). If overloading is suspected, decrease the amount of sample or compare separations with rectangular and wedge-shaped sample zones.

Check that the density of the sample does not exceed that of the top of the gradient. This can be done by allowing small drops of the sample to fall into a small volume of the starting solution in a test tube. Dilute the sample, if necessary. It is convenient, especially at first, to add about 0.2% Blue Dextran to the sample to make it visible. The resulting blue zone in the gradient marks the approximate position and width of the sample zone.†

Load the sample onto the gradient with a bent pipet (Fig. 6.7) to avoid disturbing the gradient. Make sure that tubes opposite one another are balanced according to the manufacturer's instructions‡ and start the centrifugation without delay to avoid droplet sedimentation. If not yet ready to accelerate to the operating speed, let the rotor run at a few thousand rpm.

6.2.4 Importance of Vacuum

A rotor in air tends to heat up because of "windage," that is, the friction of air on the rotor surface. Preparative centrifuges may be designed to operate at speeds up to approximately 20,000 rpm by providing powerful refrigerating systems. Much above 20,000 rpm, it becomes prohibitive to fight windage with increased refrigeration.

---

* It is worthwhile noting the actual temperature of liquids in cold rooms; certain reactions are much different at 5°C or 10°C than at 0°C.

† Blue Dextran (Pharmacia Fine Chemicals) has a mean particle weight of 200,000 μm and will sediment noticeably after approximately 10^{11} radians^2/seconds^1.

‡ The manufacturer may specify that all of the tubes be filled and attached, regardless of the number of actual samples, in order to avoid uneven stress on the rotor.

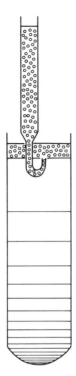

Fig. 6.7.   Use of a bent pipet for loading samples in swinging-bucket rotors. The underlying gradient is minimally disturbed if the sample is allowed to flow through a pipette with a U-shaped bend at the tip.

An ultracentrifuge, by definition, drives rotors in a vacuum chamber, so that windage is minimized; in a high vacuum the only sources of heat to the rotor are by radiation and that conducted by the drive shaft. As a consequence, the refrigerating systems of ultracentrifuges are usually light-duty machines of modest capacity. They are sufficient to chill the chamber at rest and to absorb the heat that enters the system radiatively and conductively.

If the vacuum should degrade, such as through contamination of the vacuum pump with water, the temperature of the rotor will rise uncontrollably. I have seen tubes emerge from an ultracentrifuge whose refrigerating system was operating perfectly with the plastic melted and the water boiled away. Moreover, temperature indicators of ultracentrifuges are often designed to operate by infrared sensing of the rotor surface. As little as 200 μ of air or water vapor in the chamber may so distort the reading that the temperature indicator may give a false reading and quite fail to warn of the disastrous *Wärmetod* taking place inside.

Therefore, the vacuum system of an ultracentrifuge should be checked weekly. No swinging-bucket runs should be attempted at any speed without an acceptable vacuum and no high-speed run (>40,000 rpm) should be attempted without an acceptable diffusion pump.

Note further that the properties of the gradient (especially the viscosity) are highly sensitive to temperature; so that a poor vacuum means poor repeatability of rate sedimentations.

6.2.5   To Brake or Not to Brake

At the end of a run, a decision must be made whether to decelerate a swinging-bucket or zonal rotor with the brake of the drive unit engaged or allow it to coast to rest. There are proponents of both procedures, but relatively little hard data are available. The physical problem is reasonably complicated: during deceleration, the angular momentum of the fluid must be transferred through the walls or septa of the rotor to the shaft. This transfer of momentum tends to distort isodense surfaces such that the meniscus tries to climb the surface of the leading tube wall or septum. This movement is opposed by the density gradient itself multiplied by the centrifugal field. Faster deceleration, as in braking, will of course increase the perturbing forces.

Equally good separations have been reported with and without the brake, but one may wish to test for a possible effect of braking if one requires optimum resolution from an extremely shallow gradient.

Much more evident is the commonly observed tendency of gradients to swirl during reorientation from the horizontal to the vertical position (cf. Section 6.5), which occurs between several hundred rpm and zero. The villain in this piece is the Coriolis force. The angular momentum ($L = \omega \bar{r} \bar{m}$) of the tubes spinning horizontally is rather rapidly decreased as the radius of the center of mass ($\bar{r}$) abruptly decreases during reorientation. The angular momentum of the fluid about the axis of the rotor tends to be converted into angular momentum about the axis of the tube (Fig. 6.8). Unfortunately this occurs when the stabilizing centrifugal forces are minimal. The concensus is that reorientation should be made to occur slowly.

A further approach to the problem of deceleration is the use of a double-gimbaled support for the tubes as in the high-speed rotor, formally available from Sorvall, or Leif's experimental XYZ 40 rotor (Leif *et al.*, 1972). In this design the tubes can swing in planes both parallel and perpendicular to the axis of rotation. Although this design eliminates the first source of perturba-

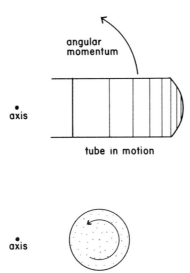

Fig. 6.8.   Transfer of angular momentum during reorientation of swinging bucket. During centrifugation (upper figure) the angular momentum is transverse to the axis of the centrifuge tube. As the bucket slows to a stop and becomes vertical (lower figure) some of the angular momentum is converted into swirling about the axis of the tube.

tion in deceleration, it introduces severe stress limitations and does not solve the problem of Coriolis mixing. Moreover, the extremely slow rate of deceleration required poses problems of programmed speed control and greatly lengthened time of centrifugation.

Low-Speed Criticals

All rotor-drive combinations have critical or resonant frequencies where the shafts tend to flex or wobble. These frequencies are determined by the mass, length, and stiffness of the rotating system, its bearings, supports, etc. In the flexible shafts of modern centrifuges, the designer has chosen to let the critical frequencies occur at low speed, where they are not dangerous. To an observer outside the centrifuge, the rather wild gyrations of the larger swinging-bucket rotors between zero and several hundred rpm can be disconcerting. The process occurs during both acceleration and deceleration. However, an observer on the rotor would not experience any unusual motion; rather, he would find that his surroundings were gyrating rather wildly. Therefore, one may balance the tubes with reasonable care and safely leave the question of low-speed criticals to the centrifuge designer.*

6.2.6   Holding Mode and Measurement of $\int \omega^2 \, dt$

Whatever the best method is of bringing a swinging-busket rotor to rest, we can agree that the tubes should not remain at rest in the centrifuge any longer than necessary. Temperature control under static conditions is poor at best; freezing lurks as a danger in many machines. Moreover, the intermittant starting and stopping of the compressor may send vibrations through the drive shaft to the waiting gradients. It is far better to plan an overnight run at reduced speed than to schedule the rotor to remain at rest in the centrifuge from midnight until morning.

Some ultracentrifuges come today with a "holding mode" option. Under "holding mode" the centrifuge is programmed to decelerate after a given interval of time or $\int \omega^2 \, dt$ not to zero, but to some preset low speed, such as 1000 rpm. At this low speed the gradients will "keep" better than at rest, since the centrifugal field continues to stabilize against perturbing forces, the temperature control of the centrifuge chamber remains efficient, and yet the positions of the separated particles remain essentially unaffected by the low speed. The operator may subsequently terminate the run at a convenient time and under a final deceleration schedule under his personal control.

6.2.7   Care of Gradients after a Run

After the centrifugation is completed, the gradients need not be treated as if they contained nitroglycerine, but resolution can be lost from vibrations, convection, and generally sloppy technique outside the centrifuge. Particle zones kept at constant temperature (usually in ice) and free from vibrations will normally show little visible deterioration over a few hours and may be returned to the centrifuge for further centrifugation, if desired. One should avoid carrying gradients down the hall or to another floor. Many workers insist that the gradient fractionating device be immediately adjacent to the centrifuge.

It is obvious that the gradients should be fractionated promptly, but the consequences of delay should be discussed. Excluding vibration and convection, we can consider how much zone broadening will occur with time through diffusion. The data of Figure 6.9 were calculated for particles with diffusion coefficients of approximately 10 Ficks (e.g., proteins of 10–15,000

---

* An early Spinco centrifuge had a stabilizing disk which automatically engaged an upper bearing to the swinging-bucket rotor below about 2000 rpm; this changed the critical frequency of the system from one below 2000 rpm to one above 2000 rpm. The rotor therefore never experienced a critical frequency.

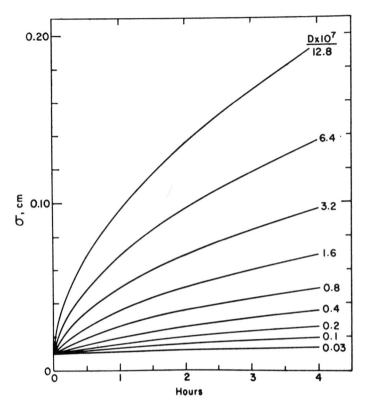

Fig. 6.9. Diffusion of particle zones with time (Vinograd and Bruner, 1966). The model employed for these calculations was a thin layer of macromolecules diffusing into an underlying solution of greater density in a slowly spinning analytical ultracentrifuge. The calculations apply equally to zones in a swinging-bucket rotor after separation but with the rotor at rest or spinning at low speed. The graph shows the σ-value of the particle distribution with respect to radius for particles with different diffusion coefficients, expressed in Ficks ($7-10$ cm^2/sec^2). The initial σ-value is 0.01 cm.

μm) ranging down to 0.1 Fick (e.g., T4 DNA). They show that if one expected knife-edge resolution (<0.1-mm zones), one had better complete the analysis within minutes, but if the zones are already on the order of 1-cm width, a delay of even a few hours is not serious for most particles.

The diffusion of particle zones in zonal rotors can be used to measure diffusion coefficients (Halsall and Schumaker, 1970) and is particularly advantageous when dealing with small amounts of material.

6.2.8   Recovery of the Gradient

Everything in density gradient centrifugation seems to be divided between two schools of thought; recovery of gradients is hardly an exception. Approximately half the research population displaces the gradient by puncturing the tube at the bottom and draining the contents, usually by displacement with a lighter liquid (Fig. 6.10); the other half displaces the gradient from the top (Fig. 6.11).

Noll (1969) has argued the virtues of bottom drainage eloquently. They include (1) generally shorter tubing connectors, (2) no density inversions, (3) a more "natural" geometry, and (4) less contamination of particulate samples with the soluble (i.e., nonsedimenting) components of the sample. He points out that added radioactively labeled species, such as amino acids, are usually small molecules and therefore nonsedimenting. Since their radioactivity may be 100 times greater than those of particles into which they become incorporated, it is clearly preferable that these not contaminate the tubing and flow-cell of the analytical system before the particles, as they would if the gradient is recovered light-end first.

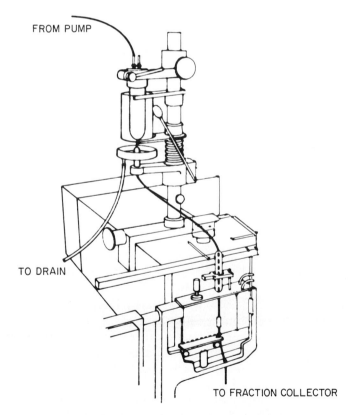

FROM PUMP

TO DRAIN

TO FRACTION COLLECTOR

Fig. 6.10. Recovery of gradients from tubes by downward displacement (Noll, 1969). The tube is punctured from below and displaced by pumping water or a light fluid from above. The gradient is led through a flow spectrophotometer to a fraction collector.

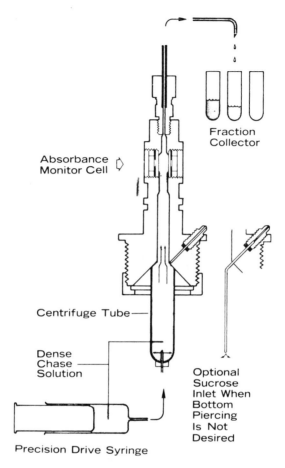

Fraction
Collector

Absorbance
Monitor Cell

Centrifuge Tube —

Dense
Chase
Solution

Optional
Sucrose
Inlet When
Bottom
Piercing
Is Not
Desired

Precision Drive Syringe

Fig. 6.11.   Recovery of gradients from tubes by upward displacement (ISCO). In Brakke's (1963) device a dense solution is introduced into the bottom of the tube. The gradient is displaced upward through a flow photometer. The flow path remains very wide up to the photometer to avoid distortions due to laminar flow.

On the other hand the lines of flow around a needle at the base of a tube are complex and, especially in the case of viscous fluids, are bound to produce some mixing across isodense surfaces. Furthermore, solids collected at the bottom of a tube may contaminate the displaced gradient in an unpredictable manner. It is also much easier to design an efficient funnel to collect the gradient at the top of a tube as in Fig. 6.11.

Two of the commercially available systems for recovering gradients are shown in Figs. 6.12 and 6.13.

Apart from top versus bottom collection, there are several other important

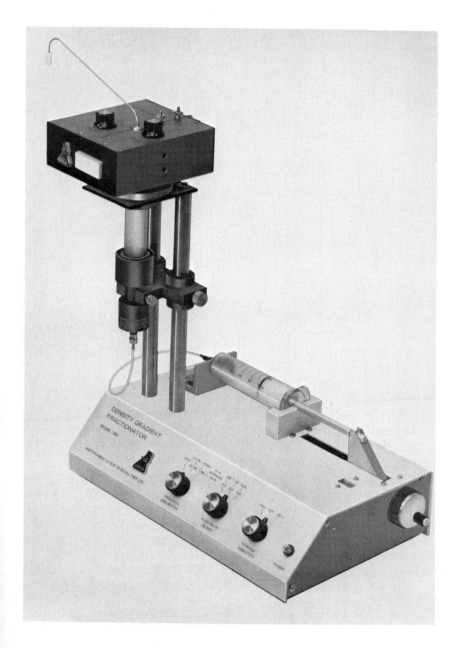

Fig. 6.12. Tube puncturing and gradient monitoring systems (ISCO). This is the commercial version of the apparatus shown in Fig. 6.11. The gradient is displaced upward by pumping a cushion fluid into the bottom of the tube. The gradient passes through a flow photometer at the top.

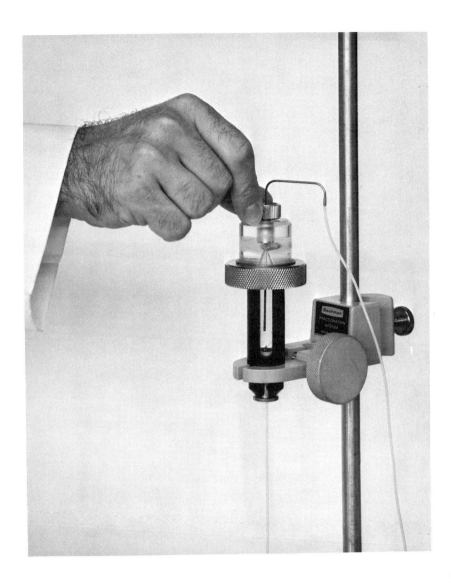

Fig. 6.13. Another tube puncturing and gradient monitoring system (Spinco Division/ Beckman Instruments). The principle is similar to that of Figs. 6.11 and 6.12, except that the gradient is displaced through a narrow bore tube before reaching a photometer (not shown).

considerations. The cross section of tubing and flow cells should be constant and free from discontinuities. One may easily demonstrate the loss of resolution in eddy currents by pumping a clear solution followed by a colored solution of a different density through the junction of two pieces of PVC tubing of different diameter (Fig. 6.14).

When a gradient is led through thin tubing the restorative forces of the density gradient are reduced to negligible proportions; the fluid then moves by laminar flow, meaning that a velocity gradient extends across the diameter of the tube from near zero at the walls to a maximum at the center (Fig. 6.15). The shape of this velocity gradient is parabolic. A zone moving through the tube will therefore be distorted. J. E. Joyce (personal communication) has calculated that the loss of resolution, while obviously a function of both diameter and length, is very nearly proportional to the volume of the tube.

Although an inference from Joyce's calculations should be that connective tubing should be as narrow as possible, Brakke (1963) has described a successful photometric scanning system that employs bulk flow through a very wide channel, which minimizes laminar flow (cf. Fig. 6.11). Brakke and Van Pelt (1968) report that the gradient can be displaced through a scanning chamber and returned to the tube repeatedly with little loss in resolution.

Jolley *et al.* (1967) describe a novel procedure for recovering the gradient as a solid plug: riboflavin and the components of acrylamide gel are in-

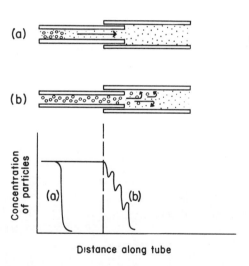

Fig. 6.14. Turbulent flow across a discontinuity. When a colored solution flows from tubing of a smaller to a larger diameter, eddy currents invariably destroy any sharp boundaries that might be present initially. In (a) a zone of particles is moving along a tube: in (b) the particle front has passed a discontinuity resulting from an increase in the size of the tubing. The lower figure shows that concentration profile resulting from eddy currents.

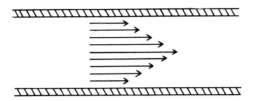

Fig. 6.15. Laminar flow in tubing. In laminar (nonturbulent) flow, fluid that is immediately adjacent to the wall moves with zero velocity, while that in the center moves with a maximum velocity.

corporated into the gradient and photopolymerized after the run. The gel may then be sliced, stained (cf. also Khandjian, 1977), or used for immunodiffusion (Quinn and Fernando, 1977).

6.2.9   Gradient Monitoring Devices

The usual object in analyzing gradients is to obtain one or more "profiles" of absorbance, enzyme activity, radioactivity, etc. Optical flow cells are commonly available for continuous recording absorbance, typically at 254, 260, or 280 nm. The principal concern with these, as noted immediately previously, is that they not compromise resolution.

Although serially arranged flow detectors would be much more efficient, existing technology largely restricts one to discrete measurements on collected fractions. Noll (1969) has described an ingenious automatic fraction collector that also processes samples for scintillometry.

We frequently need to know the parameters of the actual gradient as recovered from the rotor. This is usually achieved by refractometry* or pycnometry, as described in Section 5.4.

The size of swinging buckets limits the number of analyses that can be performed on gradient fractions, but where multiple enzyme or chemical assays are required, some sort of automatic procedure is highly desirable. With Technicon-types of segmented, continuous-flow analyzers, which are widely available in most laboratories, one should be careful that separation between adjacent samples is sufficient to preserve the original resolution. The GeMSAEC fast analyzers (Anderson, 1969) are more suitable for measurements of enzyme velocity and may be directly interfaced with automated data processing.

---

* Appendix C lists the refractive indices of gradient materials.

6.2.10 Swinging-Bucket Rotors as Analytical Instruments

When we speak of an "analytical ultracentrifuge," we mean a centrifuge where the sedimenting sample may be observed continuously (cf. Chapter 8). Any serious measure of sedimentation coefficients must be done in an analytical ultracentrifuge, but it is possible to obtain rough estimates of sedimentation coefficients from rate–zonal separations in either swinging-bucket or zonal rotors (cf. Section 7.7).

Such measurements are inherently inaccurate for several reasons: (1) sedimentation coefficients are estimated from the difference between initial and final positions of the particle, neither of which can be determined with great precision, or from the relative position of a sample and a marker; (2) the particles of interest can and probably do change their size and density during their passage through the gradient; and (3) the temperature can not be determined with great precision.

Isokinetic gradients (cf. Section 3.2.3) are easily the gradient shapes of choice for estimating sedimentation coefficients in swinging-bucket rotors. Since the distance a particle moves is proportional to time and centrifugal field or, more precisely the $\int r\omega^2 \, dt$ (cf. Figs. 3.12 and 3.13), one can estimate the sedimentation coefficient directly by measuring the distance migrated and plugging into Eqs. (3.17a) or (3.17b). A rearrangement of (3.17b) is

$$S^* = \Delta r / K_r \omega^2 \, \Delta t$$

The actual determination of Δr, which is the difference between the initial and final position of the particle, is somewhat complicated. A simple way is to fill the tube with known increments of fluid volume and measure the heights of the meniscus above the bottom of the tube. A graph of these values gives a straight line except near the bottom of the tube. The starting position is determined from the volume of the gradient plus that of the original sample. The final position is usually determined by displacing the gradient from the tube through a recording photometer. The position of a given particle may also be determined by collecting fractions and testing the fractions for enzymatic activity, radioactivity, etc.

Perhaps the simplest way of estimating sedimentation coefficients in isokinetic gradients is to use internal or external markers: particles of known sedimentation coefficients included with the sample or in other centrifuge tubes and run at the same time. Ideally, one would like to bracket an unknown particle between two markers. Indeed the closer a marker is to an unknown the less critical is the shape of the gradient. The ultimate marker is a radioactive sample which may coincide exactly with an unknown and still be detected. In this case the shape of the gradient is irrelevant to the determination of s.

The advantages of markers are obvious: sedimentation coefficients can simply be read off from a linear graph (cf. Fig. 3.12), but the inclusion of markers in the same tube may obscure the unknown particle unless the particles and the unknown are detected independently, as was noted before for radioactive labels.

Some additional considerations in estimating sedimentation coefficients from rate–zonal runs are

(1) The best temperature is 4°C, since the variation of density with fluctuations in rotor temperature is least at the point of maximum density.

(2) One should use the smallest amounts of sample consistent with detection in order to optimize resolution and minimize errors due to particle–particle interactions.

(3) The ionic strength should be kept low to avoid perturbing the physical constants of sucrose (density and viscosity) on which the isokinetic gradient is based.

Given the many analyses that can be performed with extremely small amounts of material, it follows that analytical separations in swinging-bucket rotors can serve a wide variety of purposes. The simplicity of swinging buckets and the advantages of multiple samples recommend them over zonal rotors for all but large preparative operations.

6.3 ZONAL SEPARATIONS

6.3.1 Choice of Rotor

The neophyte is presented with a bewildering set of designations for zonal rotors: B-IV, Ti-14, A-XII, B-29, RK-3, etc., sound as much like fantastic armaments of war as laboratory instruments. A brief look at the history of zonal centrifugation should clarify the picture.

In the development of zonal centrifugation at the Oak Ridge National Laboratories each rotor design was assigned a binomial consisting of a letter and a roman numeral. The A-series of rotors were to operate in centrifuges without benefit of vacuum*; B-series rotors were for ultracentrifuges; and

---

* Until the invention of the removable seal, the problems of designing zonal rotors for ultracentrifuge operations were substantially more complicated than for ordinary centrifuges; since the seal assembly had to hold a high vacuum and be free of critical frequencies over a very wide range.

the K-series were large machines for industrial-scale applications. The roman numerals were simply sequential and bore no hint of the function or characteristics of the rotor. Moreover, the smallest modification in the design would merit a new number; thus A-V, A-IX, A-XII marked one sequence of rotor development and B-VIII, B-IX, B-XVI another. Some current commercial versions of Oak Ridge rotors are shown in Figs. 5.8A and 6.16. A complete list of the Oak Ridge designations is presented in Appendix E.

When rotor designs were released to the public, the centrifuge manufacturers first reproduced the Oak Ridge instruments more or less exactly, but as the design of rotors evolved it was quite natural for the companies to issue their own designations (Table 6.2). At Spinco, for example, the popular B-XIV became the Al-14 or Ti-14 depending on whether it was fabricated of aluminum or titanium. More recently, the centrifuge manufacturers have developed new designs that do not correspond to any Oak Ridge rotor, such as the SZ-14 of Sorvall and the Z-60 of Spinco.

I proposed a system in which the volume and speed of the rotor shell were expressed in a binomial representing volume and centrifugal field (Price, 1972); thus, the Ti-14 becomes a 655-48. The response to this scheme has been less than deafening. Nonetheless, the notion of the rotor shell is not a bad place from which to consider the choice of zonal rotors. One may

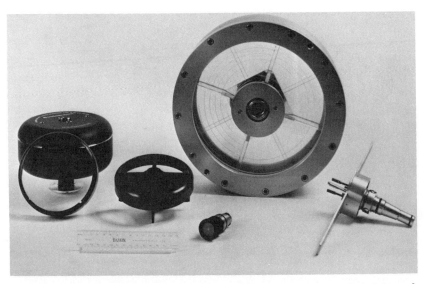

Fig. 6.16. B30A and Z-15 zonal rotors (Damon/IEC Division). The B30A (*left*) is a commercial version of the B-XXX, differing principally in the seal assembly. The Z-15 (*right*), a transparent rotor, is a descendent of the A-XII, and has in turn been modified in the Z-8 (Table 6.2).

consult Fig. 6.2 for the minimum speed needed to separate the particles of interest, then compare the column labeled g_{min} in Table 6.2 to identify the zonal rotors which may be competent for the task. The next consideration is Volume: B-XIV and B-XV types may both be suitable for the separation of a virus, but the B-XV has three times the volume of a B-XIV. I suggest trying the smaller rotor first, unless the size of sample clearly dictates otherwise (cf. Section 6.1.1). In fact, we find that the B-XIV type of rotor is easily the most popular in the laboratory because of convenience in handling, even when its high speed is not needed.

If the physical properties of the particles to be separated are known, it is possible to predict the resolution and shapes of particle zones by computer simulation (Sartory *et al.*, 1976; Steensgard and Møller, 1979).

6.3.2 Some General Considerations in Operating Zonal Rotors

In Chapter 3 it was suggested that it was a mistake to regard zonal rotors as overgrown swinging buckets, that the motion of particles in polar coordinates carried a new set of implications for optimizing resolution and capacity. Similarly the practical operation of zonal rotors calls for special techniques and offers special opportunities. The sets of procedures described here are among many acceptable variations.

One should have a supply of at least 10 m each of telescoping sizes of PVC tubing (e.g., Tygon S50 HL) as shown in Fig. 6.17. Note that PVC tubing can be firmly welded with a few drops of cyclohexanone.* The 2-mm ID tubing† should be employed to lead samples into and recover gradients from the rotor. Larger tubing may be used to carry the gradient into the rotor and still larger tubing for cooling. Several dozen quick connectors with similar internal diameters are needed in many locations. Semiball O-ring joints‡ of ST 12/5 and 12/2 and Luer-Lok joints are suitable. An indefinitely large number of hemostats, say 12, will be extremely convenient to control fluid flow and prevent embolisms. They should be about 15 cm (5.5 in.), straight, with 5-cm (2 in.) jaws.

A refrigerated water circulator will be needed; a large pail of chipped ice, water, and a good sized submersible pump (e.g., Little Giant) will serve. If tap water must be used, its pressure will have to be reduced to 0.2–0.3 kg/cm^2 (3–5 psig) to avoid bursting connections. Although not absolutely

* Polyvinylchloride glue, made from scraps of PVC dissolved in a 3:1 mixture of tetrahydrofuran and dimethylformamide, may also be used to cement PVC tubing as well as PVC rods, sheets, electrical tape, etc.
† Available in the United States on special order as 5/64 in. ID. Specify 1/4 in. OD so that it will be compatible with other tubing in the series.
‡ Kontes Glass Co., Vineland, New Jersey.

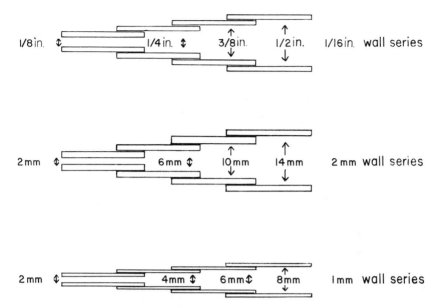

Fig. 6.17. Telescoping PVC tubing. The laboratory should maintain stocks of tubing that nicely telescope with one another. Three series suitable for zonal operations are shown below. The 2-mm wall series is a bit coarse, but it is compatible with the 1-mm series at 6-mm and 10-mm ID. In the United States $\frac{5}{16}$-in.-ID × $\frac{1}{4}$-in.-OD tubing is available on special order.

essential, a source of compressed air (or nitrogen) at about 1 kg/cm^2 (15 psig) is desirable. An extra-large sink near the centrifuge is a welcome luxury when it comes to cleaning the rotor, seal, gradient pump, lines, etc.

6.3.3 Loading the Gradient

The sequence for loading and unloading the rotor is shown in Fig. 6.18. To load the rotor, one starts it spinning at a low speed with the cover open. Depending on the system, the loading speed may be between 300 and 3000 rpm. The primary considerations are avoidance of low-speed criticals,* and generation of sufficient centrifugal field to avoid sectorial loading,† while avoiding excessive heating of the seal surfaces or shear of sensitive particles in crossing the seal.

The gradient is led through the peripheral line into the spinning rotor; the axial line is left open or the tubing immersed in a beaker of water to monitor the displacement of air. Watch most carefully for droplets of water

---

* Resonant frequencies, where the rotor wobbles.
† Uneven loading into different sectors.

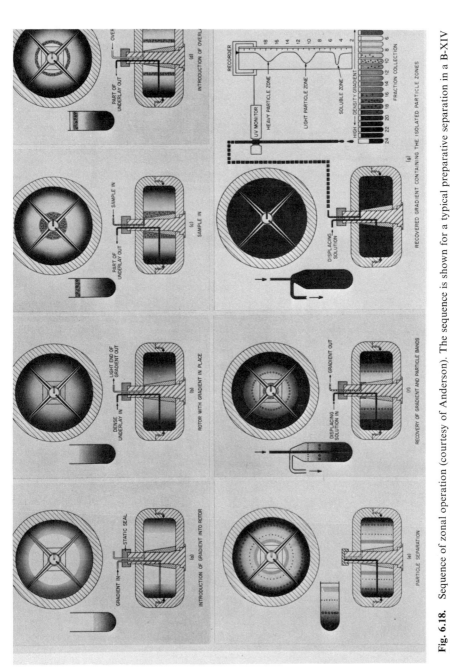

Fig. 6.18. Sequence of zonal operation (courtesy of Anderson). The sequence is shown for a typical preparative separation in a B-XIV or B-XV type of rotor. The inset in each figure shows the corresponding operation in swinging-bucket separations.

which may be carried out with the displaced air and are a sign of imperfections in the fluid seal. If more than 1 cm^3 is discharged in the course of filling the rotor, check the seals and, if necessary, replace the dynamic or static seal or both, before committing a sample to the rotor (see Section 7.6 on polishing seals).

A common schedule is to prepare the gradient at room temperature to minimize viscosity; then, while the sample is prepared, allow it to cool in the refrigerated centrifuge chamber. Approximately 1 hr should be allowed to reach temperature equilibrium. If that interval is not available, the gradient may be passed through a simple heat exchanger (Fig. 6.19). Some gradient pumps are provided with cooling jackets.

An *underlay* or *cushion* of dense solution (usually the limiting or final

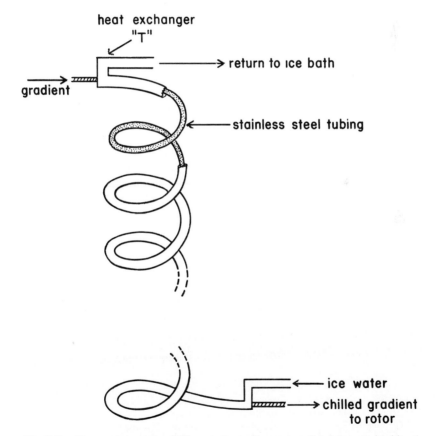

Fig. 6.19.   Heat exchanger for chilling gradients. One meter of stainless steel tubing (ca. 6 mm OD) is enclosed by 10 mm OD PVC tubing and connected at both ends through a Swage-Lok heat exchanger "T." Ice water is circulated in the direction opposite to the flow of gradient.

solution of the gradient) is often introduced under the gradient to collect particles that might penetrate through the gradient. An extra volume of underlay equal to the planned volume of sample-plus-overlay is required to displace air completely from the rotor and cause the top of the gradient to fill the axial channel of the static seal.

6.3.4   Sample Preparation and Loading

The cell brei or particle suspension should be prepared with the same considerations cited in Section 6.2.3: the sample should be free of aggregations to avoid spurious distributions of particles. The quantity of particles should be within the capacity of the gradient (cf. Section 3.2.4 and 3.3.1) and, in the case of rate separation, the volume of the sample together with the expected zone broadening should be compatible with the desired resolution.

The density of the sample can be checked by allowing small drops to fall into test tubes containing portions from the top of the supporting gradient and the bottom of the underlay. It is sometimes useful to incorporate Blue Dextran* into a final concentration of 0.2% w/v to visualize the sample more easily at this stage and later to locate the original position of the sample zone.

The sample may be placed in a hand-operated syringe or a jacketed sample addition funnel (Fig. 6.20) with a short length of 2-mm ID tubing that may be connected to the axial line of the seal. An inverse sample gradient (cf.

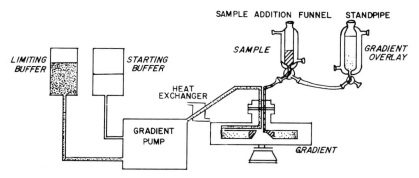

Fig. 6.20.   Sample addition funnel and standpipe. Sample may be loaded under 0.2–0.6 atm air pressure through a jacketed funnel connected to the center channel through a three-way stopcock. Overlay solution waits under pressure in an adjacent standpipe.

* Pharmacia Fine Chemicals.

Section 3.2.4 and Fig. 3.26), which may be needed in the case of concentrated samples, may be generated with a two-syringe generator (Fig. 5.4c) at the time of loading or prepared ahead of time and stored in a sample addition funnel.

Fluid is driven from the sample addition funnel under a low pressure ($0.2–0.6$ kg/cm^2) of air or N$_2$.

The peripheral line must be open since the movement of the sample into the rotor displaces underlay from the rotor. Normally the peripheral line is fed into a beaker in order to monitor any leakage across the seal or retrieve a valuable sample, in the case of catastrophic failure of the seal.

Samples may be loaded at rates up to 150 cm^3/min without obvious loss of resolution (Price and Kovacs, 1969). The overlay should chase the sample into the rotor in one continuous operation, so that no portion of the sample is exposed to excess heating in or adjacent to the seal. An arrangement that allows a rapid and continuous loading of sample and overlay is to pressurize the sample addition funnel in parallel with a standpipe containing the overlay (Fig. 6.20). A three-way stopcock at the base of sample addition funnel connects both vessels to the axial channel.

6.3.5 Role of Overlay

Samples are conventionally* pumped through the center channel so that they come to lie between the top of the gradient and the center channel (Fig. 6.18c). For several reasons it is disadvantageous to leave samples in this position: the centrifugal field is lowest near the center; the radial width of the sample is maximal; and, because of the ramps and chords that funnel fluid into the center channels, the circumferential distribution of particles in the sample zone is not uniform. To avoid these problems, chase the sample zone farther into the rotor, at least as far as the end of the ramp, by pumping a lighter fluid after it (Figs. 6.18d and 6.20). By a kind of reverse radial dilution, the sample zone becomes radially thinner the farther it is displaced into the rotor Fig. 6.21.† This decrease in zone width is especially important for optimizing resolution in rate separations, but it must be balanced against a corresponding decrease in the pathlength.

Overlays are commonly prepared simply from water or buffer, but a *gradient overlay* is beneficial to resolution by minimizing the volume of fluid that diffuses into the sample zone (Price and Kovacs, 1969).

---

* Compare the MACS system of direct sample injection (Section 7.4).

† Consider the analogy of water led from a tall cylinder to a flat dish. The volume remains the same, but the thickness of the fluid can be drastically altered. In the same way a wide sample zone becomes progressively narrower at it is displaced into the rotor by addition of overlay.

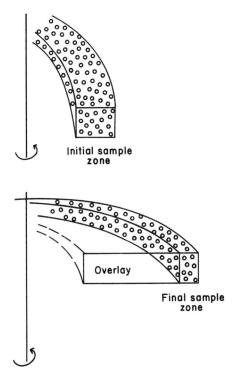

Fig. 6.21. Control of zone width by the addition of overlay. A sample zone immediately adjacent to the core is relatively wide (left). The same volume when displaced further into the rotor by the addition of overlay, becomes much thinner. One may think of this as reverse radial dilution.

6.3.6 Importance of Vacuum

Because of their simple shapes, zonal rotors suffer less heating from windage than swinging-bucket rotors, but they are just as sensitive to the poor temperature control that can result from an unsatisfactory vacuum (cf. Section 6.2.4). Just because zonal centrifugation involves working with an open chamber door for long intervals, the vacuum pump is especially susceptible to fouling from condensed water, not to mention spilled sucrose. It is essential to check the vacuum pump oil weekly.

6.3.7 Estimation of $\int \omega^2 \, dt$

As explained in Section 6.1.5, the separation achieved in a given gradient is governed by the $\int \omega^2 \, dt$. One can estimate this quantity from the value of $(\text{rpm})^2 \times$ time [cf. Eq. (6.3)], but the estimate suffers from the difficulties of estimating the integral during the acceleration and deceleration together with the inherent inaccuracies of analog tachometers and speed controls. Most modern ultracentrifuges offer digital $\int \omega^2 \, dt$ meters, which provide accurate measurements and vastly improved repeatability of rate separations in both zonal and swinging-bucket rotors.

6.3.8 Deceleration and the Holding Mode Option

Since conventional zonal rotors rely on a continuing centrifugal field to stabilize the gradient during loading and unloading, it is obviously undesirable to allow the rotor to stop during a run. For this reason it is preferable to allow a rotor to decelerate on drive with the speed control set to the loading speed of perhaps 2000 rpm rather than to decelerate on brake or coast.

A particularly convenient insurance policy against inadvertant stoppage in zonal centrifuges is a holding mode option, in which the centrifuge automatically drives down to a holding speed after a preset time or $\int \omega^2 \, dt$. This option is advantageous in swinging-bucket separations for different reasons (cf. Section 6.2.5).

6.3.9 Recovery of Gradient

When the zonal rotor has been slowed to its loading speed, the vacuum is released, the chamber opened, and the fluid seal reattached (Fig. 6.18f).

In *center unloading* (Fig. 6.18f) a chilled dense solution, usually the underlay (also called the *piston fluid*) is pumped to the edge and the gradient recovered, light end first, from the center. A pulseless, constant-speed pump should be employed. With connective tubing of 2-mm ID the gradient may be unloaded at speeds up to 60 cm³/min without significant loss of resolution (cf. also Table 6.3).

There are several disadvantages to center unloading: the underlay is almost invariably the most viscous component of the gradient, which means increased hazards from seal leakage during unloading and a bowlfull of sticky sucrose at the end of the run. Moreover, the gradient material may be costly. Rather than displace Ficoll, Metrizamide, or cesium chloride with Ficoll, Metrizamide, or cesium chloride, one may substitute a dense, water-immiscible, and nontoxic flurocarbon, such as one of the Fluorinerts* (Allington†).

Anderson, who first inflicted center unloading on an unsuspecting public, subsequently offered surcease in a rotor configuration in which gradients

---

* The 3M Manufacturing Company.
† ISCO Applications Res. Bull., No. 7.

Table 6.3.   Zone Widths of Various Sample Volumes[a]

A. Samples of 0.2% w/v Blue Dextran were inserted within a sucrose gradient of 0.2 mg/cm^6 and loaded at the center. The pumping rate was 30 cm^3/min^1, and the loading speed was 2000 rpm. The samples were then unloaded immediately either at the center or at the edge.

	Recovered zone width (ΔV in cm^3 at 0.606 peak height)	
Initial zone volume (cm^3)	Unloaded at center	Unloaded at edge
B-XXIX		
5	6.3	27.8
10	9.4	22.0
20	18.3	45.0
30	30.5	44.9
40	42.9	49.6
B-30A		
5	4.72	15.65
10	9.01	16.24
20	18.90	23.62
30	26.58	29.82
40	35.43	35.43

B. Zone widths in B-XXIX at various pumping speeds; conditions as in A, except that sample volume was 5 cm^3 throughout.

	Recovered zone width (ΔV in cm^3 at 0.606 peak height)	
Pumping speed (cm^3/min)	Center	Edge
10	6.79	22.74
30	6.35	20.23
60	7.97	17.86

C. Zone widths in the B-XXIX at the edge during loading compared to unloading. Conditions as in A, except that 5-cm^3 samples were either loaded at the center and recovered at the edge or loaded at the edge and recovered at the center. Pumping rate was 60 cm^3/min.

Direction of pumping	Recovered zone width (ΔV in cm^3 at 0.606 peak height)
Center to edge	15.06
	12.25
Edge to center	19.93
	19.34
	17.42

D. Resolution in the sample insertion channel of the Z-8 (MACS-type) rotor. Conditions the same as in A, except that sample volumes were uniformly 5 cm^3. For explanation of sample insertion channel, see Section 7.4.

Table 6.3 (Cont.)

Mode of entry	Recovered zone width (ΔV in cm^3 at 0.606 peak height)
Center channel	3.3
	3.6
	3.8
Sample insertion channel	5.5
	6.9
	4.6
	5.8

[a] Samples are unloaded at the center and edge of B-XXIX, B-30A, and Z-8 (MACS-type) rotors (Price and Kovacs, 1969; Price, 1974; Price and Casciato, 1974).

may be unloaded from the edge (Anderson *et al.*, 1967). In the **B-XXIX** prototype, now duplicated in a number of rotor systems, *edge unloading* is effected by pumping buffer or water through the center channel and collecting the gradient at the edge in great circle grooves (Fig. 6.22). This system provides resolution that is almost as good as that in center unloading (cf.

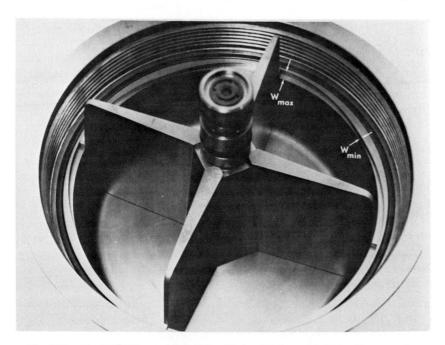

Fig. 6.22. The B-XXIX rotor (Oak Ridge National Laboratories). Gradients may be unloaded from the edge by funneling the fluid in two dimensions toward channels in the septa: along vertical ramps and horizontally along great circle grooves, which are circles whose center is displaced from the axis of the rotor.

Table 6.3). The *almost* is due to a physical inconsistency: in edge unloading a lighter solution displaces a heavier solution, which is acceptable provided the direction of the gradient and the centrifugal or gravitational field are the same. However, within edge channels and in the tubing emerging from the rotor, a density inversion is inevitable and some loss of resolution occurs.

The effects of the density inversion are inversely related to the rate of flow; indeed, resolution is improved in edge unloading by displacing the gradient very rapidly (Table 6.3).

A potential hazard of edge unloading is that the gradient is normally led through the peripheral channel of the fluid seal, which may be damaging to delicate particles. This hazard is avoided in the reversed flow adapters of the MACS system (cf. Section 7.4).

Brown *et al.* (1973) (cf. Section 9.3.3) exploited edge unloading for the screening of a wide range of particle sizes in a single gradient. In what they call *sequential product recovery*, the sample is loaded onto a gradient and spun for a given interval. The rotor is decelerated, the distal portion of the gradient unloaded from the edge, replaced with fresh gradient, and the cycle repeated at a larger value of $\int \omega^2 \, dt$. This is continued until the smallest particles are finally recovered. In this way one obtains a series of fractions

Table 6.4.   **Gradient Monitoring Devices**[a]

Quantity	Type of measurement	Comments
Optical absorption	light	May be used in UV[b] or visible[b] or in a spectral sweep
Fluorescence	light	Suitable for very low concentrations; quenching becomes important at high particle concentrations
Turbidity, light scattering	light	Can be used to estimate particle size as well as particle concentration
Radioactivity	α-, β-, or γ-rays	Quite practical for γ rays; problem of short path lengths and self absorption for α and β rays
Refractive index	light	For measuring solute concentrations (see Table 5.5)
Fluid density	resonant frequency	For measuring solute concentrations (see Table 5.5)

[a] The quantities are among those that can in principle be measured in a gradient effluent from a zonal rotor. Few of them have been adapted to the physical requirements of a compact, integrated system.

[b] Commercial devices available from IEC, Spinco, and LKB; some small modifications may be required to adapt to existing detectors or to accommodate requisite flow rates.

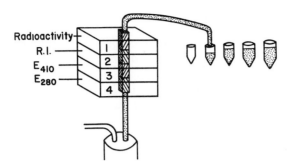

Fig. 6.23. Stacked cow cells for on-stream monitoring of gradients. With present technologies it is possible to design flow detectors for a variety of functions that would stack closely over a zonal rotor.

corresponding to different values of s. The use of equivolumetric gradient shapes in this system would simplify the estimation of s values and improve resolution over that obtained with linear gradients.

6.3.10   Gradient Monitoring Devices

The relatively limitless volume of zonal rotors greatly expands the possibilities for extracting information from the recovered gradient. Multiple, stacked flow cells are perfectly feasible (Fig. 6-23): optical absorption, refractive index, fluorescence, radioactivity, and fluid density are among the currently practical devices (Table 6.4).

The gradient is normally collected in fractions on a time, volume, or weight basis. The fraction may then be subjected to a variety of chemical and enzymological tests to yield multiple profiles. Technicon-type devices and GeMSAEC fast analyzers (Anderson, 1969) are among the most useful systems for generating repetitive data of this sort.

6.4   DATA PROCESSING

The information required for and generated from density gradient centrifugation, especially in zonal rotors, lends itself handsomely to automatic data processing. In the present state of the art each system will be peculiar to the interests and resources of the laboratory group, but some general observations may nonetheless be helpful.

6.4.1 Acquisition and Storage

Nearly all of the components of the centrifuge system and its monitoring devices produce analog signals. Although an instantaneous record of one or two such signals in the form of a strip chart recorder is useful, the quantity of data that can accumulate on strip charts quickly become unwieldy, especially if curves are to be examined closely for zone shape, distance between zones, correlation with enzyme activities, etc. One of the more generally useful approaches is to convert all signals to digital form for storage in automatic data processing equipment. This may require an analog to digital converter, although more and more laboratory instruments are available with digital displays and binary coded decimal (BCD) output.

The sampling rates required in centrifuge operations are almost trivially slow by the current state of the art; so that it is perfectly feasible to sample a dozen analog signals sequentially through a signal converter. The data can then be stored economically on paper tape, or more conveniently on magnetic tape or flexible diskettes.

Ridge (1973) has described a computerized analysis of data from a zonal centrifuge. A somewhat more comprehensive scheme, but similar in kind, is presented in Fig. 6.24.

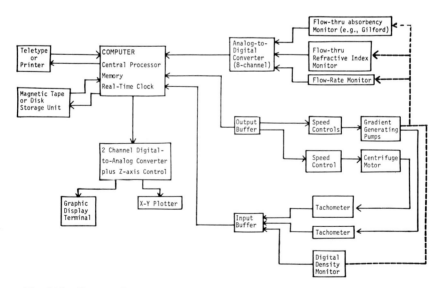

Fig. 6.24. Computerized control and analysis of centrifuge data (E. F. Eikenberry, unpublished). A hypothetical system for both controlling the speed of the centrifuge and analyzing the profiles of gradients. Storage of data on the $\omega^2 dt$ of a given run could be combined with sedimentation profiles to obtain sedimentation coefficients, etc.

6.4.2   Data Reduction

Empirical equations of data fields are available (Appendix C) that relate refractive index, concentration, viscosity, and density of most of the common gradient solutes. Given one of these quantities and the temperature of a given gradient, it becomes almost trivial to compute the actual shape of a delivered or recovered gradient.

Programs are also available (Bishop, 1966) to compute the sedimentation coefficients of ideal particles which migrate to different positions in any arbitrary gradient given the rotor, speed, time, starting radius, etc. A more ambitious program (J. E. Breillatt, personal communication) called DIFSED predicts zone position and shape following sedimentation in any given gradient.

Programs are also available (cf. Funding, 1973) for analyzing observed sedimentation profiles into a series of Gaussian distributions. Other programs can be rather readily devised to compare particle concentration with measured quantities in gradient fractions in order to report specific and total activities and concentration of the measured components along a gradient.

6.4.3   Presentation of Gradient Profiles

Although some workers may prefer to see tabulations of gradient analyses, most biologists are more comfortable with figures, that is, visualizations of the data. One of the great advances in this field are computer-controlled X–Y recorders, with which arrays of data may be plotted as curves. In contrast to the strip chart record, which must be transformed painfully point by point, the X–Y recorder programs invite the selection of any desired set of scales: the abcissa may correspond to 10 ml/cm or 100 ml/cm; the ordinates to 10,000 cpm/cm or 3 units of cytochrome oxidase/cm, etc.

In ideal cases where recovery and resolution are complete, the localization of an enzyme activity or chemical component may be so striking as to be evident in any kind of presentation. In other cases the data must be analyzed more carefully. Schneider (cf. 1972) cautions against attempts to interpret the results from fractions in which the sum of activities in the several fractions fail to equal that of the original homogenates (i.e., where recovery is other than 100%).

De Duve (1959) proposed a means of analyzing enzyme activities in experiments where activities are spread among several fractions. The activity of each fraction is divided by the protein content of the fraction to yield a quantity called the *relative specific activity*. High relative specific activity means that the fraction is enriched in the corresponding enzyme. It can easily happen that an absolutely larger portion of the enzyme activity may be found elsewhere. If, for example, most of the lysosomes of a liver sample were ruptured during homogenization, the majority of the acid phosphatase would be found in the soluble fraction, but the surviving lysosomes would nonetheless show a larger relative specific activity.

REFERENCES

List contains a number of general references not cited in the text.

Anderson, N. G. (1968). Preparative particle separation in density gradients. *Q. Rev. Biophys.* **1,** 217–263.

Anderson, N. G. (1969). Computer interfaced fast analyzers. *Science* **166,** 317–324.

Anderson, N. G., Waters, D. A., Fisher, N. D., Cline, G. B., Nunley, C. E., Elrod, L. H., and Rankin, C. T., Jr. (1967). Analytical techniques for cell fractions. V. Characteristics of the B-XIV and B-XV zonal centrifuge rotors. *Anal. Biochem.* **21,** 235–252.

Birnie, G. D. (1967). "Subcellular Components," 2nd ed. Butterworth, London.

Birnie, G. D., and Rickwood, D. (eds.) (1978). "Centrifugal Separations in Molecular and Cell Biology." Butterworths. London. 327 pp.

Bishop, B. S. (1966). Digital computation of sedimentation coefficients in zonal centrifuges. *Natl. Cancer Inst. Monogr.* **21,** 175–188.

Brakke, M. K. (1963). Photometric scanning of centrifuged density gradient columns. *Anal. Biochem.* **5,** 271–283.

Brakke, M. K. (1964). Nonideal sedimentation and the capacity of sucrose gradient columns for viruses in density gradient centrifugation. *Arch. Biochem. Biophys.* **107,** 388–403.

Brakke, M. K. (1967). Density gradient centrifugation. *Methods Virol.* **2,** 93–118.

Brakke, M. K., and Van Pelt, N. (1968). Photometric scanning of a centrifuged gradient column at several wavelengths. *Anal. Biochem.* **26,** 242–250.

Brown, D. H., Carlton, E., Byrd, B., Harrell, B., and Hayes, R. L. (1973). A rate-zonal centrifugation procedure for screening particle populations by sequential product recovery utilizing edge-unloading zonal rotors. *Arch. Biochem. Biophys.* **155,** 9–18.

Chevrenka, C. H., and McEwen, C. R. (1971). "A Manual of Methods for Large Scale Zonal Centrifugation." Beckman Instruments, Spinco Division, Palo Alto, California.

Cline, G. B., and Ryel, R. B. (1971). Zonal centrifugation. *In* "Methods in Enzymology" (W. B. Jakoby, ed.), Vol. 22, pp. 168–204. Academic Press, New York.

de Duve, C. (1959). Gradient centrifugation of cell particles. Theory and applications. *Prog. Biophys. Biophys. Chem.* **9,** 325–369.

de Duve, C. (1963). The separation and characterization of subcellular particles. *Harvey Lect.* **59,** 49–87.

Eikenberry, E. F., Bickle, T. A., Traut, R. R., and Price, C. A. (1970). Separation of large quantities of ribosomal subunits by zonal ultracentrifugation. *Eur. J. Biochem.* **12,** 113–116.

Funding, L. (1973). Analytical ultracentrifugations with zonal rotors. *Spectra 2000* **4,** 46–49.

Griffith, O. M. (1978). Rapid density gradient centrifugation using short column techniques. *Anal. Biochem.* **90,** 435–443.

Halsall, H. B., and Schumaker, V. N. (1970). Diffusion coefficients from the zonal ultracentrifuge using microgram and milligram quantities of material. *Biochim. Biophys. Acta* **39**, 479–485.

Headon, D. R., Hsiao, J., and Ungar, F. (1978). The intracellular localization of adrenal 38-hydroxysteroid dehydrogenase/Δ^5-isomerase by density gradient perturbation. *Biochem. Biophys. Res. Commun.* **82**, 1006–1012.

Hinton, R., and Dobrota, M. (1976). "Density Gradient Centrifugation." North-Holland, Amsterdam. 294 pp.

Infante, A. A., and Baierlein, R. (1971). Pressure-induced dissociation of sedimenting ribosomes: Effect on sedimentation patterns. *Proc. Natl. Acad. Sci. U.S.A.* **68**, 1780–1785.

Jolley, W. E., Allen, H. W., and Griffith, O. M. (1967). Ultracentrifugation using acrylamide gel. *Anal. Biochem.* **21**, 454–461.

Khandjian, E. W. (1977). *In situ* studies of subcellular particles immobilized in sucrose–acrylamide density gradients. *Anal. Biochem.* **77**, 376–396.

Leif, R. C., Kneece, W. C., Jr., Warters, R. L., Grinvalsky, H., and Thomas, R. A. (1972). Density gradient system. III. Elimination of hydrodynamic, wall, and swirling artifacts in preformed isopycnic gradient centrifugation. *Anal. Biochem.* **45**, 357–373.

Leighton, F., Poole, B., Baudhuin, P., Coffey, J. W., Fowler, S., and de Duve, C. (1968). The large-scale separation of peroxisomes, mitochondria, and lysosomes from the liver of rats injected with Triton WR-1339. *J. Cell Biol.* **37**, 482–513.

Martin, R. G., and Ames, B. N. (1961). A method for determining the sedimentation behavior of enzymes: Application to protein mixtures. *J. Biol. Chem.* **236**, 1372–1379.

Moore, D. H. (1969). Gradient centrifugation. *In* "Physical Techniques and Biological Research" (D. H. Moore, ed.), 2nd ed., Vol. 2, Part B, pp. 285–314. Academic Press. New York.

Morgenthaler, J.-J., and Price, C. A. (1976). Density-gradient sedimentation in silica sols. Anomalous shifts in the banding densities of polystyrene "latex" beads. *Biochem. J.* **153**, 487–490.

Noll, H. (1969). An automatic high-resolution gradient analyzing system. *Anal. Biochem.* **27**, 130–149.

Price, C. A. (1972). Zonal centrifugation. *In* "Manometric and Biochemical Techniques" (W. W. Umbreit, R. H. Burris, and J. F. Stauffer, eds.), 5th ed., Vol. 11, pp. 213–243. Burgess, Minneapolis, Minnesota.

Price, C. A. (1974). On resolution in edge-loading zonal rotors. *Anal. Biochem.* **60**, 319–321.

Price, C. A., and Casciato, R. J. (1974). Multiple alternate channel selection (MACS): New versatility for zonal rotors. *Anal. Biochem.* **57**, 356–362.

Price, C. A., and Kovacs, A. (1969). Resolution in zonal rotors. *Anal. Biochem.* **28**, 460–468.

Quinn, P. J., and Fernando, M. A. (1977). Immuno-ultracentrifugation: A combination of density gradient centrifugation and immunodiffusion. *J. Immunol. Methods* **14**, 253–255.

Reid, E., ed. (1970). "Separations with Zonal Rotors." University of Surrey, Guildford, Surrey, U.K.

Ridge, D. (1973). Automatic acquisition of data for analytical use of zonal centrifuges. *Spectra 2000* **4**, 39–43.

Ryan, N. M., and Headon, D. R. (1979). Quantification with density perturbants in density-gradient centrifugation. *Biochem. Soc. Trans.* **7**, 511–512.

Schneider, W. C. (1972). Methods for the isolation of particulate components of the cell. *In* "Manometric and Biochemical Techniques" (W. W. Umbreit, R. H. Burris, and J. F. Stauffer,eds.), 5th ed., pp. 196–212. Burgess Publ., Minneapolis, Minnesota.

St. Onge, J. M., and Price, C. A. (1975). Automatic sorting of ichthyoplankton: Factors controlling plankton density in gradients of silica. *Mar. Biol.* **29**, 187–194.

Sartory, W. K., Halshall, H. B., and Breillat, J. P. (1976). Simulation of gradient and band propagation in the centrifuge. *Biophys. Chem.* **5,** 107–135.

Steensgaard, J., and Moller, N. P. H. (1979). Computer simulation of density-gradient centrifugation. *In* "Subcellular Biochemistry" (D. B. Roodyn, ed.), Vol. 6, pp. 117–141. Plenum, New York.

Vinograd, J., and Bruner, R., (1966). Band centrifugation of macromolecules in self-generating gradients. II. Sedimentation and diffusion of macromolecules in bands. *Biopolymers* **4,** 131–156.

Wattiaux, R., and Wattiaux-De Coninck, S. (1970). Distribution of mitochondrial enzymes after isopycnic centrifugation of a rat liver mitochondrial fraction in a sucrose gradient: Influence of the speed of centrifugation. *Biochem. Biophys. Res. Commun.* **40,** 1185–1188.

7

Special Topics

7.1 CONTINUOUS-FLOW CENTRIFUGATION WITH ISOPYCNIC BANDING

Rotors for the collection of particles from large volumes of suspensions have been employed widely for many years. The prototype of continuous-flow harvesting is the Sharples centrifuge in which the suspension is led through a hollow spinning cylinder and the particles are pelleted against the wall. Zonal rotors have been designed to employ the same principle, except that the particles are sedimented into an annular density gradient at the edge of the rotor (Fig. 7.1). The particles are first trapped within the gradient and ultimately move to their equilibrium density. Therefore the particles are not only concentrated many fold from the original suspension, but recovered according to their ρ_{eq}. The process is called *continuous-flow centrifugation with banding*.

At first glance it seems that continuous-flow centrifugation would be incompatible with the fluid seals that were discussed with regard to preparative zonal centrifugation. The standard zonal seal admits fluid to or from two locations; thus, fluid can be introduced or withdrawn from the center or the edge. In continuous-flow zonal centrifugation one must not only introduce and recover a gradient, but one must also introduce a particle suspension and discharge a spent supernatant at two additional locations and in directions different from the desired movement of the gradient. How does one achieve these functions within a single, two-channel seal? The problem is presented in a highly schematic form in Fig. 7.2.

The problem has in fact been solved in several different ways. The first

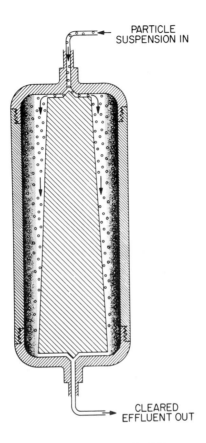

PARTICLE
SUSPENSION IN

CLEARED
EFFLUENT OUT

CONTINUOUS FLOW
(OPERATING SPEED BETWEEN
2000 AND 35,000 rpm)

Fig. 7.1. Continuous-flow in a zonal rotor (Courtesy of Oak Ridge National Laboratories). A particle suspension flows past a thin, annular gradient at the edge of the rotor. The particles are trapped in the gradient and the spent supernatant is discharged. This is a generalized K-type rotor.

solution ultimately became the B-XVI rotor* (Fig. 7.3). The B-XVI was a core modification of the B-IV (Fig. 7.4). Both are spindle-shaped rotors of prodigious complexity which most of us would cheerfully forget.

The operation of the B-XVI is shown in Fig. 7.5. A standard two-way fluid seal does double duty by an internal valving arrangement. The gradient may be loaded and unloaded with the rotor at rest, when the top of the rotor is

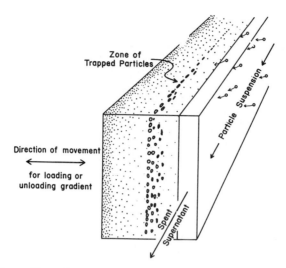

Fig. 7.2. The problem of continuous-flow zonal centrifugation. Imagine a zonal rotor unfolded into a rectangular solid. A gradient must be introduced into and recovered from the rotor by moving fluid in two directions; the rotor must also admit a particle suspension and discharge a spent supernatant along directions perpendicular to the gradient.

also the top of the gradient. Above 2000 rpm the top and bottom of the rotor are the entry and exit points for the flowing suspension and supernatant. Alternatively, air may be injected to block the inner, continuous-flow channel, so that the gradient may be unloaded dynamically.

The living descendants of the B-XVI include the enormous K-type rotors, the smaller RK's and J-1; the CF-32; JCZ; and CF-6 (Table 7.1). The K, RK (Figs. 7.6 and 7.7), and the J rotors differ fundamentally from the B-XVI in that flowing suspension passes through much simpler single-pass seals at the top and bottom of the rotor. The reliability of the seals at high speed is much improved, but the operation is otherwise similar to that of the B-XVI (Fig. 7.8). The meter-long K's are employed industrially for the large-scale purification of viruses for vaccine production (cf. Section 9.4.3); the others are generally suitable for the research laboratory.

The CF-32 (Fig. 7.9) and JCZ (Fig. 7.10) are core modifications of the Ti-15 and JZ rotors; they retain the basic two-way seal design of the B-XVI and their mode of operation is similar (Fig. 7.5).

The CF-6 (Fig. 7.11) solves the logistics of continuous-flow centrifugation

---

* This has been designated in successive versions as the B-VIII, B-IX, and B-XVI. Although a number of laboratories found the B-XVI to be a uniquely serviceable instrument, the stringent requirements of the upper bearing were a frequent source of difficulty. The shipment of a number of the rotors to the Soviet Union was regarded by some observers as a bold stroke in the Cold War.

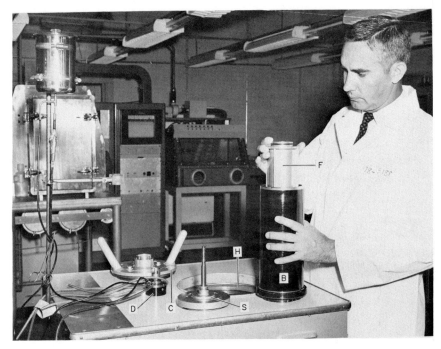

Fig. 7.3.   The B-XVI continuous-flow rotor (Courtesy of Oak Ridge National Laboratories). The partially disassembled rotor is shown in the laboratory of the Molecular Anatomy Program. Pictured are the special cover (C) which screws into a hole (H) in the lid of the rotor chamber, the damper bearing (D), the rotor cover and spindle (S), the B-IV shell (B), and B-XVI continuous-flow core (F).

by having four separate channels: one open, circular groove carries the gradient to the edge of the rotor; another leads the particle suspension into the rotor; a drain tube carries off the supernatant; and a single-pass seal collects the gradient at the end of the run (Fig. 7.12).

Still another solution to the routing of fluids in continuous-flow centrifugation is the MACS system (cf. Section 7.5); interchangable seal adapters, which are described more fully in Section 7.5, connect alternately to gradient channels or to continuous-flow channels. A prototype continuous-flow version of the Z-15 rotor employing the MACS system is shown schematically in Fig. 7.13.

Cline (1971), provided more detailed information on the operation of K- and RK-rotors than is available for any other flow-band system. The following pointers on continuous-flow procedures are largely excerpted from his work (Cline, 1971; cf. also Cline and Ryel, 1971; Cline and Dagg, 1973).

Choice of rotor.   The rotor must be fast enough so that the particles of

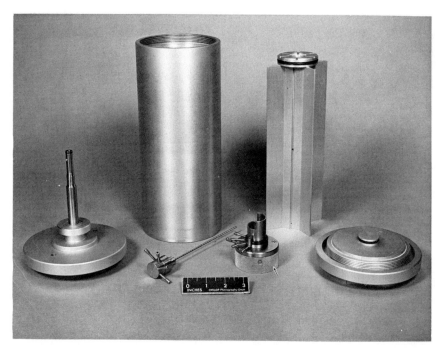

Fig. 7.4. The B-IV rotor (Courtesy of Oak Ridge National Laboratories). The rotor is shown outside of the centrifuge. Normally only the damper bearing (arrow) and upper seal package protrude from the cover of the rotor chamber. The various pieces of tubing connect to oil and coolant as well as the axial and peripheral channels.

interest can be cleared from the flowing stream. The efficiency or *fractional clean-out* f_c

$$f_c \equiv \frac{\text{initial concentration} - \text{concentration in effluent}}{\text{initial concentration}}$$

is a resultant of rotor speed, the sedimentation of the particle in the suspending medium, and the residence time, which is dependent on the geometry of the rotor. Perardi and Anderson (1970), for example, find that clean-out with the original tapered cores is less than with a straight cylindrical core, presumably because the suspension in the latter case flows in a thin film between the core and the density gradient. Although residence time is decreased, the radial distance the particles must traverse before becoming trapped in the gradient is also minimized.

Sartory (1970) derived Eq. (7.1) to describe clean-out in a rotor with zero taper as a function of several parameters.

$$f_c = \frac{4 \times 10^{-16} \pi^3 r^2 (\text{rpm})^2 l S_{T,M}}{Q} \tag{7.1}$$

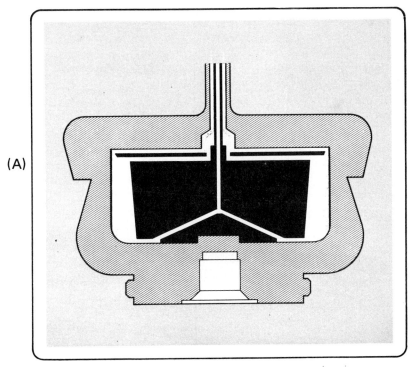

(A)

Fig. 7.5. Mode of operation of the B-XVI, CF-32, and JCZ continuous-flow rotors (Griffith, 1975). (A) Loading the rotor. The rotor is accelerated to about 2000 rpm and completely filled through the edge line with three steps, the most dense solution serving as a cushion; the middle step is selected to be near the banding density of the particles. Diffusion quickly smooths the steps to a continuous gradient within the narrow annular space of the rotor. Buffer or water is then pumped through the center channel. The hydrostatic pressures within the rotor force the light, buffer solution through the lower of the two edge channels shown in the diagram. The rotor is then accelerated to the desired operating speed with buffer continually flowing through the rotor. (Otherwise, expansion of the rotor during acceleration will draw air into the rotor and create air locks.) (B) Sample flow. At the desired operating speed the flow of buffer is replaced by the particle suspension. The flow rate is adjusted to clean out 90–99% of the smallest particles at the selected speed (Fig. 7.15). Slower flow rates can result in sectorial loading with corresponding loss of resolution and capacity. (C) Unloading the rotor. The rotor is decelerated to 2000 rpm. A small volume of air is then pumped through the edge line, which establishes an air lock isolating the lower edge channel. A displacing solution equal to or denser than the cushion is then pumped through the edge line to unload the gradient as in conventional zonal rotors.

where r is the radius of the rotor, l the path length of the particle suspension in contact with the gradient, $S_{T,M}$ the actual sedimentation coefficient under local conditions, and Q the volume of suspension entering the suspension in cm^3/min. We are to assume that fluid flow is laminar and that it occurs without Coriolis acceleration. The wearing of spiral grooves in the surface of the core of K-type rotors suggests that this assumption is not valid.

(B)

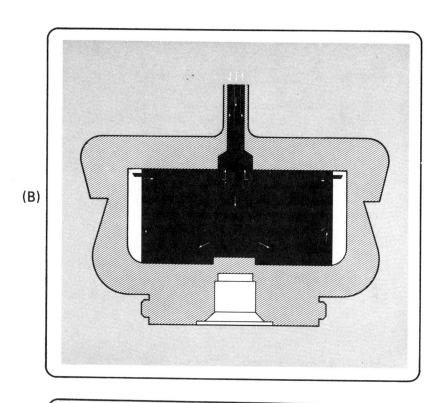

(C)

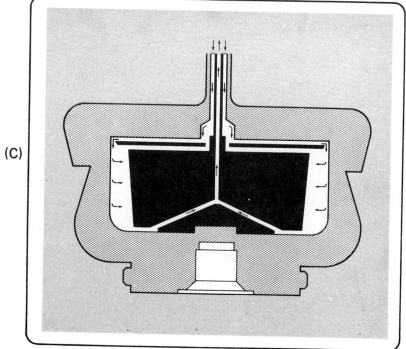

Table 7.1. Characteristics of Continuous-Flow Zonal Rotors

Manufacturers and designation	Gradient volume (cm³)	Maximum speed		Radius at edge	g_{max}	Flow path length (cm)	Drive unit
		rpm	ω^2				
IEC CF-6	515	6,000	3.95×10^5	14.7	5,930	92.3	PR-2, PR-6, PR-6000
Sorvall SZ-14 GK	770	18,000	3.5×10^6	9.5	34,000	2.9	RC-5
Spinco JCF-Z	400	20,000	4.39×10^6	8.9	40,000	8.9	J-21 Interchangeable core in JCZ-Z; recommended for particles >400 S
Spinco CF-32 Ti	300	32,000	1.12×10^7	8.9	102,000	7.3	L-series
Electro-Nucleonics							
K-3	3200	35,000	1.34×10^7	6.6	90,000	76.2	Interchangeable cores in K-series
K-10	8000	35,000	1.34×10^7	6.6	83,500	76.2	bowl and drive unit
K-11	380	35,000	1.34×10^7	6.6		76.2	
Electro-Nucleonics							
RK-3	1600	35,000	1.34×10^7	6.6	90,000	38.1	Interchangeable core; in RK bowl
RK-10	3980	35,000	1.34×10^7	6.6	90,000	38.1	and drive unit
RK-11	190	35,000	1.34×10^7	6.6	90,000	38.1	
MSE B-20 Ti	325	35,000	1.34×10^7	8.9	122,000	6.7	Superspeed 65 and 75, interchangeable with B-15
Electro-Nucleonics							
J-1	780	55,000	3.32×10^7	4.4	150,000	38.4	RK

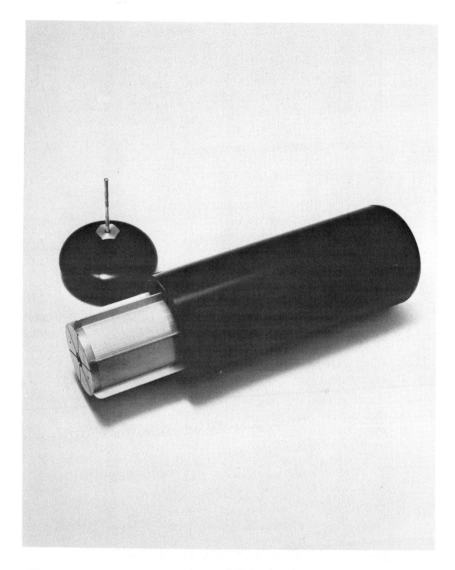

Fig. 7.6. The RK rotor (Electro-Nucleonics). The partially disassembled rotor shows the RK-core with 6 septa; above is the top cap and spindle.

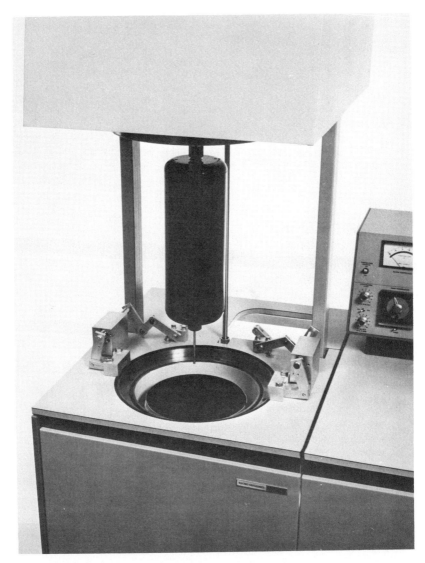

Fig. 7.7.   The Model K zonal centrifuge (Electro-Nucleonics). A K rotor is suspended over the rotor chamber, revealing the lower spindle. The rotor is driven by a turbine at the top. The control console stands at the right.

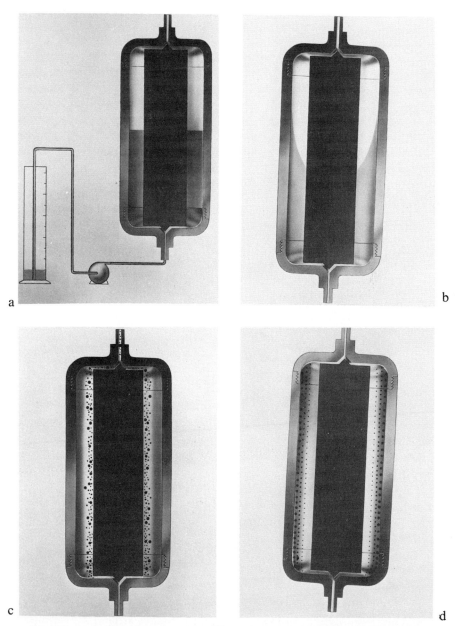

Fig. 7.8. Operation of K-type rotors (Electro-Nucleonics). (a) The density gradient is loaded at rest, usually with a simple step gradient. (b) The rotor is slowly accelerated while the gradient reorients from a horizontal to a vertical configuration. (c) When the rotor has reached operating speed the particle suspension is pumped in at the top, across the gradient, and the supernatant drawn off the bottom. (d) Centrifugation is continued at the end of the run to ensure that the particles have reached their equilibrium density. (e) The rotor is decelerated slowly and smoothly and the gradient reorients. (f) and (g) With the rotor at rest the gradient may be unloaded, the absorbance measured, and fractions collected. (*Continued*)

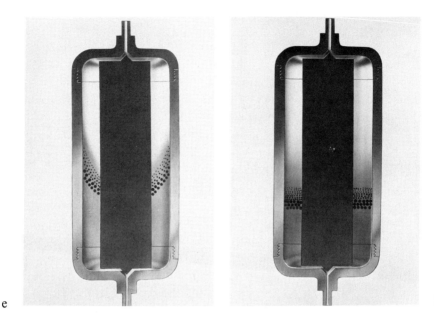

e   f

g

Fig. 7.8.   *Continued*

In the CF-6, to take a different example, residence time is lengthened and clean-out optimized by causing the suspension to flow around the periphery of a large, flat cylinder, rather than across the vertical dimension (Fig. 7.12a).

Because of the great differences in rotor geometry, clean-out cannot be simply compared among rotors by reference to any single parameter. Computed conditions for approximately 100% clean-out for the J-1 and CF-32 rotors are presented in Figs. 7.14 and 7.15. Figure 7.16 shows a similar

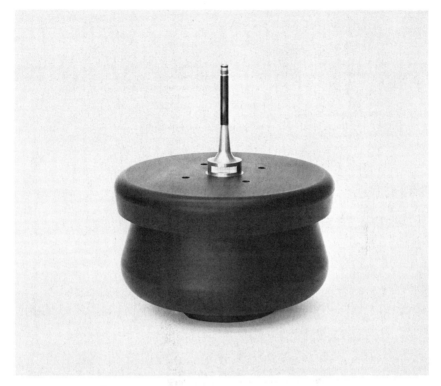

Fig. 7.9. The CF-32 rotor (Spinco Division, Beckman Instruments). The shell of the rotor is the same as that of the popular Ti 15; the core, the top cap, and spindle are diffcrent. The operation of the CF-32 is shown in Fig. 7.5. The damper bearing and upper seal assembly, not shown, are similar to those of the B-IV (Fig. 7.4) and JCZ (Fig. 7.10).

set of curves for the CF-6. For any given particle there is a playoff between rotor speed and sample flow rate.

Gradient shape. The gradient can be designed exactly as that for isopycnic separations (cf. Section 3.3). Since the radial path is rather short, CF rotors are commonly loaded with step gradients, which then rapidly become smoothed through diffusion.

Since fresh sample is constantly flowing across the gradient, solute diffusion is a major consideration. Cesium chloride, for example, diffuses so rapidly that a gradient is measurably flattened between loading and immediate unloading. Such a gradient will therefore degrade rapidly during continuous-flow harvesting. An additional and undesirable consequence of gradient wash-out is that the sample downstream will be more dense than that upstream, which is equivalent to asking that the sample flow uphill (i.e.,

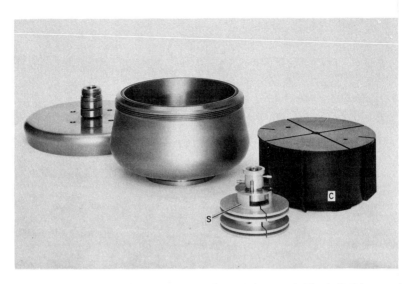

Fig. 7.10. The JCZ rotor (Spinco Division, Beckman Instruments). The shell of the rotor is the same as the JZ; the core (C) and fluid seal assembly (S) are modifications of the B-IV (Fig. 7.4) and the CF-32. A simplification in the JCZ is that the centrifuge system is not dependent on the maintenance of a high vacuum.

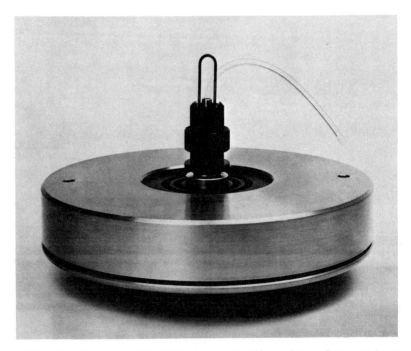

Fig. 7.11. The CF-6 rotor (IEC Division, Damon). This continuous-flow rotor has an unusually long flow-path (92 cm) due to flow around the circumference of the rotor. This feature produces more efficient clean-out than would otherwise be realized from its relatively low speed. Operation of the CF-6 is shown in Fig. 7.12.

210

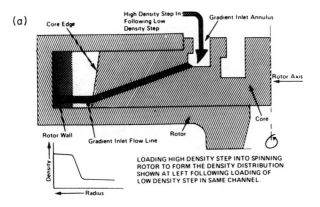

(a)

Core Edge

High Density Step In Following Low Density Step

Gradient Inlet Annulus

Rotor Axis

Core

Rotor Wall   Gradient Inlet Flow Line   Rotor

LOADING HIGH DENSITY STEP INTO SPINNING
ROTOR TO FORM THE DENSITY DISTRIBUTION
SHOWN AT LEFT FOLLOWING LOADING OF
LOW DENSITY STEP IN SAME CHANNEL.

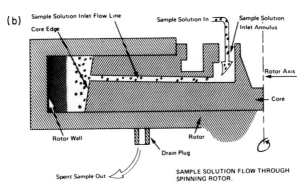

(b)

Sample Solution Inlet Flow Line

Core Edge

Sample Solution In

Sample Solution
Inlet Annulus

Rotor Axis

Core

Rotor Wall   Rotor

Drain Plug

Spent Sample Out

SAMPLE SOLUTION FLOW THROUGH
SPINNING ROTOR.

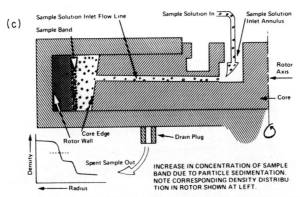

(c)

Sample Solution Inlet Flow Line

Sample Band

Sample Solution In

Sample Solution
Inlet Annulus

Rotor
Axis

Core

Core Edge
Rotor Wall   Drain Plug

Spent Sample Out

INCREASE IN CONCENTRATION OF SAMPLE
BAND DUE TO PARTICLE SEDIMENTATION.
NOTE CORRESPONDING DENSITY DISTRIBU-
TION IN ROTOR SHOWN AT LEFT.

Fig. 7.12 Operation of the CF-6 rotor. There are two channels for the movement of fluid into the rotor and two separate channels for the disharge or recovery of fluid out of the rotor. The sequence of operations is shown in transverse section in (a) through (d). (a) A step or preformed gradient is introduced through an outer groove. (b) and (c) A particle suspension flows through an inner groove and around the circumference of the gradient. The spent fluid escapes through a drain hole in the bottom. (d) At the end of the run the gradient is recovered through a single-pass dynamic seal at the center as a result of displacement by dense solution flowing to the edge.

211

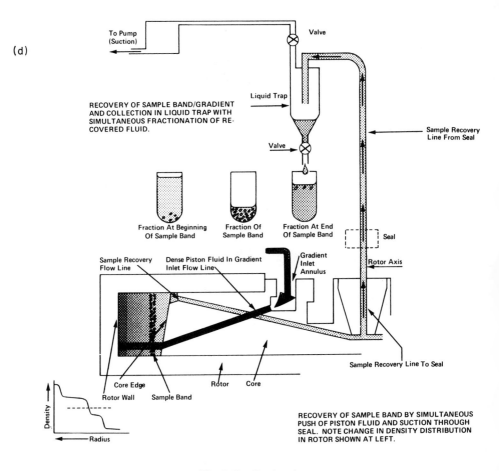

(d)

RECOVERY OF SAMPLE BAND/GRADIENT AND COLLECTION IN LIQUID TRAP WITH SIMULTANEOUS FRACTIONATION OF RECOVERED FLUID.

RECOVERY OF SAMPLE BAND BY SIMULTANEOUS PUSH OF PISTON FLUID AND SUCTION THROUGH SEAL. NOTE CHANGE IN DENSITY DISTRIBUTION IN ROTOR SHOWN AT LEFT.

Fig. 7.12   *Continued*

there must be an expenditure of work to match the added rotational inertia). This added work appears as a substantial back pressure resisting the flow of sample.

Solute diffusion can be lessened by increasing the viscosity in the gradient. This may be achieved by adding sucrose or polymers and by lowering the temperature.

Reorienting gradient techniques.   K-Type rotors are loaded and unloaded at rest; thus the gradient reorients during acceleration and deceleration (cf. Harvey, 1970). At one time Cline (1971) recommended an acceleration rate of about 3 rpm/sec up to 5000 rpm, at which time reorientation of isodense surfaces is complete, but more recently practitioners have adopted a wider latitude in the choice of ramp speeds.

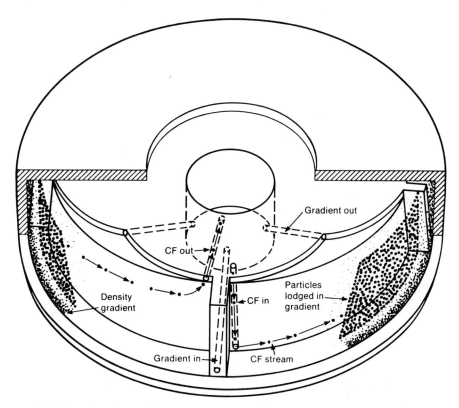

Fig. 7.13. A continuous-flow Z-15 rotor employing the MACS system. The cut-away view shows a continuous-flow core with two sets of channels. One seal adapter connects in the central cavity to the "gradient in" and "gradient out" channels; another seal adapter connects to the continuous–flow "CF in" and "CF out" channels. The selectivity of the seal adapters is based on the specific vertical level of each channel terminus in the central cavity (cf. Section 7.5).

Sample size and flow rates. As noted before, sample volumes are limited by flow rates and the time during which a gradient remains stable to wash-out. As an order of magnitude, however, one can note that influenza virus is routinely processed in 200-liter quantities in the K-2 rotor (Sorrentino *et al.*, 1973) and that algal plankton are cleared by the relatively low-speed CF-6 at flow rates of 400 cm^3/min (Price *et al.*, 1974).

Separation of particles sensitive to shear. We (Price *et al.*, 1973a) observed that chloroplasts are sheared during flow across dynamic seals of small bore. Where the integrity of a particle might be threatened by such shear forces, one should look carefully at seal diameters (cf. Table 7.1).

Application. As indicated in calculations of clean-out (Fig. 7.14–7.16), continuous-flow zonal rotors may be used for the concentration and purifi-

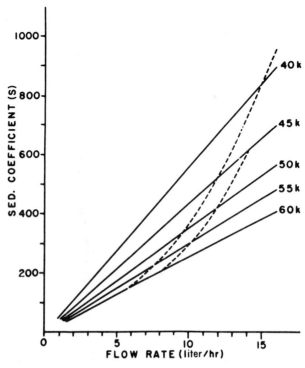

Fig. 7.14. Clean-out in the J-1 rotor (Cline, 1971). Calculated values for the clean-out of particles as a function of flow rate at different rotor speeds. The dotted lines show the maximal flow rates when flow is from bottom to top (top line) and from top to bottom (bottom line).

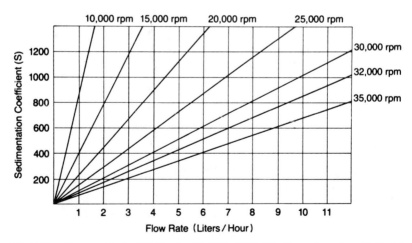

Fig. 7.15. Clean-out in the CF-32 rotor (Griffith, 1975). The figure shows hypothetical flow rates calculated to achieve 99% clean-out in the geometry of the CF-32 rotor. Clean-out in the JCF-Z rotor is very similar.

214

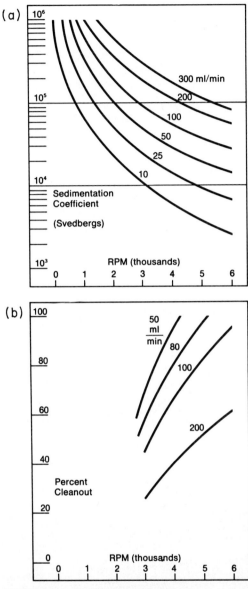

Fig. 7.16. Clean-out in the CF-6 (IEC/Damon). (a) The curves show the speed along the abcissa required to produce 93% clean-out of particles of different sedimentation coefficients. The several curves are for different flow rates. The arrow shows that particles of 25,000 S should be 93% retained in the rotor when the rotor speed is 3500 rpm and the flow rate of the particle suspension is 50 ml per minute. (b) The expected clean-out of polystyrene latex as affected by rotor speed and flow rate. The polystyrene particles have a mean diameter of 1.011 μm, a density of 1.047 gm/cm^3, and a computed sedimentation coefficient of 25,800 S. The arrow shows that these particles should be 93% retained when the rotor speed is 3500 rpm and the flow rate is 50 cm^3/min.

215

cation of whole cells down to particles the size of ribosomes. The most spectacular applications have been in the industrial-scale preparation of viruses for vaccine production. A gradient profile of a harvest of influenza virus is shown in Fig. 9.14 and electron photomicrographs of the crude and purified virus are shown in Fig. 9.15. Gradient fractions containing Tussock moth polyhedrosis virus purified in the K-II rotor are shown in Fig. 7.17.

Continuous-flow zonal centrifugation can also be used for the harvest of large quantities of membrane-bound organelles, such as mitochondria (Barnett and Brown, 1967) and chloroplasts (Brown *et al.*, 1970; Price *et al.*, 1973a). The chloroplasts are also resolved into intact and stripped organelles (Fig. 7.18).

In addition to the large volumes of sample that may be processed in continuous-flow zonal rotors, there are several intrinsic advantages to the method. One is that the integrity of fragile particles is better preserved in a gradient than when they are pelleted against a solid surface. Another is that the gradient affords purification by isopycnic separation and that further

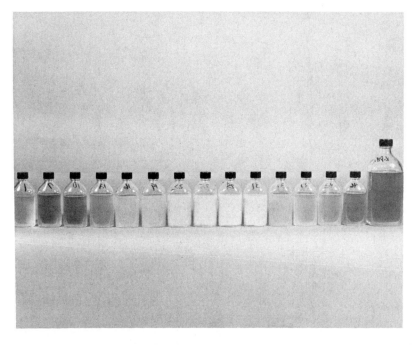

Fig. 7.17. Gradient fractions from a separation of polyhedral virus (J. E. Breillatt, unpublished). The crude virus is obtained as an autolysate of corpses of infected Tussock moth and centrifuged along a sucrose gradient in the K-II rotor. Each of the smaller bottles contains 250 cm^3. The virus is visible as a milky suspension in fractions 19–31.

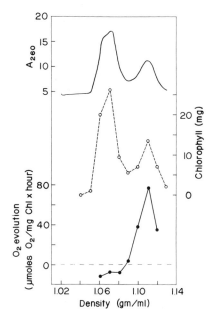

Fig. 7.18. Harvest and resolution of intact chloroplasts by continuous-flow centrifugation (Morgenthaler *et al.*, 1975). Spinach chloroplasts were harvested on a gradient of colloidal silica in the CF-6 rotor. The more dense band on the right contains almost exclusively intact chloroplasts, as indicated by the rate of CO_2-dependent O_2 evolution (lower curve).

purification with respect to s is achieved, because small particles largely escape the rotor in the spent effluent. The extent of purification with respect to s is estimated by examination of clean-out curves. Finally, the short sedimentation distance required to trap the particles means that for a given speed, clean-out is an order of magnitude better than in those continuous-flow rotors that rely on pelleting.

7.2 FLOTATION

Ogston (1963) proposed an *infracentrifuge*, in which particles would be accelerated from the edge to the center. The principle was to employ a rotor with negative radius. An alternate procedure might be to drive the centrifuge at imaginary velocities, such as $1000i$ rpm. In either case the value of $r\omega^2$ and consequently dr/dt in the basic sedimentation equation [Eq. (1.1)] becomes negative.

The same effect can be achieved with less violence to the laws of physics by working on the density factor $(\rho_p - \rho_m)$. If the density of the medium ρ_m

is made greater than the particle density ρ_p, the particles will tend to float toward the center of the rotor. A traditional protocol for analyzing serum lipoproteins consists in the differential centrifugation of sera in solutions of successively increasing density. Lipoproteins of successively higher density are thus floated to the surface. In this way hematologists designate *low density lipoproteins* (LDL), *high density lipoproteins* (HDL), and *very high density lipoproteins* (VHDL) (Havel *et al.*, 1955).

Beckman/Spinco have designed their Type 25 rotor specifically for the differential flotation of lipoproteins. It is an angle rotor and holds 100 tubes at 25° from the vertical.

Wilcox and Heimberg (1968) have adapted density gradient centrifugation to the analysis of serum lipoproteins by loading samples at the edge of a B-XXIX rotor containing a gradient of sucrose and potassium bromide. They demonstrated that the traditional serum lipoprotein fractions could be recovered from different positions in the gradient and in addition that several of them showed marked heterogeneity (cf. Fig. 9.22). One can also use swinging bucket or vertical rotors (cf. Terpstra *et al.*, 1981).

As in sedimentation, one can employ either rate–zonal or isopycnic flotation. There are, moreover, two significant tactical advantages of flotation over sedimentation: the sample starts at the edge of the rotor where the *centripetal* field is maximal and, provided the particles are compatible with the gradient solute, rather larger values of $|\rho_p - \rho_m|$ can be produced for flotation than for sedimentation.

7.3   GRADIENT CENTRIFUGATION IN ANGLE AND VERTICAL ROTORS

Density-gradient centrifugation developed in swinging-bucket rotors and was extended to zonal rotors, but Flamm *et al.* (1966) showed that a certain class of separations can be performed advantageously in the much more common angle rotors.

Meselson *et al.* (1957) discovered a gold mine of information on DNA by discovering how to separate and measure different species of these nucleic acids according to their equilibrium densities in the analytical ultracentrifuge. The separation occurs in *sedimentation equilibrium gradients* (cf. Sections 3.3.C and 8.3) of cesium and rubidium salts, in which the radial distribution of the solute is determined by an equilibrium of diffusion and sedimentation. The general principle is applicable to the preparative separation of species of DNA, where one may recover the physically separated DNAs, as well as to their analysis.

Although swinging-bucket rotors have been used for the preparative separation, there are constraints on self-generated equilibrium gradients which limit the usefulness of these rotors. Specifically, the gradient of density is rigorously determined with respect to radius such that different species of DNA band very closely to one another (Fig. 9.16). The resolution of bands is correspondingly limited. Flamm *et al.* (1966) pointed out that the generation of equilibrium gradients and the separation of DNAs could take place more rapidly in angle rotors, where the radial path over which equilibrium must occur is much shorter. More importantly, the geometry is such (Fig. 9.17) that the volumetric distance among bands is greater in angle rotors than in swinging-bucket rotors of the same total volume. Since the volumes of zones do not change during reorientation, the improved separation is retained upon reorientation and recovery. The utility of their procedure has been widely recognized and is now standard for the preparative separation of nucleic acids (cf. Section 9.5.1).

A few refinements:

(1) The reorientation of the gradient should take place slowly by allowing the rotor to coast to rest to minimize smearing of the gradient by shear (cf. Section 7.5).

(2) Viscosity increases the shear forces and the need for slow reorientation.

(3) The geometry of the angle rotor strongly influences the amplification of volumetric separation; a steep angle as in the Spinco No. 50 rotor (Table 7.2) is highly advantageous.

If a steeply inclined rotor is advantageous, why not go all the way and have a vertical rotor? DuPont–Sorvall asked that question a few years ago and

Table 7.2. Characteristics of Some Vertical and Small-Angle Rotors Useful for Density-Gradient Centrifugation

Manufacturer and designation	Place by volume	Maximum speed (rpm)	g_{max}	Angle to vertical	Radial path length (mm)
Spinco VTI50	8 × 38.5	50,000	241,200	0	25.4
Spinco VAL-26	8 × 38.5	26.000	70,000	0	25.4
Spinco JV-20	8 × 38.5	20,000	41,000	0	25.4
Sorvall TV-850	8 × 36	50,000	236,547	0	25.4
Sorvall SV-288	8 × 36	20,000	40,310	0	25.4
Spinco 30.2	20 × 10.5	30,000	94,500	14	31
Spinco 21	10 × 94	21,000	59,200	18	60
Sorvall TV-865B	8 × 17	65,000	399,765	0	
Spinco VTI65	8 × 5.1	65,000	401,700	0	12.7
Spinco VTI-80	8 × 5.1	80,000	510,000	0	12.7
Sorvall SV-80	16 × 5	19,000	40,980	0	
Sorvall TV-865	8 × 5	65,000	400,000	0	12.7

answered it with a series of rotors in which the tube cavities are indeed vertical (cf. Table 7.2). They were followed shortly by Beckman–Spinco. Sedimentation equilibrium is achieved even more rapidly in vertical rotors than in rotors with small angles and the amplification upon reorientation is somewhat greater. There are some small disadvantages in that special plugs or sealed tubes are required to retain the liquid, a program of slow acceleration and deceleration is required to prevent swirling, there are greater possibilities for wall effects, and the range of densities within a tube may be too small.

Vertical rotors may also be used for rate separations (cf. Section 9.5.2) with the attendant advantages of decreasing the time required to complete a separation. However, the increase in zone width that almost invariably accompanies rate separations (cf. Section 3.2.4) is also amplified during reorientation of the gradient; as a consequence, the time saved must be traded for a loss of resolution.

7.4   MULTIPLE-ALTERNATE-CHANNEL-SELECTION (MACS)

Among the B-XIV and B-XV types of zonal rotors (Table 6.2) are three types of removable seals: in the original Oak Ridge design, the dynamic seal remains on the rotor (Fig. 7.19a); in the Spinco and IEC versions both the dynamic and static seal are removed after the rotor is loaded.* In the IEC design, shown in Fig. 7.19b, the axial and peripheral channels of the fluid seal communicate with the center and edge channels of the rotor core through a conical seal adapter. It seemed to us (Price and Casciato, 1974) that, since the connections between seal adapter and core are determined wholly by the vertical level at which the channels are drilled, one had almost total liberty in the actual selection of which core channels should connect with those of the fluid seal.

The first application of this bit of serendipity was a *reverse flow* seal adapter (Fig. 7.20). In this case the edge channel of the rotor core is led to the axial channel of the fluid seal, a decided advantage in the edge unloading of particles sensitive to shear.

A more radical departure was the construction of a third channel for the direct injection of sample at a predetermined radius (Fig. 7.21). The advantage in this case is that no extra underlay is required to fill the rotor prior to loading the sample and overlay (cf. Fig. 6.22). Resolution with direct sample injection is almost as good as with conventional loading (Table 6.3).

* Indeed, one might call them removable, removable seals; for they have the additional advantage that the Rulon seal member may be changed during a run if trouble should develop.

(a)

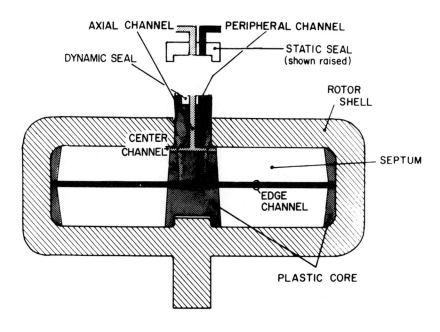

(b)

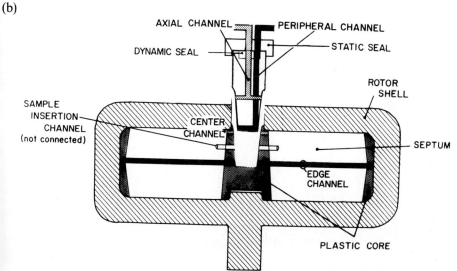

Fig. 7.19. Oak Ridge and IEC-types of removable seal adapters (Price and Casciato, 1973). (a) In the original Oak Ridge design of the B-XIV and B-XV types of rotors, the dynamic, Rulon seal remains on the spinning rotor after loading is complete; the static seal is lifted off and replaced with a vacuum cap. (b) In the IEC (shown here) and Spinco versions, the dynamic seal is also removed after the rotor is loaded, and replaced with a vacuum cap.

221

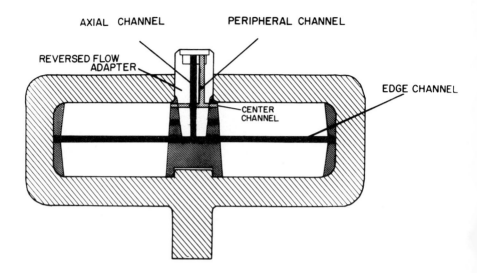

Fig. 7.20. Reverse-flow seal adapter (Price and Casciato, 1974). In an application of the MACS principle, the edge channel of the core connects with the axial channel of the seal while the center channel of the core connects with the peripheral channel of the seal. This reversal from the usual arrangement shown in Fig. 7.1b is achieved by employing an alternate seal adapter.

The general principle of multiple alternate channel selection (MACS) is simple: the two channels of the fluid seal may be connected to any pair of channels within the core through the choice of interchangeable seal adapters. Among the current or contemplated applications are a semibatch harvesting system (Fig. 7.22), in which a third channel feeds sample and displaces spent supernatant through an outlet just above a thin annular gradient; a continuous-flow system in which the gradient and sample flow through two completely independent pairs of channels (Fig. 7.13). Zonal rotors capable of handling multiple samples are also possible.

The ultimate goal is that a single rotor shell could be used to serve a wide variety of purposes, perhaps all centrifuge operations, through the use of different cores and seal adapters.

7.5   REORIENTING GRADIENT CENTRIFUGATION

The most irascible components of early zonal centrifuges were the fluid seals. At the same time that Anderson and co-workers were trying to build

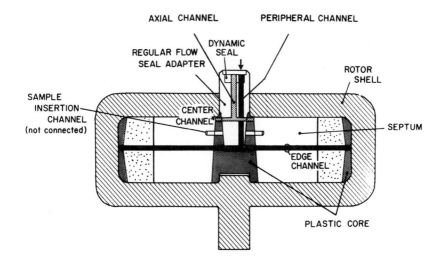

(a)

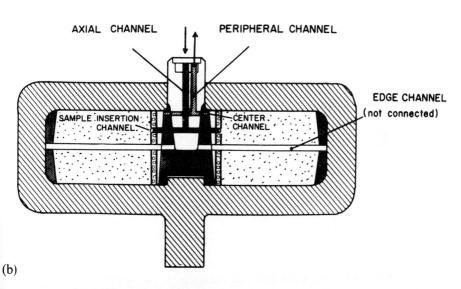

(b)

Fig. 7.21. Direct sample injection by means of MACS (Price and Casciato, 1974). The core contains a third channel which opens into the rotor cavity at a predetermined radius. (a) The gradient is introduced either with a conventional seal adapter or with one connecting the edge to periphery and the sample injection channel to the axis of the seal. (b) The sample is injected by means of another seal adapter which connects the sample injection channel to the axis and the center channel to the periphery. The sample may be preceded by an overlay through the same connections.

223

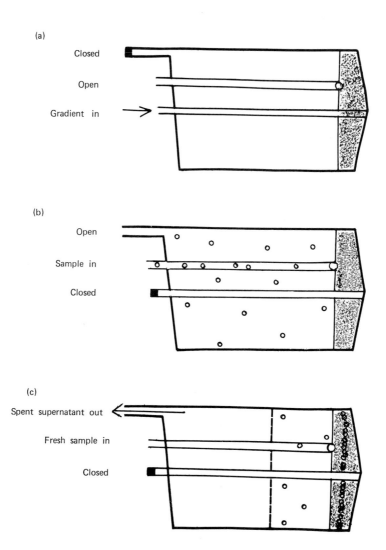

(a)

Closed

Open

Gradient in

(b)

Open

Sample in

Closed

(c)

Spent supernatant out

Fresh sample in

Closed

Fig. 7.22. Semibatch harvesting by means of MACS (C. A. Price and R. J. Casciato, unpublished). The core contains a third channel which opens into the rotor cavity a short distance from the curvature of the rotor near the edge. (a) A thin, annular gradient is first constructed outboard of the third channel. (b) The remainder of the rotor is filled with the particle suspension to be harvested by means of a seal adapter that connects the third channel of the core to axial channel of the seal and the center core channel to the periphery of the seal. The seal is removed and the rotor accelerated until the particles are cleared into the gradient. (c) The rotor is decelerated and the same seal adapter attached. A fresh volume of particle suspension is loaded into the rotor displacing the spent supernatant. The process is then repeated through additional cycles of (b) and (c). At the end of the run the particles are centrifuged to their equilibrium density in the gradient and unloaded.

more reliability into fluid seals, they also gave thought to eliminating them altogether. In an early study Anderson *et al.* (1964) considered the feasibility of filling a rotor at rest with a gradient, accelerating it to speed, decelerating, and unloading the rotor at rest.

When a gradient at rest is set in motion, fluid dynamics require simply that the meniscus be perpendicular to the summation of forces on the liquid. Considering a continuous gradient, one may visualize an infinite number of isodense surfaces, each of which must everywhere be perpendicular to the vectorial sum of the centrifugal and gravitational fields

$$\mathbf{F} = \mathbf{G} + \mathbf{r}\omega^2 \tag{7.2}$$

Equation (7.2) reduces to a paraboloid of revolution

$$\mathbf{Z} = \frac{\omega^2\mathbf{r}^2}{2\mathbf{g}} + \mathbf{Z}_0 \tag{7.3}$$

The actual slope of the surface of the paraboloid varies strongly with the angular velocity ω. If one views a gradient confined in a cylinder (Fig. 7.23), the isodense surfaces are of course horizontal at rest. As the speed increases, the gradient is depressed in the center while the isodense lines slope upward toward the lateral walls. Above a certain critical speed, the isodense lines intersect the top and bottom surfaces of the cylinder. The gradient then becomes completely transformed from a horizontal into a vertical orientation. Deceleration follows the reverse process.

As we observed (Anderson *et al.*, 1964; Price and Bostian 1964), the gradient is subjected to substantial shear during reorientation. Unless the process occurs very slowly, the gradient experiences unacceptable mixing.

Nonetheless reorienting gradient works and has had a number of useful applications. Density gradient centrifugation in angle rotors (cf. Section 7.3) relies on this process for the recovery of the gradients, as does continuous-flow centrifugation is B-XVI and K-type rotors (Harvey, 1970; cf. Section 7.1).

DNA is especially sensitive to shear, which occurs to an unacceptable degree when DNA is pumped across fluid seals of conventional diameter (cf. Section 7.7). The B-XXXIII, a reorienting gradient version of the B-XV, has been used successfully for the rate separation of high-molecular-weight DNA (Lett *et al.*, 1970). The A-XVI has been used for collecting nuclei (Elrod *et al.*, 1969).

Another rotor, the SZ-14 (Sheeler and Wells, 1969) (Fig. 7.24),* is designed to be used in the reorienting gradient mode, but the sample is normally loaded dynamically. The operation is shown in Fig. 7.25. A substantial economy has been achieved by dispensing with the fluid seal, but the principal advantage is in minimizing shear forces on delicate particles. Resolution in

* DuPont Instruments/Sorvall Operations.

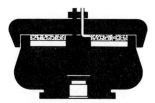

1. Density gradient and sample loaded in horizontal layers
   (Rotor at rest)

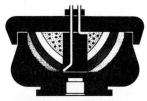

2. Layers reorient
   (Acceleration)

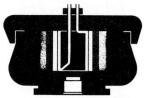

3. Layers vertical—separation of particles takes place
   (Rotor at speed)

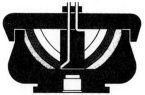

4. Layers reorient
   (Deceleration)

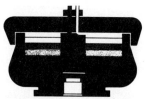

5. Density gradient and separated particles ready
   for unloading (Rotor at rest)

Fig. 7.23. Gradient reorientation (Spinco–Beckman). The sequence shows the process of gradient reorientation in a JZ rotor with a modified core.

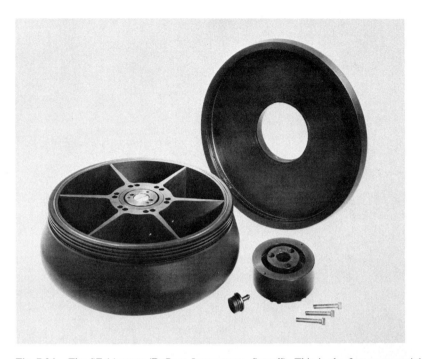

Fig. 7.24. The SZ-14 rotor (DuPont Instruments–Sorvall). This is the first commercial rotor to be designed exclusively for the reorienting gradient mode; it is normally used in a hybrid mode that nonetheless avoids extreme shear. The rotor has a six-chambered core. A clear plastic distributor is used in place of the fluid seal. The centrifugal field in the distributor serves to apportion sample equally among the six compartments. The arrow labeled core opening indicates the outlet of a channel from the distributor to one of the compartments.

the SZ-14 and other reorienting gradient systems is said to be inferior to that of dynamically unloaded rotors, but quantitative comparisons are not available.

The JCF-Z (Spinco) rotor has an interchangeable core designed for the reorienting mode (Table 6.2). The design and operation are very similar to the SZ-14. Griffith and Wright (1972) have reported semiquantitative comparisons of resolution in the reorienting and dynamic modes in the same rotor shell. They show a very similar pattern of particle zones in a fractionation of rat liver, but the results were obtained with step gradients, which tend to minimize zone broadening and at the same time lead to an undertermined degree of cross contamination between adjacent zones.

One can imagine qualitatively that a gradient will be perturbed most where the largest changes in the shape of an isodense layer occur, and that this will

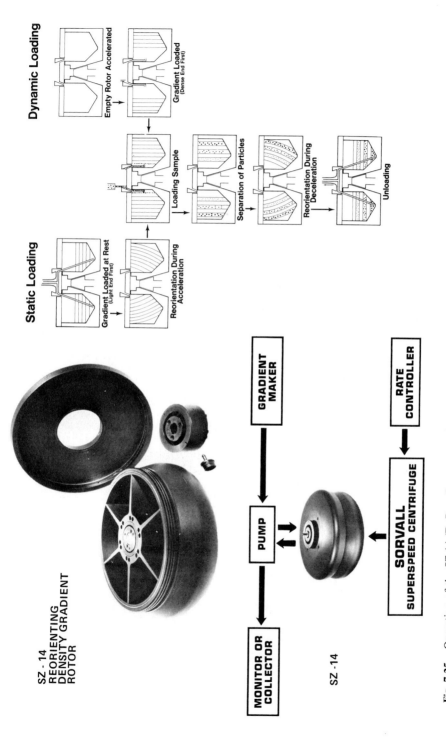

Fig. 7.25. Operation of the SZ-14 (DuPont Instruments–Sorvall). The gradient may be loaded at rest ("static loading") or dynamically ("dynamic loading."). The sample could be loaded at rest (not shown), but it is normally added dynamically. Dynamic loading minimizes the danger of sectorial loading errors. The base of the rotor is in the form of a V-shaped groove, which facilitates funneling of particle zones during unloading.

be near the middle of the gradient. Hsu and Anderson (1969) have computed these perturbations quantitatively. Hsu *et al.* (1979) have determined the effects of reorientation on resolution.

7.6 SEALS: POLISHING AND MAINTENANCE

Most zonal rotors depend on fluid seals composed of a rotating member made of Rulon* and a static member usually made of stainless steel. Single-pass seals, those which contain a single fluid channel, as in K-type rotors, present few problems. The seals of B-XIV and B-XV types of rotors with their twin channels can be another story: the smallest dent, scratch, or asymmetry on the Rulon surface can cause leakage between the axial and peripheral channels or, less likely, between the peripheral channel and the exterior.

Once a Rulon seal has been properly polished, it will last for months of daily use. A well used seal begins to leak because the Rulon member wears ruts into the static seal. Moreover, in most current commercial seal assemblies the Rulon is kept nicely enclosed, protected from finger nails. These assemblies need only be thoroughly soaked or rinsed at the end of the run to remove sucrose and salts, and perhaps lubricated.

Should the seal begin to fail, first examine the static seal face. If it is grooved, the seal face must be discarded or refaced by a machinist with access to instruments for determining optical flatness. If the static seal is sound, the integrity of the Rulon seal may be suspected. It may be polished on a large slab of plate glass by carefully rotating the surface with a sequence of polishing grits ending in levigated alumina (Table 7.3). Move frequently to a fresh spot on the glass to ensure continuing flatness and avoid asymmetrical pressure, especially rolling along the edges.

Table 7.3. Abrasives for Polishing Rulon Seals

Abrasives are listed in increasing order of fineness. Available from Edmund Scientific Company, Barrington, New Jersey, U.S.A.

No. 80 Alundum*
No. 220 Alundum
Barnsite
Rouge
Cerium oxide

* Use very sparingly and only for deep cuts.

* A compound of Teflon and iron powder; trademark of E. I. du Pont.

When properly polished and installed, the seal should pass no more than occasional bubbles through the axial channel during the loading of a gradient; in the aggregate no more than a few tenths of a milliliter should be tolerated. A seemingly modest leak permits a great deal more fluid to cross over when the sample is backed in or during edge unloading, because the pressure across the seal is then greatly increased.

Sometimes a new Rulon seal needs to be polished in order to bring its performance to an acceptable level.

7.7 ESTIMATION OF SEDIMENTATION COEFFICIENTS

We have frequently repeated the generalization that rate separations operate principally to separate particles of different sizes or sedimentation coefficients. A corollary of this statement is that one should be able to deduce the equivalent sedimentation coefficient s^* from the distance that a particle moves in a given gradient.

Bishop (1966) has developed a Fortran computer program for estimating s^* values of particles recovered from any arbitrary gradient. Her strategy was to treat each gradient fraction as a homogeneous slice and then to compute the s^* that a particle would need in order to traverse each of the preceding slices under the conditions of centrifugation.

Since the distance sedimented would also be a function of the density of the particles ρ_p, Bishop also developed a graphical plot of possible values of s^* for different ρ_p (Fig. 1.8). Although the Bishop program offers the greatest generality, there are other means of estimating s^* values for certain specific gradients.

Funding (1973) has developed an Algol program for estimating s^* values in isokinetic gradients in zonal rotors. Since the radial movements of particles in isokinetic gradients are in direct proportion to their s^* values and the $\int \omega^2 dt$, the mathematics are uncomplicated.

The equivolumetric gradient shape provides a still simpler means of estimating s^* values. Here the volumetric distance from the sample zone (i.e., the fraction number itself) is directly proportional to s^* and to the $\int \omega^2 dt$. The factor of proportionality is the equivolumetric gradient constant [Eq. (3.20) and Appendix D3,4].

---

* The sedimentation coefficient that an ideal particle would need in order to move to the same position.

7.8 TRANSPARENT ROTORS

Direct and continuous knowledge of a process is enormously more informative than data obtained from a single point in time. Imagine the poverty of precision and accuracy if the measurement of the sedimentation coefficient of a protein had to rely on a single photograph of the analytical cell of an ultracentrifuge.

Almost from the beginning of the development of zonal centrifuges, Anderson planned for transparent zonal rotors. He specifically conceived of a rotor volume held between two Plexiglas end caps (Fig. 7.26). Because of stress limitations, these would be restricted to low speeds, and therefore are found exclusively among the A-series of rotors (Appendix E). The A-XI rotor (Fig. 7.27) was an attempt at a purely analytical zonal rotor with the cells reduced to two sector-shaped compartments.

The first commercially practicable transparent zonal rotor was the A-IX (Fig. 7.26), which was quickly modified to correct a stress problem and became the A-XII. It was designed to fit (but barely) into the centrifuge chamber of the PR-2 drive unit (IEC). It contains 1300 cm^3 and an internal radius of 18 cm. The MSE version of the A-XII can be driven to 5000 rpm (Table 6.2).

The whole idea of transparent rotors is to be able to see the entire sedimentation process (cf. Fig. 7.28). In this sense the A-XII has been a success: one can optimize rate separations with many fewer tries than in opaque rotors, provided the particle zones are visible, and we even demonstrated how the rotor, fitted with a travelling microscope (Fig. 7.29 and 7.30) could be used for the direct estimation of sedimentation coefficients of large particles (Price and Hirvonen, 1967). Anderson et al. (1966) described a photoelectric scanning system for the A-XII in which a light source and detector are arranged to sweep across the radius of the rotor (Fig. 7.31a). Some results with the scanner are shown in Fig. 7.31b.

Although the relatively low speed of the A-XII has restricted its use to large particles, it is an excellent rotor for the resolution of nuclei (Fig. 9.6) and the size fractionation of whole cells (cf. Sections 9.2.1 and 9.2.3). Faster transparent rotors, the Z-8 and Z-15 (IEC) and HS (MSE) (Table 6.2), broaden the range of amenable particles to include lysosomes and others down to about 10 million dalton.

The disadvantages of current transparent rotors are their high cost (50% greater than B-type rotors) and their relative complexity. Were it commercially feasible to redesign them today, one should doubtless envision an ease of assembly and disassembly quite similar to that of the B-XIV and B-XV types.

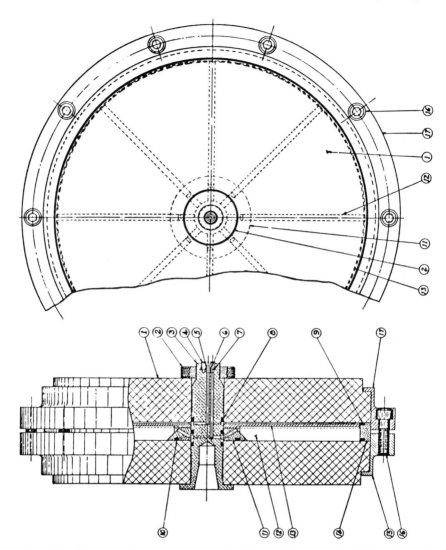

Fig. 7.26. Diagram of the transparent zonal A-IX rotor (Courtesy of Oak Ridge National Laboratories). The rotor volume is contained between plexiglass end caps (1). The sandwich is held together by aluminum rims (17). Although this relatively early rotor contained a number of features which were later modified, it provided a clear demonstration of the zonal principle. With relatively small modification, the A-IX became the A-XII.

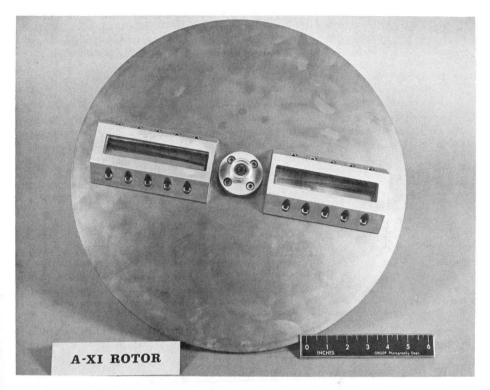

Fig. 7.27. The A-XI zonal rotor (Courtesy of Oak Ridge National Laboratories). The sedimentation of relatively large particles could be observed in the oppositely placed sector shaped compartments.

Although it would seem feasible to simply install sapphire windows in a B-XV, there would be an unavoidable loss of strength and consequent derating. What is really needed is an analytical–preparative system; that is, an electrooptical system compatible with an ultracentrifuge drive and a rotor or series of rotors to match. Unfortunately no one in the near future is likely to commit the funds required for that kind of endeavor.

7.9 ENVIRONMENTAL GRADIENTS

The concept of *environmental gradients* was first proposed by Anderson (1970) as part of a larger strategy of gradient solubilization. Particles are carried through the density gradient by rate sedimentation (Fig. 7.32). The superimposed environmental gradient is selected to solubilize the particles

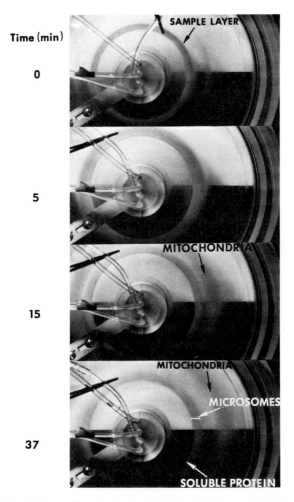

Fig. 7.28. Sedimentation of mitochondria in the A-XII rotor (R.E. Canning, unpublished). A clarified brei of liver was loaded onto a sucrose gradient in an A-XII rotor, accelerated to approximately 5000 rpm and photographed at intervals of time.

or components of the particle somewhere within the gradient by depolymerization, extraction, etc. The centrifugal field is chosen so that the resulting monomers or micromolecules once formed will not migrate sensibly during the centrifugation. However, heterogeneous particles in the original sample will have moved to different regions of the gradient before shedding their micromolecules or dissolving into them. The location of micromolecules in

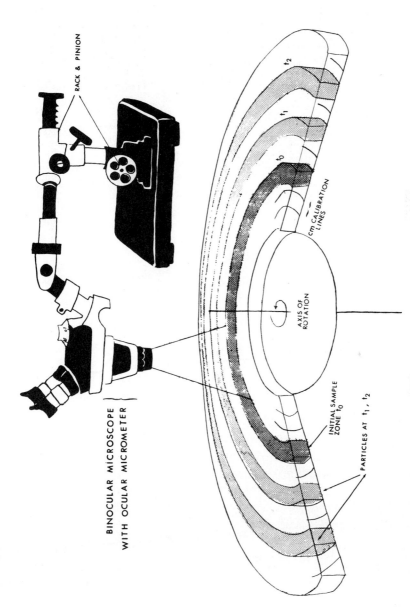

Fig. 7.29. Scheme for the measurement of sedimentation rates in the A-XII zonal rotor (Price and Hirvonen, 1967). Arcs were scribed at intervals of 1 cm in the core of the A-XII. A traveling microscope fitted with an optical micrometer focused on the bands of particles in the rotor; a zoom lens permitted the micrometer scale to correspond to an integral number of centimeters. In this way the position of a sedimenting band could be precisely measured.

RACK & PINION

BINOCULAR MICROSCOPE
WITH OCULAR MICROMETER

t_2

t_1

t_0

cm CALIBRATION
LINES

AXIS OF
ROTATION

INITIAL SAMPLE
ZONE t_0

PARTICLES AT t_1, t_2

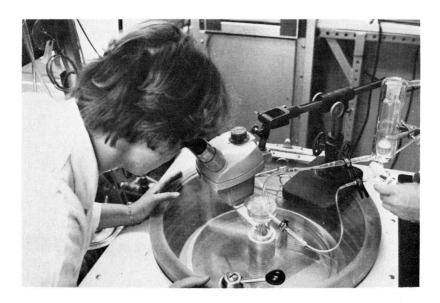

Fig. 7.30. Arrangement for measuring sedimentation rates in the A-XII. The physical arrangement is the same as that diagrammed in Fig. 7.29.

the recovered gradient should reflect either heterogeneity among particles or differential dissociation of components attached to a particle.

One application of environmental gradient centrifugation is the gradient resolubilization of viruses precipitated in polyethylene glycol. The suspension of particles is then sedimented through a reverse gradient of polyethylene glycol imposed on a sucrose density gradient. At low sedimentation rates different viruses become soluble at those concentrations of polyethylene glycol in which they are barely soluble (Clark and Lister, 1971). In a similar application Breillatt centrifuged precipitated tRNA in a gradient of cetyl trimethylammonium bromide in sucrose with an imposed gradient of NaCl (Fig. 7.33). The tRNA resolubilizes at critical concentrations of salt.

One caveat with this method: the rate of sedimentation of the particles must be slow enough that physical equilibrium between monomer and polymer or micromolecule and crystal is maintained at all times; otherwise the macromolecules will be spread over large regions of the gradient.

7.10   STERILIZATION

One frequently needs to work under sterile conditions, either for the protection of the sample or of the operator. The second case, more a question of containment, is a large and complex problem under continuing investigation (cf. Cho *et al.*, 1966). It should suffice to note here that the conventional zonal seals produce a fine aerosol, which presents a serious hazard during loading and unloading of pathogenic material.

Most of the components and accessories of zonal systems can be heat sterilized, but the consequences may be messy: the bonds between metal and PVC tubing typically loosen at sterilizing temperatures and the tubing turns opalescent, more or less reversibly. Bonds may be reinforced with tie wraps.*

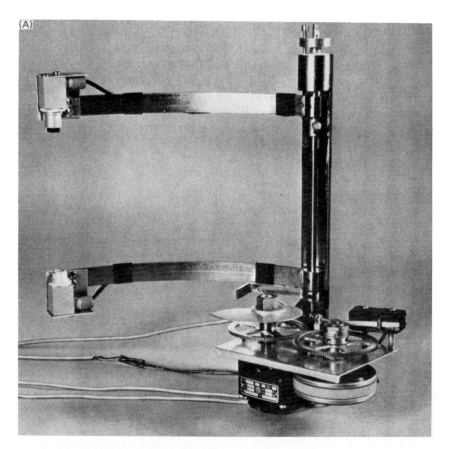

Fig. 7.31. Photoelectric scanning of transparent, A-type rotors (Courtesy of Oak Ridge National Laboratories). (A) Canning designed this device to scan the A-XII zonal rotor. The photocell at the end of the upper arm looks through the rotor to a pencil-shaped beam of light shining from the end of the lower arm. (B) A photometric trace of sedimenting ragweed pollen.

* A common item among commercial electricians.

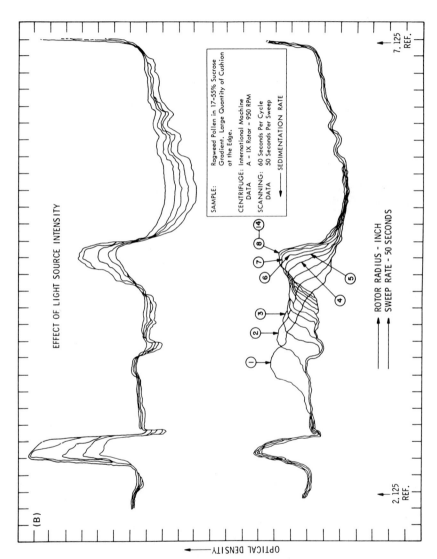

Fig. 7.31. *Continued*

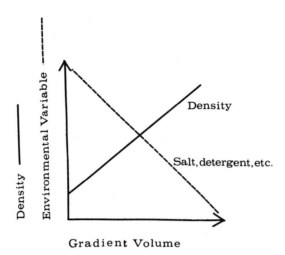

Fig. 7.32. Environmental gradients (after N. G. Anderson, 1970). A gradient of some chemical activity is imposed on a density gradient in order to immobilize or transform selectively a mixture of particles. The dotted line might represent such items as pH, salt, or detergent.

Most gradient materials may be heat sterilized, although sucrose will caramelize when heated in the presence of certain salts. Alternatively, solutions and tubing may be treated with diethyl pyrocarbonate, which decomposes to ethanol and water upon heating to 100°C for 5 min. Filtration through sterile membrane filters, usually of 0.45 μm porosity, is an alternate treatment for liquids.

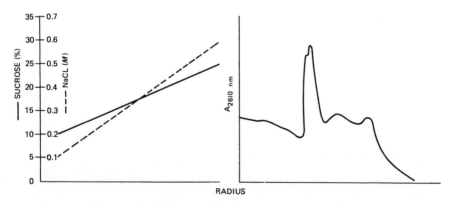

Fig. 7.33. Gradient resolubilization of tRNA (J. E. Breillatt, unpublished). (Left) A gradient of NaCl (dotted line) is superimposed on a density gradient of cetyl trimethylammonium bromide in sucrose (solid line). The sample consisted of precipitated, crude tRNA. Different species of tRNA became soluble at different concentrations of salt. (Right) Absorbancy profile of the recovered gradient.

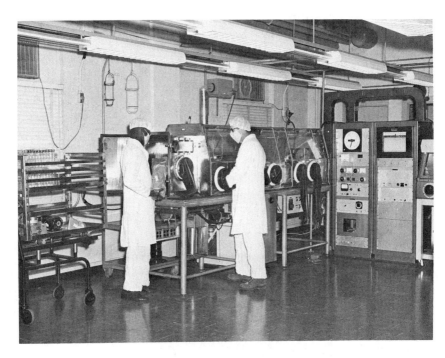

Fig. 7.34. Physical containment facility for centrifuge operations (Courtesy of Oak Ridge National Laboratories). A Model L centrifuge, whose base is visible behind the technician on the right, is surmounted by a glove box. Apparatus and materials can be sterilized in a pass-through sterilizer before leaving the enclosure.

If sterilization of rotors and tubing is to be done routinely, it will become worthwhile to outfit a sterilizer, perhaps a discarded one, for gas sterilization. Mixtures of ethylene oxide in CO_2 are commonly and conveniently employed.

There is widespread fear of the danger of explosions of ethylene oxide, but this is not a hazard with the commercial mixtures of ethylene oxide designated for sterilizing. A contained centrifuge facility at the MAN program laboratory at Oak Ridge is shown in Fig. 7.34.

7.11   OTHER USES OF DENSITY-GRADIENT CENTRIFUGATION

The rate of spreading of zones in the zonal centrifuge may be used to measure the *diffusion coefficients* of macromolecules (Halshall and Schumaker, 1970). The gradient and centrifugal fields in this case serve simply to maintain a thin zone of particles in a liquid. The method has advantages over conventional methods for measuring diffusion coefficients in the extremely small amounts of sample required. Analysis of rate sedimentation in otherwise identical gradients of sucrose in H_2O and D_2O will yield the $s_{20,w}$ and ρ_p (Sadler, 1979). If one also knows the Stokes radius, which may be obtained by gel filtration, the molecular weight and frictional coefficient may also be computed. Finally, if one is dealing with a hydrophobic protein maintained in solution with a detergent, the same data yield the amount of detergent bound to the protein.

Nieuwenhuysen (1979) described the effects of solvation on the buoyant density of sedimenting particles. He warns that large errors in the estimation of sedimentation coefficients can occur when measurements are conducted in gradients that are strongly dehydrating, such as those of sucrose.

Anderson and Breillatt (1971) adsorbed antigens and antibodies to polystyrene latex beads and observed changes in the banding densities of the beads. The procedure is sufficiently sensitive to permit measurements of the densities of the antigens and antibodies, to separate beads with the antigen attached from those with unbound antibody, and to calculate equilibrium constants between antigen and antibody (Genung and Hsu, 1978).

REFERENCES

Anderson, N. G. (1970). Method of centrifugal separation and recovery of chemical species utilizing a liquid medium. U.S. Patent 3,519,400.

Anderson, N. G., and Breillatt, J. P. (1971). Isopycnometric weighing of antibodies and antigens using polystyrene latex beads. *Fed. Proc., Fed. Am. Soc. Exp. Brol.* **30,** 594 abs.

Anderson, N. G., Barringer, H. P., Cho, N., Nunley, C. E., Babelay, E. F., Canning, R. E., and Rankin, C. T. (1966). The development of low-speed "A"-series zonal rotors. *In* "The Development of Zonal Centrifuges" (N. G. Anderson, ed.) National Cancer Institute Monograph No. 21, pp. 113–136. USDHEW, Bethesda, Maryland, 526 pp.

Anderson, N. G., Price, C. A., Fisher, W. D., Canning, R. F., and Burger, C. L. (1964). Analytical techniques for cell fractions. IV. Reorienting gradient rotors for zonal centrifugation. *Anal. Biochem.* **7,** 1–9.

Barnett, W. E., and Brown, D. H. (1967). Mitochondrial transfer ribonucleic acids. *Proc. Natl. Acad. Sci. U.S.A.* **57,** 452–458.

Bishop, B. S. (1966). Digital computation of sedimentation coefficients in zonal centrifuges. *Natl. Cancer Inst. Monog.* **21,** 175–188.

Brown, D. H., Barnett, W. E., Harrell, B. W., and Brantley, J. N. (1970). Large-scale preparation of chloroplasts by continuous-flow centrifugation in the K-X zonal rotor. *In* "Microsymposium on Particle Separation from Plant Materials" (C. A. Price, ed.), Oak Ridge Natl. Lab. pp. 17–22. Natl. Tech. Inf. Serv., Springfield, Virginia.

Cho, N., Barringer, H. P., Amburgey, J. W., Cline, G. B., Anderson, N. G., McMauley, L. L., Stevens, R. H., and Swartout, W. M. (1966). Problems in biocontainment. *Natl. Cancer Inst. Monogr.* **21,** 485–502.

Clark, M. F., and Lister, R. M. (1971). The application of polyethyleneglycol solubility–concentration gradients in plant virus research. *Virology* **43,** 338–351.

Cline, G. B. (1971). Continuous sample flow density gradient centrifugation. *In* "Progress in Separation and Purification" (E. S. Perry and C. J. Van Oss, eds.), pp. 297–324. Wiley, New York.

Cline, G. B., and Dagg, M. K. (1973). Particle separations in the J- and RK-types of Flo-Band zonal rotors. *In* "Advances With Zonal Rotors" (E. Reid, ed.), Vol. 3, pp. 61–273. Longmans, Green, New York.

Cline, G. B., and Ryel, R. B. (1971). Zonal centrifugation. *In* "Methods in Enzymology" (W. B. Jakoby, ed.), Vol. 22, pp. 168–204. Academic Press, New York.

Elrod, L. H., Patrick, L. C., and Anderson, N. G. (1969). Analytical techniques for cell fractions. XIII. Rotor A-XVI, a plastic gradient-reorienting rotor for isolating nuclei. *Anal. Biochem.* **30**, 230–248.

Flamm, N. G., Bond, H. E., and Burr, H. E. (1966). Density-gradient centrifugation of DNA in a fixed angle rotor. A higher order of resolution. *Biochim. Biophys. Acta* **129**, 310–317.

Funding, L. (1973). Analytical ultracentrifugations with zonal rotors. *Spectra 2000* **4**, 46–49.

Genung, R. K., and Hsu, H.-W. (1978). Interaction of antibody with antigen immobilized on polystyrene latex beads: Characterization by density gradient centrifugation. *Anal. Biochem.* **91**, 651–662.

Griffith, O. M. (1975). "Techniques of Preparative, Zonal, and Continuous-Flow Ultracentrifugation." Beckman Instruments, Inc., Spinco Division, Belmont, California.

Griffith, O. M., and Wright, H. (1972). Resolution of components from rat liver homogenate in reorienting density gradients. *Anal. Biochem.* **47**, 575–583.

Halsall, H. B., and Schumaker, V. N. (1970). Diffusion coefficients from the zonal ultracentrifuge using microgram and milligram quantities of material. *Biochim. Biophys. Acta* **39**, 479–485.

Harvey, D. R. (1970). Reorienting gradient technique for continuous-flow centrifugation. *Anal. Biochem.* **33**, 469–471.

Havel, R. J., Eder, H. A., and Bragdon, J. H. (1955). The distribution and chemical composition of ultracentrifugally separated lipoproteins in human serum. *J. Clin. Invest.* **34**, 1345–1353.

Hsu, H. W., and Anderson, N. G. (1969). Transport phenomena in zonal rotors. II. A mathematical analysis of the areas of isodensity surfaces in reorienting gradient systems *Biophys. J.* **9**, 173–188.

Hsu, H.-W., Brantley, J. N., and Breillatt, J. P. (1979). Transport phenomena in zonal centrifuge rotors. XII. Dispersion in reorienting self-generating density gradients. *Sep. Sci. Technol.* **14**, 69–77.

Lett, J. T., Klucis, E. S., and Sun, C. (1970). On the size of the DNA in the mammalian chromosome. Structural subunits. *Biophys. J.* **10**, 277–292.

Meselson, M., Stahl, F. W., and Vinograd, J. (1957). Equilibrium sedimentation of macromolecules in density gradients. *Proc. Natl. Acad. Sci. (U.S.A.)* **43**, 581–583.

Morgenthaler, J.-J., Marsden, M. P. F., and Price, C. A. (1975). Factors affecting the separation of photosynthetically competent chloroplasts in gradients of silica sols. *Arch. Biochem. Biophys.* **167**, 289–301.

Nieuwenhuysen, P. (1979). Density-gradient-sedimentation velocity of solvated macromolecules: Theoretical considerations about the buoyancy factor. *Biopolymers* **18**, 277–284.

Ogston, A. G. (1963). A survey of the uses of the ultracentrifuge in biological research. *In* "Ultracentrifugal Analysis in Theory and Experiment" (J. W. Williams, ed.), pp. 263–272. Academic Press, New York.

Perardi, T. E., and Anderson, N. G. (1970). K-series centrifuges. Effect of core taper on particle capture efficiency. *Anal. Biochem.* **34**, 112–122.

Price, C. A., and Bostian, G. (1964). Development of reorienting gradient centrifugation using the A-XIII rotor. *Oak Ridge Natl. Lab.* [*Rep.*] *ORNL* **ORNL-3656**, 15–22.

Price, C. A., and Casciato, R. J. (1974). Multiple alternate channel selection (MACS): New versatility for zonal rotors. *Anal. Biochem.* **57**, 356–362.

Price, C. A., and Hirvonen, A. P. (1967). Sedimentation rates of plastids in an analytical zonal rotor. *Biochim. Biophys. Acta* **148**, 531–538.

Price, C. A., Breden, E. N., and Vasconcelos, A. C. (1973a). Isolation of spinach chloroplasts in the CF-6 continuous-flow zonal rotor; implications for membrane-bound organelles. *Anal. Biochem.* **54**, 239–246.

Price, C. A., Mendiola, L. R., and Morgenthaler, J.-J. (1973b). Sedimentation behavior of Euglena chloroplasts in isosmotic gradients of Ficoll. *Fed. Proc., Fed. Am. Soc. Exp. Biol.* **32**(3).

Price, C. A., Mendiola-Morgenthaler, L. R., Goldstein, M., Breden, E. N., and Guillard, R. R. L. (1974). Harvest of planktonic marine algae by centrifugation into gradients of silica in the CF-6 continuous-flow zonal rotor. *Biol. Bull. (Woods Hole, Mass.)* **147**, 136–145.

Sartory, W. K. (1969). Instability in diffusing fluid layers. *Biopolymers* **7**, 251–263.

Sartory, W. K. (1970). Fractional celanout in a continuous-flow centrifuge. *Sep. Sci.* **5**, 137–143.

Sheeler, P., and Wells, J. R. (1969). A reorienting gradient zonal rotor for low-speed separation of cell components. *Anal. Biochem.* **32**, 38–47.

Sorrentıno, J., Metzgar, D. P., and Bolyn, A. E. (1973). Purification of influenza vaccine on a commercial scale using density gradient centrifugation. *Spectra 2000* **4**, 205–210.

Terpstra, A. H. M., Woodward, C. J. M., and Sanchez-Muniz, F. J. (1981). Improved techniques for the separation of serum lipoproteins by density gradient ultracentrifugation: Visualization by prestaining and rapid separation of serum lipoproteins from small volumes of serum. *Anal. Biochem.* **111**, 149–157.

Wilcox, H. G., and Heimberg, M. (1968). The isolation of human serum lipoproteins by zonal ultracentrifugation. *Biochim. Biophys. Acta* **152**, 424–426.

8

Analytical Centrifugation in Density Gradients (by Eric F. Eikenberry)

The objective of analytical centrifugation is the accurate measurement of one or more physicochemical properties of the solute particles contained in the sample. The most precise measurements of this type may be made in the analytical centrifuge, which permits continuous optical observation of the sample during centrifugation. To achieve this, the sample is contained in a special cell equipped with transparent windows. Calibrated, precision optical systems permit measurement of absorbance, refractive index, or refractive index gradient of the sample solution. Because the primary aim is a measurement, emphasis is placed on the use of minimal amounts of material contained in small sample volumes and generally no attempt is made to recover separated or purified material.

In this chapter, the discussion focuses on the use of density gradient techniques in the analytical centrifuge. Zonal rotors with transparent plastic endplates may also be used as analytical rotors. In these rotors one measures the radial position of a zone by means of a traveling microscope. This information may be used to estimate a sedimentation coefficient as well as to determine visually when a desired separation has been achieved. The separated material in this case is readily recovered. Analytical zonal centrifugation is discussed in Chapter 7.

The majority of experiments performed in the analytical centrifuge may be grouped in four basic types: boundary sedimentation, sedimentation–diffusion equilibrium or approach to equilibrium in a two-component system, band sedimentation, and sedimentation–diffusion equilibrium in a density gradient. The theoretical background for these analyses is presented in Chapters 3 and 4. In the discussion that follows, the term "macromolecules" means any molecular species, mixture of species, or indeed any collection of particles.

Boundary sedimentation.   In this type of experiment an initially uniform suspension of macromolecules is centrifuged at sufficiently high speed that the sedimenting motion of the particles predominates over their tendency to diffuse. Thus, a boundary is formed at the meniscus of the fluid column and moves toward the bottom of the cell during the course of the experiment. The motion of the boundary may be used to determine the sedimentation coefficient of the particles, while the shape of the boundary can give information concerning the homogeneity of the particles in the sample (cf. Fig. 2.3).

Sedimentation–diffusion equilibrium in a two-component system. If the centrifuge is operated at a much lower speed than is required for a boundary sedimentation experiment, the effects of diffusion will become significant. If the experiment is sufficiently prolonged, equilibrium is established between centrifugal transport of the macromolecules by sedimentation and centripetal transport by diffusion. The distribution of the molecules at equilibrium is a function of the molecular weight of the molecules (cf. Section 4.3.7). This technique is in fact used as a precise method for the determination of molecular weights. A related technique is that of *approach to equilibrium* in which information regarding the molecular weight of a species is extracted from measurements of the concentration distribution as a function of radius and time before equilibrium is attained.

Band sedimentation. This technique, which is the analytical version of the widely used zone sedimentation technique (Chapter 6), is discussed in Section 8.2.

Sedimentation–diffusion equilibrium in a density gradient.   This technique is discussed in detail in Section 8.3.

The generation and utilization of density gradients is of explicit importance only in band sedimentation and sedimentation–diffusion equilibrium in a density gradient, which are the primary subjects of this discussion. Small density gradients must also be present both in boundary sedimentation and in sedimentation–diffusion equilibrium. Indeed, the presence of these small density gradients is of vital importance to the stability of the fluid column in these experiments. However, generation of the density gradients is incidental to the experimental procedure and is not generally of any concern to the experimenter. Further discussion of boundary sedimentation and sedimentation–diffusion equilibrium may be found in Schachman (1959). Yphantis (1964), Van Holde (1971), and Williams (1979).

8.1 THE HARDWARE OF ANALYTICAL CENTRIFUGATION

8.1.1 Cells and Rotors

The sample for analytical centrifugation is contained in a cell such as that illustrated in Fig. 8.1. The cell housing and associated hardware serve to hold the two windows forcibly against the centerpiece. The resulting sealed cavity is the sample compartment. When the cell is properly installed in the rotor with the cell axis parallel to the axis of rotation, the sample compartment is an accurate cylindrical sector centered on the axis of rotation. The assembled cell may be filled through a small hole in the center of the centripetal side of the cell housing.

A variety of centerpieces is available. The one illustrated in Fig. 8.1 is a standard, single-sector centerpiece, which has a 4° sector angle, a thickness of 12 mm, and a capacity of approximately 0.7 cm³. When filled completely, the height of the fluid column, measured along a radius of the rotor, is also 12 mm. A double-sector centerpiece is favored for many types of experiments. One compartment is filled with the sample solution while the other

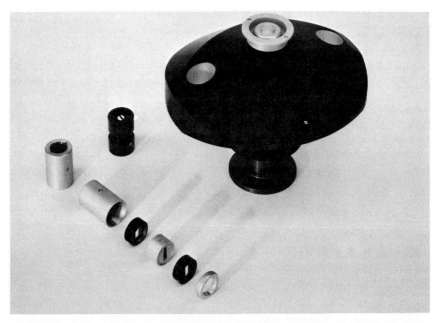

Fig. 8.1. Rotor and cell of an analytical ultracentrifuge (Beckman–Spinco). The An-D rotor operates in the Model E Analytical Ultracentrifuge. An analytical cell, shown disassembled at lower, left, fits in the circular holes on either side of the rotor. This cell contains a standard single-sector centerpiece.

compartment is used as a reference and is filled with solvent. Each compartment has a sector angle of 2° and a capacity of approximately 0.35 cm³.

The windows of analytical cells are usually made of quartz. However, sapphire may be employed when the mechanical distortion caused by the centrifugal field must be minimized for optical reasons. Sapphire windows are especially useful in interference photography. A further improvement in optical quality can be obtained by using plane-polarized illumination in conjunction with sapphire windows (Williams, 1979).

Figure 8.1 illustrates a standard two-cell rotor. This rotor, in the aluminum version, may be used at speeds up to 60,000 rpm, while the titanium version is rated for a maximum of 70,000 rpm. At 70,000 rpm an acceleration of approximately 387,000 g is obtained at the base of the fluid column. Other rotors are designed to hold four or six cells, but are restricted to lower speeds.

8.1.2 Optical Measurements

The optical systems in analytical centrifuges have been devised to measure continuously any of three solution parameters as a function of radius in the rotor, namely (1) absorbance, (2) refractive index gradient, and (3) refractive index difference. These functions are performed, respectively, by the ultraviolet (UV)-adsorption optical system, the Schlieren optical system, and the Rayleigh interference system. Of these, only the absorption system is important for density gradient work; in comparison, measurements based on refractive index generally lack sensitivity and are subject to strong interference by the density gradients. These systems and other means of making optical measurements in analytical centrifugation have been reviewed by Schachman (1959) and Tanford (1961).

The absorption optical system displays the solution absorbancy, usually in the UV region of the spectrum, as a function of radius in the rotor. When the experimental material contains compounds that have a high extinction coefficient, this system is considerably more sensitive than the systems which measure refractive index changes. In addition, measurements based on absorption can usually be selective for the macromolecular component under investigation with minimal interference from other components that may be present in the solution. In contrast, refractive index measurements are not selective.

Data may be recorded photographically or by use of a photoelectric scanner system. If the record is made photographically, the positions of bands or boundaries may be measured on the film with the aid of a microdensitometer. Figure 8.2 shows a typical film record from a UV-absorption system for a band sedimentation experiment. This optical system utilizes the

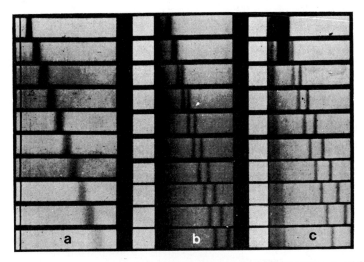

Fig. 8.2. Band sedimentation of viruses (Vinograd *et al.*, 1963). A 30-mm band-forming centerpiece was used and photographs were taken in the UV at 16-min intervals. The meniscus is at the left. (a) Southern bean mosaic virus sedimented in 1 M NaCl, .04 M NaPO$_4$, pH 6.9. The virus was loaded in a zone of 50 mm^3 and the rotor speed was 12,590 rpm. (b,c) Resolution of two forms of λ-phage, wildtype and a more slowly sedimenting mutant, by band sedimentation in CsCl. The sample zone was 25 mm^3. (b) Bulk solution $\rho = 1.25$, 12,590 rpm: (c) $\rho = 1.34$, 20,410 rpm.

light from a mercury vapor lamp which is filtered to isolate the emission line at 254 nm.

The photoelectric scanner system measures the difference in absorbance between the solution and the reference solvent which are contained respectively in the two compartments of a double-sector cell. The result is that one obtains the equivalent of a double-beam absorbance measurement. The output consists of a chart recording of the relative absorbance as a function of radius in the rotor (cf. Schachman and Edelstein, 1966; Williams, 1979). This chart record is very similar to that obtained from a microdensitometer scan of a film record (except that the film is a negative image), but the precision of the measurements from the scanner is greatly improved over those from film. Figure 8.3 illustrates a scanner record from an experiment similar to the one shown in Figure 8.2. The scanner system also possesses considerable advantages in reproducibility and speed of operation. Further, the scanner system is used in conjunction with a monochromator; so that the wavelength of the illumination can be chosen to suit a particular experiment.

The absorption optical system requires solute concentrations sufficient to give a differential absorbance in the range of approximately 0.05 to 1.0 at the wavelength chosen. This system is especially useful in band sedimentation experiments and in sedimentation–diffusion equilibrium in density gradients.

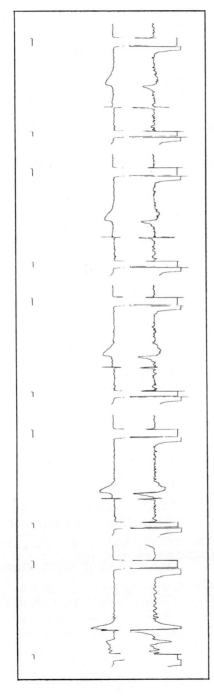

Fig. 8.3. Photoelectric scanner record of band sedimentation of λ-phage DNA (Chevrenka and Elrod, 1971). A band of λdg DNA was layered over 0.1 *M* NaCl in a band-forming centerpiece and sedimented at 30,000 rpm. The cell was scanned at 265 nm at 8-min intervals. The upper trace is the absorbance and the lower trace is its first derivative. The meniscus can be seen as a stationary vertical line about one-third the distance from the left of each frame.

8.2   ANALYTICAL BAND SEDIMENTATION IN DENSITY GRADIENTS

The technique of band sedimentation in self-generating density gradients utilizing a special band-forming centerpiece was developed for the analytical centrifuge by Vinograd et al. (1963). Although this method is completely analogous to zone sedimentation in preparative centrifugation the term band sedimentation is commonly used. In this technique a small volume of a suspension of macromolecules is deposited on the surface of a sedimentation medium which contains a shallow density gradient. This deposition occurs automatically at the beginning of the experiment shortly after the rotor begins to turn. The sedimentation medium, which is also called the sedimentation solvent, serves to stabilize the fluid column against convection and provides an ionic environment and solution density which may be controlled to enhance the desired separation. The macromolecules sediment outward from the sample lamella through the density gradient and separation of components takes place in accordance with differences in the sedimentation coefficients of the macromolecular species in the sample.

Band sedimentation offers several advantages in comparison to the traditional boundary sedimentation technique.

(1) Very small amounts of material are required.

(2) Resolved components are physically separated from each other and therefore do not have the opportunity to interact. Since nonsedimenting material is left behind on the top of the fluid column, the method is free from the Johnston–Ogston effect, in which the sedimentation coefficient of a macromolecule is reduced by the presence of a slower sedimenting species.

(3) The sedimentation medium may be chosen arbitrarily, subject to the requirements of forming the density gradient. Dialysis is not required to adjust the small-molecule content of the sample.

(4) With UV-absorption optics, which are ideally suited for use in band sedimentation, the motion of a band is much easier to follow and evaluate than the motion of a boundary.

Disadvantages of the technique are that more manipulations are required in setting up the experiment than in boundary sedimentation analysis and convective disturbances occasionally occur in the density gradient which necessitate the repetition of the experiment.

Band sedimentation is especially applicable to the study of nucleic acids, viruses, and other nucleoprotein particles (Vinograd and Bruner, 1966; Burton and Sinsheimer, 1965). This method may also be applied to proteins, but the results are less satisfactory because of spreading of the bands caused by diffusion (Vinograd et al., 1963).

8.2.1 Method

Three types of modified single-sector centerpieces for use in band sedimentation have been described by Vinograd *et al.* (1965). These are designated types I, II, and III, and are illustrated in Fig. 8.4. They differ chiefly in the method of transfer of the sample from the sample well to the top of the density gradient. In the type I centerpiece transfer takes place through the narrow channel cut in the face of the centerpiece which is pressed against the upper cell window. Transfer in the type II centerpiece takes place through a gap between the face of the centerpiece and the window. This gap is maintained by placing a gasket between the two parts during assembly of the cell. In the type III centerpiece transfer takes place through the upper channel when displacing fluid from the gradient enters the lower channel under the influence of the centrifugal field. The type I centerpiece is well suited to general work, whereas type III is useful with somewhat viscous solutions, such as DNA, under conditions in which the density difference between the medium and the solution is large. Type II is the easiest to make, but in use it usually results in some mixing of the sample with the gradient during transfer.

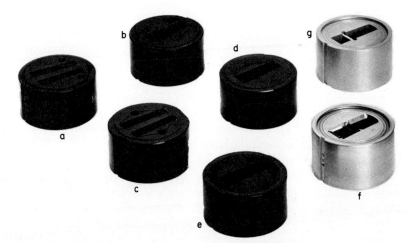

Fig. 8.4. Centerpieces for band sedimentation (Beckman–Spinco). (a) band-forming, type I, double sector; (b) band-forming, type I, single sector; (c) band-forming, type III, double sector; (d) band-forming, type III, single sector; (e) band-forming, type II; (f) mechanical separation, moving partition; and (g) mechanical separation, fixed partition centerpieces.

In use, the cell is partly assembled with the centerpiece and lower window in place in the cell housing. The sample, usually between 10 and 50 mm^3 in volume, is placed in the sample well, and assembly of the cell is completed. The cell is then filled through the normal filling hole with the sedimentation medium. The level of filling is determined by the requirement that the transfer of the sample, which is caused by hydrostatic pressure, must take place when the rotor is accelerated. Surface tension of the liquids in the narrow channels prevents any premature mixing. Sample transfer normally takes place when the rotor speed reaches 500–2000 rpm. The transfer may be monitored conveniently with the Schlieren optical system because a sharp gradient in refractive index is characteristic of the boundary between the sample and the medium.

8.2.2 Sample Requirements

The necessary concentration of macromolecules in a sample for band sedimentation analysis is determined by the requirement that the band be discernible by the optical system throughout the experiment. With absorption optics this implies that the extinction coefficient, as well as the sedimentation coefficient and the diffusivity of the macromolecules must be taken into account. Sample volumes as mentioned previously are generally in the range of 10 to 50 mm^3. The smaller volumes give sharper initial bands, but tend to aggravate problems with convective instabilities in the fluid column (cf. Section 8.2.3). A practical optimum concentration is that which will give an absorbance of approximately 0.5 at the band maximum. To compensate for diffusion, an initial concentration somewhat higher than this is usually chosen.

With samples which have strongly concentration-dependent sedimentation coefficients, such as native high-molecular-weight DNA, it is useful to reduce the sample concentration below this optimum. It is possible to obtain useful results with an absorbance at the band maximum as low as 0.05. For native DNA a minimum of approximately 0.1 μg of material is required.

The density of the sample must be such that an adequate stabilizing density gradient is formed when the sample is transferred to the top of the column of sedimentation medium. This requires that the concentration in the sample of low-molecular-weight solutes, such as salt, must be low in comparison to the concentration in the medium. This is discussed further in Section 8.2.3.

8.2.3 The Density Gradient

The stabilizing density gradient in band sedimentation is formed in two different ways: (1) by diffusion of low-molecular-weight solutes into the sample lamella; and (2) by redistribution of low-molecular-weight solutes in the centrifugal field. The former is called the *diffusion gradient*, the latter is the *field gradient*. The diffusion gradient is formed very quickly after the sample is layered onto the sedimentation medium, but it is confined to the upper part of the fluid column. Thus, the diffusion gradient is responsible for stabilizing the motion of the band during the early part of the experiment. The field gradient is formed first at the top and bottom of the fluid column and moves gradually toward the center. While the diffusion gradient tends toward zero with increasing time, the field gradient increases throughout the experiment, tending asymptotically to the equilibrium distribution of the low-molecular-weight solute. Thus, the field gradient becomes especially important when the sedimenting band of macromolecules is in the lower portion of the fluid column. In band sedimentation, both the diffusion and the field gradients are small in magnitude compared with the preformed density gradients commonly used in preparative density-gradient centrifugation.

The magnitude of the diffusion gradient is directly proportional to the volume of the sample and to the density difference between the sample and the sedimentation medium. The density difference between the sample and the medium is generally caused by a difference in the concentration of a single low-molecular-weight compound such as NaCl, CsCl, KCl, or D_2O. With these rapidly diffusing substances, a density difference of 0.02 to 0.04 gm/cm^3 between the sample and the medium is generally sufficient to stabilize the bands from a 10-mm^3 sample. A larger sample volume allows the density difference to be smaller.

If a higher-molecular-weight solute, such as sucrose, is used in the medium, the diffusion gradient is formed more slowly. In this case, it may be necessary to use a lower rotor speed than when a salt is used. This is done to prevent the sedimenting band from overrunning the diffusion gradient.

As in preparative density gradient centrifugation, the proper choice of the density of the sedimentation medium can enhance the resolution of components with differing buoyant densities. Concentrated salt solutions are very useful in this regard because they tend to promote unfolding of high-molecular-weight polymers and to reduce the interactions among molecules, and because a wide range of densities is available. If low ionic strength is required, D_2O may be used as the sedimentation medium for samples constituted in H_2O. Alternatively one may use organic solutes such as sucrose to form the medium.

8.2.4 Measurements

Two factors considerably simplify the interpretation of the results from band sedimentation experiments: (1) the sample concentration is usually very low; and (2) the density gradient is very shallow. The low sample concentrations typically used frequently allow a measured sedimentation coefficient to be interpreted directly as $s°$, the sedimentation coefficient at infinite dilution, without the necessity of performing measurements at several concentrations and extrapolating the results to infinite dilution. Because the sedimenting bands generally are nearly symmetrical, one can estimate sedimentation coefficients simply from the positions of the concentration maxima of the bands.

The estimate of the sedimentation coefficient $s°$ may be obtained through use of Eqs. (4.9) or (4.13). The use of these equations requires that the variation of the density of the solvent as a function of radius be negligible. The very shallow density gradients used in band sedimentation usually allow this assumption to be made and while yielding reasonably precise results. Although the gradient of density may be neglected, the magnitude of the density is not negligible and the value $s°$ obtained must be corrected to standard conditions for comparison with other values by the use of Eq. (4.11). The assumption that the gradient of density is negligible is invalid in a case in which the quantity $(1 - \bar{v}\rho)$ is very close to zero (i.e., in a case in which the particle density nearly matches the solvent density). In such a case numerical integration of Eq. (4.14) is required to estimate accurately the sedimentation coefficient.

The assumption that the sample particles sediment essentially at infinite dilution becomes questionable in the case of strongly interacting molecules, such as DNA strands, which give highly concentration-dependent sedimentation coefficients. This problem may be ameliorated by working with carefully chosen extremely low concentrations and by using a long path-length cell. Special cells with path lengths of 30 mm (measured parallel to the axis of rotation) as compared to the usual 12 mm allow the sample concentration to be reduced by a factor of 2.5 while maintaining the same degree of optical detectability of the bands. The 30-mm cells require the use of a special rotor and, for precise work, a refocusing of the optical system.

Concentration dependence causes the sedimentation coefficient to decrease at increasing concentrations of the sample. Since the velocity of sedimentation is proportional to the sedimentation coefficient, concentration dependence causes a sedimenting band to spread toward the front (i.e., away from the center of the rotor) and to sharpen at the back. Thus bands of such materials tend to become asymmetrical with a tail in the direction of sedimentation. This appearance may also be caused by an inadequate density gradient which fails to support properly the sedimenting band. These cases may be distinguished by experiments in which more concentrated sedimentation media are used in order to increase the magnitude of the density gradient. Broad bands may also be caused by heterodispersity in the sample; this, of course, is not a fault. However, these three causes of band spreading may be difficult to distinguish experimentally.

8.3 SEDIMENTATION–DIFFUSION EQUILIBRIUM IN A DENSITY GRADIENT

This technique resolves a sample into components of differing buoyant densities. The term "buoyant density" means the fluid density in which the sample particles manifest no tendency either to float or to sediment. Thus, the buoyant density is defined operationally in terms of experimental observations. This parameter is also referred to as the equilibrium density or the isodensity of the particle, and is equivalent to the reciprocal of the partial specific volume in the particular solvent used in the experiment. The observed buoyant density is profoundly influenced by various components of the medium (cf. Section 8.3.4); hence use of the term particle density is inappropriate, as that connotes a property of the particles alone.

Resolution into components according to buoyant density is accomplished in a density gradient formed by a low-molecular-weight solute at sedimentation equilibrium (cf. Section 4.3.8). Particles in such a gradient tend to move to that position in the gradient at which the sedimenting force vanishes and, hence, will form a zone or band at their isopycnic position in the gradient. The resolving power of this procedure can be very great. The difference in buoyant density between two high-molecular-weight DNAs may readily be quantified with a precision better than 1 mg/cm^3 in replicated determinations.

This technique may be used to (1) measure the absolute buoyant density of a macromolecular species; (2) measure the buoyant density of a macromolecular species relative to the density of a known marker; (3) analyze a mixture of macromolecules of differing densities; (4) estimate molecular weight; or (5) estimate partial specific volume and preferential hydration. The preparative application of this method is discussed in Section 7.3.

This technique has been most widely applied to the analysis of nucleic acids, especially DNA (see, e.g., Meselson and Stahl, 1958; Szybalski, 1968; Dawid et al., 1970; Brown et al., 1971). Proteins and glycoproteins may be banded at equilibrium in gradients of mineral salts, but form very wide bands because of their comparatively low molecular weights [Eq. (4.33)] (Ifft, 1969; Creeth and Denborough, 1970; Adams and Schumaker, 1970; Lundh, 1977). Chromatin has been banded at low ionic strength in gradients of chloral hydrate (Hossainy et al., 1973).

8.3.1 Method

For this application a standard single or double-sector cell is chosen which allows a fluid column height of 12 mm to be used. The cell is filled with a uniform solution containing the gradient-forming solute (generally a simple salt such as CsCl) and the particles to be analyzed. The centrifuge is operated at 30,000–45,000 rpm until equilibrium is attained, generally about 20–30 hr. The lower rotor speeds require longer times to reach equilibrium. The higher rotor speeds give sharper bands, but the gradient of density is steeper, which causes the bands to be closer together. Accordingly, there is no best rotor speed, and the speeds used in various laboratories are largely based on custom.

Data are recorded using UV-absorption optics with either photographic film or the photoelectric scanner. The latter necessitates the use of a double-sector cell. Absorption optics are a must in this case because the density gradients manifest huge changes in refractive index, while zones of particles are nearly invisible refractometrically. Figure 8.5 shows a photograph in UV light of DNA at equilibrium in a gradient of CsCl.

8.3.2 Choice of Solute

Values of $1/\beta^0 = (1/\omega^2 r)dp/dr$ Eq. (4.31), Ifft, 1969; Sharp and Ifft, 1979, and Appendix C16] are used to predict and interpret the results of sedimentation equilibrium in density gradients. The choice of solute is made on the basis of the solubility and biological integrity of the particles to be separated along with the requirement that the solute be capable of achieving a solution density greater than the buoyant density of the solvated particle. Some prior knowledge of the expected buoyant density is required or one must perform preliminary trial and error experiments to find it. In general, there is no theoretical basis for predicting this density. In addition the choice of solute affords the resolution between particles of similar density according to Eq. (4.34). Once the choice of solute is made, Eq. (4.32), together with a choice of initial solute concentration, may be used to predict where in the fluid a column the material under investigation will band, a consideration which also affects the speed chosen for the centrifuge. It may be noted that higher speeds produce steeper, longer gradients which may be useful if the buoyant density of the particles is imprecisely known. The initial solute concentration is usually chosen to give an initial density equal to the expected buoyant density. This choice serves to band the material near the center of the fluid column. A critical examination of pressure effects requires that this location be varied during the course of the experiments to permit extrapolation to zero pressure. Finally Eq. (4.33) may be used to predict the width of the bands.

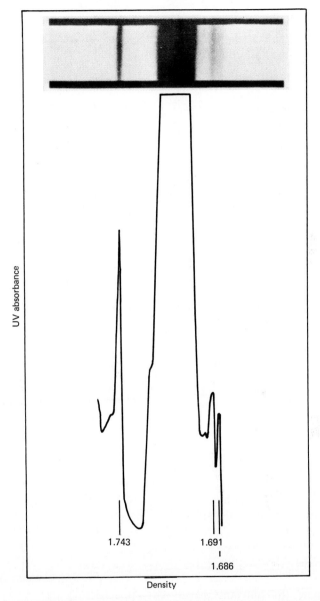

Fig. 8.5.   Equilibrium density sedimentation of DNA from *Euglena* (Edelman *et al.*, 1965). Deoxyribonucleic acid was extracted from whole cells and spun to equilibrium in CsCl in an analytical cell of the Model E. The photograph at the top of the figure was taken in the UV; the trace below is a densitometer scan of the photograph. The band at 1.743 cm^3 is a density standard; the main band, greatly overloaded, corresponds to nuclear DNA; and several satellite bands at lower densities correspond to chloroplast and mitochondrial DNAs.

The time required to achieve equilibrium in these experiments can be very long using as starting conditions a uniform suspension of all ingredients. The time may be reduced drastically by using very short fluid columns [Eq. (4.29)]

8.3.3 Sample Requirements

The primary constraint on the sample is that there be sufficient absorbance to be detected. Since this is a true equilibrium technique, there are no problems with overloading, and convective stability is ensured by the strong density gradient. The amount of sample required is in turn dependent on the molecular weight of the sample because the width of the band at equilibrium is inversely proportional to the square root of the molecular weight of the macromolecules (Eq. 4.33). For a single species of high-molecular-weight DNA, $0.25-0.5$ μg suffices to give a strong band; one-tenth of this can be detected readily.

The gradient-forming solute may be introduced into the sample in the dry form or as a saturated stock solution. The most commonly used gradient-forming solutes are CsCl and Cs_2SO_4, both of which are able to give aqueous solutions of comparatively high density. The density of the sample solution is adjusted so that the macromolecules band in the central portion of the fluid column, which implies that the initial density of the uniform solution should approximately match the buoyant density of the macromolecules. The density of the sample may be estimated refractometrically, pycnometrically, or with a digital density meter (Elder; 1979), either before the experiment or afterward. In the latter case it is necessary to remix thoroughly the contents of the cell before making the determination. The required initial density depends both on the macromolecular species to be banded and on the ionic content of the gradient. In CsCl, for example, DNAs from various sources have buoyant densities in the range of about 1.69 to 1.74 gm/cm^3, while in Cs_2SO_4, DNA bands in the range of 1.42 to 1.455 gm/cm^3. Figure 8.6 illustrates the range of densities found for various types of DNA in both CsCl and Cs_2SO_4.

8.3.4 Measurements

To estimate the buoyant density of a macromolecular species from equilibrium density gradient data, it is necessary to have a calibration of the gradient in terms of solution density as a function of radius. This is discussed in Section 4.3.8 and in detail by Szybalski (1968). The problems in deducing an absolute density calibration are considerable because of the presence of both a compositional and a compressional component in the density gradient, and because it is difficult to make direct measurements on the solution during the centrifugation. Szybalski (1968) discusses in detail the procedure for making an absolute calibration based on knowledge of the average density of the sample solution, measured either before or after the experiment.

The calibration of the composition density gradient [cf. Eq. (4.32)] is based on

$$\rho(r) \approx \rho_i + [\omega^2/2\beta(\rho_i)](r^2 - r_i^2) \qquad (8.1)$$

where $\rho(r)$ is the solution density as a function or radius r, ρ_i the initial (uniform) density of the sample, ω the angular speed of the rotor, and r_i the isoconcentration radius at which $\rho(r_i) = \rho_i$. The quantity $\beta(\rho)$ is defined in Section 4.3.8. The isoconcentration radius is given to a first order approximation by

$$2r_i^2 \approx r_b^2 + r_m^2 \qquad (8.2)$$

where r_b is the radius to the base of the fluid column and r_m the radius to the meniscus.

Equations (8.1) and (8.2) do not account for the effects of compression on the physical density gradient. The absolute density of a particle is found after banding it in several different gradients with different ρ_i so that the band occupies different positions in the fluid column and thus experiences different parts of the density gradient. The results are then extrapolated to zero pressure to compensate for the compression gradient. A procedure for the approximate calibration of analytical density gradients has been given by Jeffrey (1968).

Estimation of the buoyant density of a macromolecule relative to the known (and assumedly accurate) density of a marker is much simpler, and this is the procedure commonly used. Equation (8.1) may be solved to give the density difference between two positions r_1 and r_2 in the form

$$\rho(r_1) - \rho(r_2) \cong [\omega^2/2\beta(\rho_i)](r_1^2 - r_2^2) \qquad (8.3)$$

If the bands of the unknown and of the standard are relatively close together, the pressure correction may be safely ignored. If the bands are widely separated, accurate estimates require that several experiments with different ρ_i be performed in order to establish the density differences at zero (i.e., atmospheric) pressure. The density differences thus obtained may readily attain a precision of 1 mg/cm^3.

For work with DNA, the standard reference is *Escherichia coli* DNA which has a buoyant density of 1.7035 gm/cm^3* in CsCl and a density of

---

* Some authors give the density of DNA from *E. coli* as 1.7100 gm/cm^3 in CsCl. This discrepancy is discussed by Szylabski (1968). In general, the absolute densities of reference DNAs are not known with high precision, but differences in buoyant densities obtained by this technique are quite accurate.

1.4260 gm/cm^3 in Cs$_2$SO$_4$. DNA from *Micrococcus lysodeikticus* is frequently used as a secondary standard where *E. coli* DNA would band too close to the unknown. *M. lysodeikticus* DNA has a density of 1.7245 gm/cm^3 in CsCl and 1.435 gm/cm^3 in Cs$_2$SO$_4$.

The amount of material in a band may be estimated directly from the integral of the absorbance profile of the band provided that the extinction coefficient of the particles is known. Bands of high-molecular-weight substances are generally quite narrow, so that it is not necessary to correct for the sectorial shape of the cell in estimating the content of a single band. The sectorial correction is important for comparison of the areas of bands from different parts of the fluid column.

Density heterogeneity of the sample may be estimated from the profile of the band at equilibrium. Alternatively, if it is known that the sample is completely homogeneous, the molecular weight may be estimated from the width of the Gaussian band (cf. Section 4.3.8). In both of these procedures it is imperative that equilibrium be attained completely before measurements are attempted.

8.3.5 Factors Affecting the Buoyant Densities of Particles

The observed buoyant density of a species of particle depends on the composition of the particle and on the constitutents of the solution which form the density gradient. If the properties of DNA are used as a specific example, it is observed that the buoyant density in CsCl is higher than that in Cs$_2$SO$_4$, as was mentioned previously. The density of DNA increases with increasing content of G–C base pairs. Figure 8.6 shows that the extent of methylation or glucosylation of DNA also affects its density: methylation decreases the density of DNA, while glucosylation increases the density in Cs$_2$SO$_4$, but decreases the density in CsCl.

In gradients of CsCl, DNA which is highly enriched in ^{15}N and ^{13}C can easily be distinguished from its ^{14}N and ^{12}C counterpart. Similarly, the incorporation of dense base analogs, such as 5-bromo- or 5-iodouracil into DNA increases its buoyant density. Experiments utilizing these types of density labels have been instrumental in determining the mode of DNA replication in bacteria and viruses (cf. Meselson and Stahl, 1958).

Buoyant densities are also affected by pH. In the case of DNA, high pH causes denaturation and strand separation with a consequent increase in density. In some cases this allows the complementary strands of the DNA to be separated. Heavy metal ions such as Ag$^+$ or Hg^{2+} can bind reversibly to DNA with a resultant large increase in density (cf. Brown *et al.*, 1971). DNA can also bind a variety of antibiotics (e.g., actinomycin, chromomycin, olivomycin, or mithramycin) and dyes (e.g., ethidium bromide or propidium

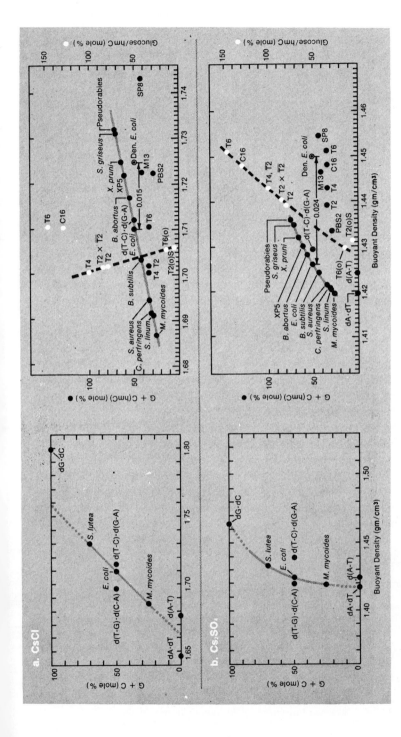

Fig. 8.6. Buoyant densities of DNAs in (a) CsCl and in (b) Cs_2SO_4 as a function of $G+C$ content (Szybalski, 1968). The abscissa shows the densities obtained from equilibrium density sedimentation in gradients of CsCl or Cs_2SO_4. The left ordinate and black does show the content of $G+C$ in the DNAs as mole%. Striking departures from an otherwise positive, linear relation are produced by glucosylation (right ordinate and white dots).

iodide) which alter the buoyant density. Single-stranded DNA is able to bind selectively to synthetic polymers such as polydeoxyribo- or polyribo-nucleic acids. This binding causes a characteristic shift in the buoyant density of the DNA, which may be useful in effecting a particular separation. Synthetic polymer binding can be used to separate and purify the strands of double-stranded DNA subsequent to thermal or chemical denaturation.

Ribonucleic acid is too dense to be banded in CsCl, although DNA–RNA hybrids may be banded satisfactorily. Some types of single-stranded RNA such as R17 phage RNA and ribosomal RNA, can be banded at equilibrium in Cs_2SO_4 gradients, but problems with precipitation of the RNA prevent application of this approach to a wider range of RNAs. Nucleoprotein particles, such as those derived from ribosomes, may be banded in CsCl subsequent to treatment with formaldehyde or glutaraldehyde. These agents have the effect of cross-linking the constituents so that the particles do not dissociate in the high salt environment (Baltimore and Huang, 1968). The percentage of protein in the particles may be estimated from the observed buoyant density in CsCl, ρ_{eq}, according to the empirical formula (Hamilton, 1971)

$$\% \text{ protein} = \frac{1.87 - \rho_{eq}}{0.0040\,\rho_{eq}}.$$

The buoyant density of the RNA moiety is increased somewhat by the presence of the aldehyde. Other approaches to the equilibrium centrifugation of RNA have included experiments at high temperature and the use of multicomponent solvents (cf. Szybalski, 1968).

In contrast to the narrow bands given by high-molecular-weight nucleic acids at equilibrium in density gradients, proteins give comparatively wide bands, sometimes reaching to the ends of the fluid column. This property has been exploited by Lundh (1977) to obtain molecular weight, partial specific volume, and a measure of preferential hydration of human transferrin by sedimentation equilibrium in short-column density gradients of an iodinated organic salt.

REFERENCES

Adams, G. H., and Schumaker, V. N. (1970). Equilibrium banding of low-density lipoproteins. I. Determination of gradients, *Biochim. Biophys. Acta* **202**, 305–314.

Baltimore, D., and Huang, A. S. (1968). Isopycnic separation of subcellular components from poliovirus-infected and normal HeLa cells. *Science* **162**, 572–574.

Brown, D. D., Wensink, P. C., and Jordan, E. (1971). Purification and some characteristics of 5S DNA from Xenopus laevis. *Proc. Natl. Acad. Sci. U.S.A.* **68**, 3175–3179.

Burton, A., and Sinsheimer, R. L. (1965). The process of infection with bacteriophage 174. VII. Ultracentrifugal analysis of the replicative form. *J. Mol. Biol.* **14**, 327–347.

Chevrenka, C. H., and Elrod, L. H. (1972). "A Manual of Methods for Large-Scale Zonal Centrifugation." Beckman Instruments, Palo Alto, California, 85 pp.

Creeth, J. M., and Denborough, M. A. (1970). The use of equilibrium-density-gradient methods for the preparation and characterization of blood-group-specific glycoproteins. *Biochem. J.* **117**, 879–891.

Dawid, I. B., Brown, D. D., and Reeder, R. H. (1970). Composition and structure of chromosomal and amplified ribosomal DNA's of Xenopus laevis. *J. Mol. Biol.* **51**, 341–360.

Edelman, M., Schiff, J. A., and Epstein, H. T. (1965). Studies of chloroplast development in Euglena. XII. Two types of satellite DNA. *J. Mol. Biol.* **11**, 769–774.

Elder, J. P. (1969). Density measurements by the mechanical oscillator. *In* "Methods in Enzymology" (C. H. W. Hirs and S. N. Timasheff, eds.), Vol. 61, pp. 12–25. Academic Press, New York.

Hamilton, M. G. (1971). Isodensity equilibrium centrifugation of ribosomal particles; the calculation of the protein content of ribosomes and other ribonucleoprotein particles from buoyant density measurements. *In* "Methods in Enzymology" (K. Moldave and L. Grossman, eds.), Vol. 20, Part C, pp. 512–521. Academic Press, New York.

Hossainy, E., Zweidler, A., and Bloch, D. P. (1973). Isopycnic banding of chromatin in chloral hydrate gradients. *J. Mol. Biol.* **74**, 283–289.

Ifft, J. B. (1969). Proteins at sedimentation equilibrium in density gradients. *In* "A Laboratory Manual of Analytical Methods of Protein Chemistry" (P. Alexander and H. P. Lundgren, eds.), Vol. 5, pp. 151–223, Pergamon, Oxford.

Jeffrey, P. D. (1968). Calculation of equilibrium density gradients. *Biochim. Biophys. Acta* **158**, 295–298.

Lundh, S. (1977). A new approach to analytical density gradient centrifugation. Simultaneous determination of molecular weight, specific volume, and preferential hydration of human transferrin. *J. Polymer Sci.* **15**, 733–748.

Meselson, M., and Stahl, F. W. (1958). The replication of DNA in E. coli. *Proc. Natl. Acad. Sci. U.S.A.* **44**, 671–682.

Schachman, H. K. (1959). "Ultracentrifugation in Biochemistry," pp. 32–55. Academic Press, New York.

Schachman, H. K., and Edelstein, S. J. (1966). Ultracentrifuge studies with absorption optics. IV. Molecular weight determinations at the microgram level. *Biochemistry* **5**, 2681–2705.

Sharp, D. S., and Ifft, J. B. (1979). Density gradient proportionality constants, density distributions, and pressure effects for three salt solutions. *Biopolymers* **18**, 3043–3065.

Szybalski, W. (1968). "Equilibrium Sedimentation of Viruses, Nucleic Acids and Other Macromolecules in Density Gradients." Fractions, No. 1. Beckman Instruments, Palo Alto, California.

Tanford, C. (1961). "Physical Chemistry of Macromolecules," pp. 317–390. Wiley, New York.

Van Holde, K. E. (1971). "Physical Biochemistry," pp. 79–121. Prentice-Hall, Englewood Cliffs, New Jersey.

Vinograd, J., and Bruner, R. (1966). "Band Centrifugation in Self-Generating Density Gradients." Fractions, No. 1. Beckman Instrument Co., Palo Alto, California.

Vinograd, J., Bruner, R., Kent, R., and Weigle, J. (1963). Band centrifugation of macromolecules and viruses in self-generating density gradients. *Proc. Natl. Acad. Sci. U.S.A.* **49**, 902–910.

Vinograd, J., Radloff, R., and Bruner, R. (1965). Band-forming centerpieces for the analytical ultracentrifuge. *Biopolymers* **3**, 481–489.

Williams, Jr., R. C. (1979). Advances in sedimentation equilibrium. *In* "Methods in Enzymology" (C. H. W. Hirs and S. N. Timasheff, eds.), Vol. 61, pp. 96–103. Academic Press, New York.

Yphantis, D. (1964). Equilibrium ultracentrifugation of dilute solutions. *Biochemistry* **3**, 297–317.

9

Protocols for the Separation and Analysis of Some Specific Particles

Protocols for the separation of a number of particles representing a wide range of particles and techniques are presented in the following discussion. Isopycnic sedimentation in swinging buckets presents few technical problems; those that do arise are usually specific to the particle in question. For this reason I have chosen examples largely involving other procedures.*

9.1 WHOLE ORGANISMS

Microbial cells are usually harvested by simple centrifugation or, when large volumes are involved, by continuous-flow sedimentation in the Szent-Györgyi–Blum or Sharples systems, but there has not appeared to be much need for the resolving power of density gradients. One exception is the fractionation of ichthyoplankton into fish eggs, fish larvae, and invertebrates (Bowen *et al.*, 1972). Since, however, the practical exploitation of this procedure employs sedimentation at 1 *g* (Price *et al.*, 1977) rather than centrifugation, it is beyond the scope of this volume.

A general occasion requiring density-gradient centrifugation arises with

---

* The following references contain compilations of techniques and protocols for still other particles: Birnie (1972), Birnie and Rickwood (1978), Catsimpoolas (1977), Chermann and Lavergne (1973), Chevrenka and McEwen (1971), Cline and Ryel (1971), Fleischer and Packer (1974, 1979a,b), Moore (1969), Peeters (1979), Pertoft and Laurent (1977), Price, (1970), Reid (1973, 1979a,b), Rickwood (1976), and Wolff (1975).

the problem of separating microorganisms from one another or from other particulate material, as in the case of the syphilis pathogen from tissue fragments (Russell *et al.*, 1967) and marine algae from nonliving particulates in ocean water, which is the first example in this section. Still another general situation is the resolution within a population of organisms according to size or density. The separation of neoplastic mast cells according to their stage of development is described in Section 9.2.

Other examples of the collection or resolution of microorganisms are cited in Table 9.1.

9.1.1 Harvest of Marine Phytoplankton

Marine microalgae occur at very low dilution, in thousands per milliliter in nature and rarely more than a million per milliliter in the laboratory. Simple sedimentation in bottles may result in large fractional losses by the restirring that is caused by Coriolis forces during deceleration and the organisms may suffer irreversible damage upon hard pelleting. Moreover ocean water contains many particulates, such as silt and the debris of dead

Table 9.1. Separation of Microorganisms by Density-gradient Centrifugation

Organism	Method	Reference
Yeast	Rate–Zonal	Lieblová *et al.*, 1964, Sebastian *et al.*, 1971, Halvorson *et al.*, 1971
Algae	Isopycnic	Sitz *et al.*, 1970
Algae	(a) Isopycnic	Sorokin, 1963
	(b) Continuous-flow with isopycnic banding	Price *et al.*, 1974
Algae and cyanobacteria	Isopycnic	Price *et al.*, 1978, 1982
Bacteria from phage	Flotation	Juhos, 1966
Bacterium megaterium (vegetative from sporulating cells)	Isopycnic	Tamir and Gilvarg, 1966
Plankton from fresh water	Continuous-flow with isopycnic banding	Lammers, 1971
Escherichia coli	(a) Rate–Zonal	Maruyama and Yanagita, 1956
	(b) Continuous-flow with isopycnic banding	Cline and Dagg, 1973
Chlamydia trachomatis	Rate–Zonal	Maruyama and Yanagita, 1956
	Continuous-flow with isopycnic banding	Cline and Dagg, 1973
Treponema pallidum	Continuous-flow with isopycnic banding	Thomas *et al.*, 1972

organisms, so that a resolution of particulates offers potential advantages. Lammers (1971) was the first to employ continuous-flow zonal rotors for natural waters across sucrose gradients was not successful with seawater. Most marine phytoplankton penetrate the most concentrated sucrose solutions and the high osmotic pressures in the gradient are lethal to the organisms. The problem, therefore, was to find a gradient material that was sufficiently dense, compatible with marine microalgae, and compatible with seawater. The only substance that meets these requirements is Percoll, a silica sol whose surface has been modified with polyvinylpyrrolidone (cf. Section 5.1.3). The following procedure, employing gradients of Percoll, is suitable for the collection of algae from laboratory cultures or from seawater (Price *et al.*, 1978, 1982). It can also be adapted for the collection of microalgae from volumes of 200 liters of seawater in continuous-flow zonal systems (cf. Price *et al.*, 1974).

Rotors. Any rotor accommodating 100-cm^3 swinging-bucket tubes, such as the IEC No. 269 or Sorvall HL8, is suitable. Samples of about 1 liter can be analyzed in specially constructed buckets (Price *et al.*, 1982), provided that acceleration and deceleration are carefully controlled.

Although the gradient solutions are stable at room temperature or below, Percoll is not stable with high concentrations of salts at high temperatures. In order to have components that can be heat sterilized, divide the gradient solutions into Percoll- and salt-containing stock solutions.

10 × Magnesium–Tris–Seawater (Mg–Tris–SW): Dissolve 15.25 gm MgCl$_2 \cdot$ 6H$_2$O, 20.15 gm Tris base, and 13.2 gm Tris $\cdot$ HCl in filtered seawater and dilute to 500 cm^3 with filtered seawater.

1.11 × Sorbitol: Dissolve 101.2 gm sorbitol in deionized water and dilute to 1 liter.

1.11 × Percoll–sorbitol: Dissolve 101.2 gm sorbitol and dilute to 1 liter in Percoll.

(Solutions of 10 × Mg–Tris–SW, 1.11 × sorbitol, and 1.11 × Percoll–sorbitol may be heat sterilized separately or stored frozen.)

Starting solution: Mix 90 cm^3 1.11 × sorbitol with 10 cm^3 10 × Mg–Tris–SW.

Final solution: Mix 90 cm^3 1.11 × Percoll–sorbitol with 10 cm^3 10 × Mg–Tris–SW.

Sample. Use 80 cm^3 of an algal culture in seawater.

Gradient. A linear gradient of 10 cm^3 followed by 5 cm^3 of final solution as a cushion is pumped into 100-cm^3 centrifuge tubes under 80 cm^3 of an algal sample.

Temperature. Use the same temperature as original sample.

Centrifugation. Accelerate very slowly allowing approximately 3 min to reach 200 rpm; then accelerate immediately to 2000 rpm. Typical microalgae will band isopycnically in 5–10 min; small forms, such as coccoid cyanobacteria, require 20 min. Decelerate immediately to 200 rpm, then slowly to rest.

Recovery.   The bands of algae can be recovered by conventional means or by special adaptors (cf. Fig. 9.1) that permit displacement from the bottom of the tube by pumping water to the top.

Analysis of fractions.   All kinds of microalgae and cyanobacteria tested will band in these Percoll–sorbitol gradients except coccolithophores.* The

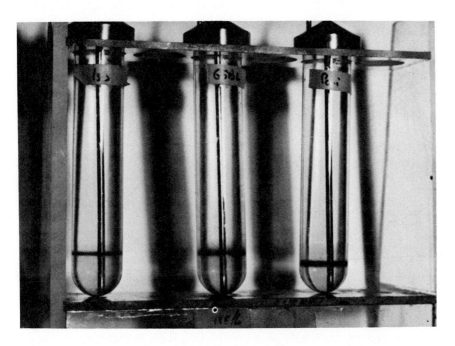

Fig. 9.1.   Sedimentation of marine microalgae in density gradients of Percoll (Price *et al.*, 1982). The conditions of separation are described in Section 9.1. Algal cultures (85 cm^3) were placed in 100-cm^3 centrifuge tubes, stainless steel adapters fitted onto the tubes, and 15 cm^3 of a gradient of Percoll in SSW was pumped through the central tube to the bottom. After spinning at 2000 rpm for 10 min, the organisms can be seen banded in the gradients. The different cultures are: Iso, *Isochrysis galbana*; GSBL, *Gymnodinium nelsoni*; and Peri, *Peridinium sp.*

* Percoll with densities up to 1.21 gm/cm^3 may be prepared by ultrafiltration. Such preparations, which we have dubbed "suPercoll," can be employed in place of Percoll for some of the more dense forms of algae, but the gradients are still insufficiently dense to float coccolithophores.

bands are typically rather narrow and appear to be specific for algal types. A sensitive test for the algae in the recovered gradient is the fluorescence of their chlorophyll *in vivo*. The gradient stream may thus be monitored by passage through a flow fluorometer. The algae may be recovered from the gradient fractions by diluting the fractions with equal volumes of starting solution and centrifuging gently.

Algae from large volumes of seawater may also be recovered by continuous-flow zonal centrifugation in these same gradients (cf. Price *et al.*, 1974).

9.2 WHOLE CELLS

Density gradient centrifugation is very widely used for the isolation of cells from animal tissues and blood. That the methods are not completely satisfactory is indicated by the continuous stream of articles reporting improvements in the methodology (cf. Catsimpoolas, 1977). Ficoll, metrizamide, Percoll, and albumin give gradients that are isosmotic or nearly so and each have their partisans. One or another will give superior resolution or recovery for a given set of cells, but it has been impossible to predict the ideal system in advance.

There are two striking applications of density gradient centrifugation of cells that involve more than just the preparation of specific kinds of cells: Lipsich *et al.* (1979) separated cytoplasts (enucleated cells) from intact or reconstructed (renucleated) cells. This greatly facilitates the detection and isolation of successful renucleation events. In the second application, non-secreting mutants of yeast are selected from secreting wild types by their banding position in density gradients (Novick *et al.*, 1980).

9.2.1 Separation of Rat Liver Cells
in Percoll Gradients (Pertoft *et al.*, 1977)

Background and Principles.   Vallee *et al.* (1947) reported that leukocytes could be separated from whole blood by sedimentation in a step gradient of serum albumin. Continuous and step gradients of albumin were subsequently used widely for this purpose, but albumin solutions have a disadvantage of high viscosity, high cost, and variability of different lots of albumin. Mateyko and Kopac (1963) recommended silica sols (Ludox, Section 5.1.3) for isopycnic banding of tissue culture cells. Subsequently Pertoft and his group (Pertoft, 1966, 1969, 1970; Pertoft *et al.*, 1968, 1977) pursued an imaginative and thorough study of silica sols as gradient materials for a variety of animal cells and subcellular particles. One of their findings was that the toxicity of different silica sols of the Ludox series could be decreased by the addition of various polymers to the sols. The endpoint of this strategy was the invention of a modified silica sol in which polyvinylpyrrolidone formed a covalently closed sheath around the silica particles (cf. Pertoft and Laurent, 1977). The material, marketed under the name "Percoll" (Pharmacia) (cf. Section 5.1.3), is markedly less toxic and markedly more resistant to gelation than any of the unmodified silica sols.

Pertoft (cf. Pertoft and Laurent, 1977) has shown that gradients of Percoll, in common with other silica sols, can be generated by subjecting the sols to high-speed centrifugation (e.g., 20,000 g for 15 to 45 min) (cf. Section 5.3).

In this protocol cells from rat liver are resolved on gradients of Percoll in Eagle's "minimum essential medium" (MEM).

Rotor. Any swinging-bucket rotor accepting 100 cm^3 tubes.

Solutions

Starting Solution. Percoll diluted to $\rho = 1.03$ gm/cm^3 in Eagle's MEM (Eagle, 1959).

Limiting Solution. Percoll diluted to $\rho = 1.10$ gm/cm^3 in Eagle's MEM.

Sample. Parenchymal and nonparenchymal cell fractions were obtained from perfused rat livers labeled with [^{125}I]-albumin or [^{125}I]-asialoceruloplasmin and suspended in Eagle's MEM + calf serum to concentrations of 4×10^6 and 2×10^6 cells per cem^3, respectively. Sample volumes were 15 cm^3.

Gradient. Linear gradients of 80 cm^3 are generated from 40 cm^3 each of the Starting and Limiting solutions.

Temperature. 4°C.

Centrifugation. 30 min at 800 g.

Results. The gradient fractions were analyzed for radioactivity, cell number, and density. The results (Fig. 9.2) show a resolution of Kupffer cells, hepatocytes, and phagocytes.

Comment. The viability of cells separated in Percoll gradients appears to be at least as good as in any other medium (Pertoft *et al.*, 1977). Superior resolution has often been reported (cf. Table 9.2). As a consequence, Percoll may become the most generally useful gradient material for cell separations.

9.2.2 Antibody-Producing Cells from Spleen (Gorzynski *et al.*, 1970)

Background. Spleen cells can be shown to produce specific antibodies by several immunochemical tests, including the formation of plaques. Previous workers reported heterogeneity in the equilibrium densities of such cells in gradients of albumin, but the data have been variable. Gorczynski *et al.* (1970) showed by studies with Ficoll gradients that the reported

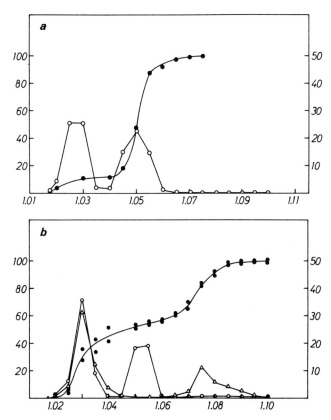

Fig. 9.2.   Separation of rat liver cells on Percoll gradients (Pertoft *et al.*, 1977). The conditions of separation are described in Section 9.2.1. Abcissae are densities of each fraction in gm/cm³; left ordinates are cell counts (○) as percentage of total cells recovered; right ordinates are radioactivity (●) as percentage of total radioactivity recovered. Livers were labeled with ^{125}I-albumin. (a) Nonparenchymal cell fraction. (b) Parenchymal cell fraction. Results of identical experiment but with cells from liver labelled with [^{125}I]-asialoceruloplasmin are superimposed (Δ).

heterogeneity is really due to differential responses to gradients of osmotic pressure that normally accompany albumin gradients.

Principles.   This method relies on isopycnic sedimentation in Ficoll gradients.

Rotor.   A SW-25 or any swinging-bucket rotor capable of 3800 *g* is required.

Solutions

Ficoll stock: Ficoll (Pharmacia) is mixed 36% w/w in distilled water,

Table 9.2. Some Other Separations of Animal Cells by Density-Gradient Centrifugation

Tissue	Method	Reference
Blood	(a) Summaries of various methods	Cutts, 1970
	(b) Continuous-flow with banding in self-generated gradients	Buckner *et al.*, 1968
	(c) Isopycnic banding in Percoll gradients	Pertoft *et al.* (1979)
Lymphocytes	(a) Isopycnic banding in albumin gradients	Shortman, 1968
	(b) Rate–zonal sedimentation in gradients of blood serum	Phillips and Miller, 1970
	(c) Isopycnic banding in Ficoll gradients	Nanni *et al.*, 1969
	(d) Isopycnic banding in Percoll gradients	Pertoft (1979)
Oyster hemocytes	Isopycnic banding	Cheng *et al.* (1980)
Insect hemocytes	Isopycnic banding in Ficoll gradients	Peake (1979)
Liver	Isopycnic banding in silica gradients	Pertoft, 1969
Hepatotocytes	Isopycnic banding in Metrizamide gradients	Mayer *et al.* (1977) Conn *et al.* (1977)
Leydig cells	Isopycnic banding in Percoll gradients	Schumaker *et al.* (1978)
Mucosal cells	Isopycnic banding in Ficoll step gradients	Scott *et al.* (1978)
Aortic cells	Isopycnic banding in Metrizamide gradients	Haley *et al.* (1977)
Islet cells	Isopycnic banding in Percoll gradients	Pertoft *et al.* (1979)
Mast tumor cells	Isopycnic banding in silica gradients	Pertoft, 1970
Various animal cells in tissue culture	Isopycnic banding in silica gradients	Mateyko and Kopac, 1963
Artificial mixtures	(a) Rate–zonal sedimentation in Ficoll gradients	Boone *et al.*, 1968
	(b) Computer program for predicting resolution in Ficoll gradients	Pretlow and Boone, 1969

deionized by stirring at 4°C with 100 gm of a mixed ion-exchange resin [AG-501-X8(D), Bio-Rad] for 4 hr with one repeat exchange. The suspension was filtered through gauze to remove the resin, through membrane filters to sterilize, and stored at 4°C.

Gradient components. The Ficoll stock was diluted with buffer and spleen cells to the desired starting and limiting concentrations. All gradient solutions were buffered 10 mM in sucrose, 3 mM in KH_2PO_4, 15 mM in 2-naphthol-6,8-disulfonic acid dipotassium salt. Osmotic pressure was adjusted with NaCl after calculating the contribution of the added solutes and assuming an effective molecular weight of 400,000 for Ficoll (36% w/w Ficoll corresponds to 1.4 mosmolal). The starting and limiting solutions were 14 and 20% w/w Ficoll, respectively, with densities of 1.05 and 1.09 g/cm^3, respectively. Both solutions were 294 mosmolal. The concentration of spleen cells was the same in the starting and limiting solutions.

Sample. Spleen cells from mice immunized with sheep red blood cells were suspended by gentle aspiration in 1 ml of buffered medium.

Gradient. Tubes for SW-25 rotor are filled by pumping 15 cm^3 each of the starting and limiting solutions in a linear gradient.

Centrifugation. Samples are centrifuged 1 hr at 3800 g (5000 rpm).

Recovery. The gradient is recovered by upward displacement with dimethylphthalate ($\rho = 1.14$ gm/cm^3).

Results. Although the nucleated spleen cells are recovered over a density range extending from 1.05 to nearly 1.1 gm/cm^3, cells producing antibodies, detected here as plaque formation (19 S–PFC), are confined to a narrower region. In isotonic gradients (Fig. 9.3) the cells band in a single zone centered on 1.062 gm/cm^3. In the osmotic gradient, however, the cells resolve into three distinct zones.

9.2.3 Resolution of Neoplastic Mast Cells into Stages in the Mitotic Cycle (Warmsley and Pasternak, 1970)

Background and Principles. In 1956 Maruyamo and Yanagita showed that an exponentially growing population of *Escherichia coli* could be resolved into small and large cells by rate–zonal sedimentation in a sucrose gradient, but the cells were damaged by the concentrated sucrose. Lieblová *et al.* (1964) employed an inert gradient medium, dextran, to resolve yeast cells into size classes. Such type fractionations have become the method of choice for studying cells in different mitotic stages and initiating synchronous cultures (cf. Probst and Maisenbacher, 1975).

Rotors. An MSE No. 62301 swinging-bucket or A-XII zonal rotor may be employed.

Gradients (linear)

Swinging bucket: Starting solution, 20 cm^3 5% w/v Ficoll in Fischer's medium*; limiting solution, 20 cm^3 10% w/v Ficoll in Fischer's medium.

Zonal: Starting solution, 500 cm^3 2% w/v Ficoll, 50 mM Tris–HCl pH 7.4, and 0.9% w/v in NaCl; limiting solution, 500 cm^3 10% w/v Ficoll, 50 mM Tris–HCl pH 7.4, and 0.9% w/v in NaCl; underlay, approximately 300 cm^3 15% w/v sucrose†; overlay, 80 cm^3 50 mM Tris–HCl pH 7.4 in 0.9% NaCl.

* Grand Island Biological Company, Grand Island, New York.

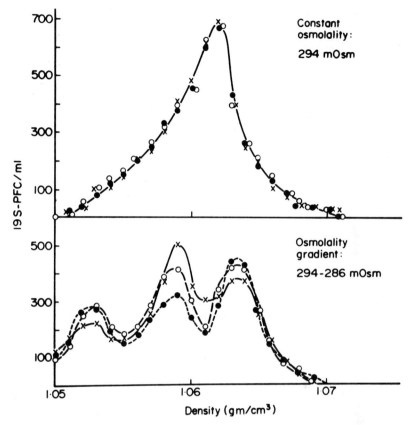

Fig. 9.3. Isopycnic sedimentation of spleen cells on Ficoll gradients (Gorczynski *et al.*, 1970). Spleen cells from mice immunized with sheep red blood cells were either constant with respect to osmotic pressure (upper figure) or contained a small osmotic gradient (lower figure). The ordinate is the number of 19S-plaque forming cells per ml and the abcissa is the density of the recovered fractions. The different symbols are from separate experiments.

Sample.   Neoplastic mast cells (P 815 Y and HC) pretreated with ^{3}H-thymidine were washed twice with cold Fischer's medium and resuspended as follows:

   Swinging bucket: Cells $(50–100 \times 10^6)$ resuspended in 1 cm^3 of Fischer's medium, and stirred slightly.

   Zonal: $0.5–1 \times 10^9$ cells in 25 cm^3 of 1% w/v Ficoll, 50 mM Tris–HCl pH 7.4, and 0.9% NaCl.

---

† The underlay of sucrose diffuses into a Ficoll gradient very rapidly; it is much better to use the limiting solution as a cushion or a method of inserting the sample that does not require displacing the gradient (cf. Section 7.4).

Temperature.   4°C.
Centrifugation.
  Swinging bucket: 5–7 min at 80 g_{av} then unloaded from the bottom.
  Zonal: 12–15 min at 500 rpm, then unloaded at 300 rpm from the center by displacement with underlay at 70 cm^3/min.
Results.   Fractions recovered from the swinging-bucket gradients were analyzed for cell number, cell volume and amount of [^{3}H]DNA (Fig. 9.4). The corresponding analyses of zonal fractions are shown in Fig. 9.5. It is clear from the comparison that zonal centrifugation, in addition to handling 10 times as many cells, has resolved them over almost twice the range of cell size; the spread among adjacent fractions is also much less.

9.3   MEMBRANE-BOUND ORGANELLES

9.3.1   Resolution of Mammalian Nuclei According to Ploidy
(Johnston *et al.*, 1968)

Background and principles.   The nuclei of many mammalian tissues, especially liver, are heterogeneous with respect to size and ploidy. Although conventional differential centrifugation yields fairly pure preparations of nuclei,* there is no discrimination with respect to size.
  Nuclei are among the densest organelles in the cell [ρ_{eq} (sucrose) $\cong$ 1.35

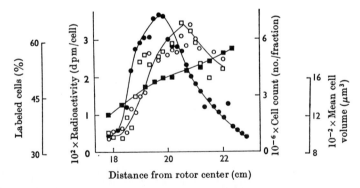

Fig. 9.4.   Rate sedimentation of mast cells in a swinging bucket rotor (Warmsley and Pasternak, 1970). Cells were separated according to size in a Ficoll gradient. Fractions were analyzed for cell number (●), mean cell volume (■), content of ^{3}H in DNA (0), and the percentage of cells labelled with ^{3}H determined autoradiographically (□).

---

* Nonetheless, Hinton *et al.* (1970) used such crude suspensions of nuclei as starting material for isolating plasma membranes.

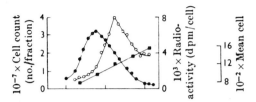

Fig. 9.5. Rate sedimentation of mast cells in a zonal rotor (Warmsley and Pasternak, 1970). Separation is identical to that in Fig. 9.4, except that sedimentation carried out in a zonal rotor. Note that the resolution with respect to cell size is substantially greater than in the swinging bucket rotor. Fractions were analyzed for cell number (●), mean cell volume (■), and content of [^{14}C]DNA (○).

gm/cm^3], a property that has been exploited in purification by pelleting nuclei through a cushion of dense sucrose; but this same property limits the application of isopycnic methods of separation.

Johnston *et al.* (1968) have utilized rate–zonal methods to resolve the nuclei of rat and mouse liver into diploid, tetraploid, and octaploid fractions.

Rotor. A-XII (MSE).

Solutions

Disruption medium: 0.32 M sucrose, 3 mM MgCl$_2$, pH 7.4, obtained by addition of solid NaHCO$_3$.

Suspending solution: 15% w/w sucrose mM MgCl$_2$ pH 7.4.

Cushion: 2.4 M sucrose mM MgCl$_2$ pH 7.4.

Starting solution: 20% w/w sucrose mM MgCl$_2$ pH 7.4.

Limiting solution: 50% w/w sucrose mM MgCl$_2$ pH 7.4.

Underlay: 55% w/w sucrose.

Overlay: 10% w/w sucrose.

Sample. The livers from three adult mice (approximately 6 gm wet weight) were disrupted in 0.32 M sucrose solution and centrifuged into a cushion of 2.4 M sucrose, and the pellet of crude nuclei resuspended in 10–20 cm^3 of 15% w/w sucrose.

Gradient. Load at 600 rpm 1000 cm^3 linear with volume, 500 cm^3 starting solution, 500 cm^3 limiting solution, approximately 300 cm^3 underlay (just displace top of gradient from rotor), 10–20 cm^3 sample introduced through the center, followed by approximately 70 ml overlay through the center to displace sample zone to $r = 6$ cm.

Temperature. 5°C.

Centrifugation. Centrifuge for 1 hr at 4000 rpm. Unload from the center at 600 rpm by pumping underlay to the edge at 50 cm^3/min. Collect 13-cm^3 fractions.

Results. The profile of apparent absorbancy (Fig. 9.6) shows three distinct sedimenting zones labeled 1, 2, and 3. Zone 1 can be divided into

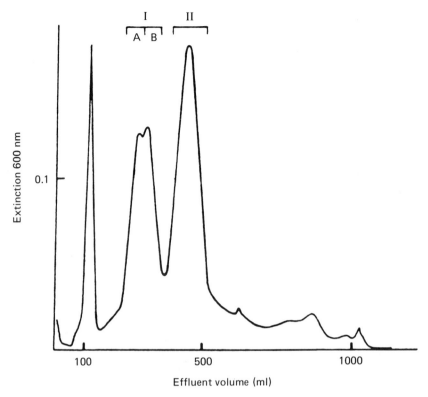

Fig. 9.6.   Rate–zonal sedimentation of mouse liver nuclei (Johnston *et al.*, 1968). The ordinate is nonspecific absorption at 600 nm, which is a measure of particle concentration. The abcissa is gradient volume. The slowest moving zone (I) contained diploid nuclei from paren-chymal and nonparenchymal cells. The most prominent zone (II) just beyond 400 ml contained tetraploid nuclei. The third zone contained octaploid, and the smaller, still more rapidly sedmenting zones contained nuclei of ploidy up to 16.

two nearly equal components, labeled A and B. Microscopic examination shows zone 1 to consist of diploid nuclei. Johnston *et al.* (1968) reported that the slower moving nuclei in A are "probably derived from non-parenchymal cells, of volume approximately 100 μm^3 with about 20% of prolate spheroids. Zone 1B has [parenchymal] nuclei of volume 150 μm^3, all of which are spherical."

The nuclei of zone 2 are tetraploid and are approximately 320 μm^3; zone 3 contains octaploid nuclei of approximately 700 μm^3.

Within the zones Johnston *et al.* (1968) reported a further resolution with respect to their competence to synthesize RNA and DNA.

The microscopic appearance of comparable fraction of rat liver nuclei is shown in Figure 9.7. Mathias (1973) has presented additional findings with the separated nuclei.

Other methods. Mathias and Wynther (1973) have employed Metrizamide (Appendix C12) and Hendricks (1972) has used silica sols for isopycnic separation of nuclei.

9.3.2 Spinach Chloroplasts (Morgenthaler *et al.*, 1974)

Background and principles. Chloroplasts as usually prepared are mixtures of intact chloroplasts, characterized by intact external membranes and an electron-dense stroma, and stripped thylakoids, that have lost most of their stroma and appear dark and granular under phase-contrast microscopy. Because the thylakoids retain most of the chloroplast pigments and some partial reactions of photosynthesis, the unfortunate term of "class II chloroplasts" has been applied to them.

Granick (1938) showed that an osmoticum, such as sucrose, is essential to the preservation of chloroplast structure. Leech (1964) employed an isopycnic separation in a density gradient of sucrose to separate intact chloroplasts from stripped thylakoids, but the high osmotic pressures generated in a sucrose gradient inactivated the photosynthetic CO_2-fixation system. Isosmotic Ficoll gradients were less damaging than sucrose (Vasconcelos *et al.*, 1971), but full recovery of photosynthetic activity was only achieved with the design of suitable gradients of silica described here.

Rotor. SW27, SB110, HS4, etc. (cf. Table 6.1).

Solutions.

Grinding–resuspension medium (G–R mix): 0.33 M sorbitol, 2 mM Na_2EDTA, 1 mM $MgCl_2$, 1 mM $MnCl_2$, 1 mM $Na_4P_2O_7$, 5 mM araboascorbic acid, 50 mM HEPES/NaOH pH 6.8.

Ludox Mix: 100 cm^3 purified Ludox AM, 3 gm PEG (Carbowax 6000), 1 gm bovine serum albumin, 1 gm Ficoll.

Starting Solution: 10 cm^3 Ludox Mix in G–R mix.

Final Solution: 80 cm^3 Ludox Mix in G–R mix.

Gradient. The volumes are suitable for two gradients of 32 cm^3 each or 6 gradients of 10.5 cm^3 each.

Sample. Blend 12 gm of diced spinach leaves in 60 cm^3 of the G–R mix for two intervals of 5 and 3 sec. Strain through one layer of Miracloth and centrifuge from 0 to 6000 rpm and return to rest in the shortest possible time. The pellet is resuspended in 1 cm^3 of G–R mix by aspiration.

Temperature. 4°C,

Centrifugation. Spin for 15 min at 7000 rpm.

Results. Stripped chloroplasts are recovered at 1.075 gm/cm^3 (Figure 9.8) and intact chloroplasts with full photosynthetic activity at 1.15 gm/cm^3.

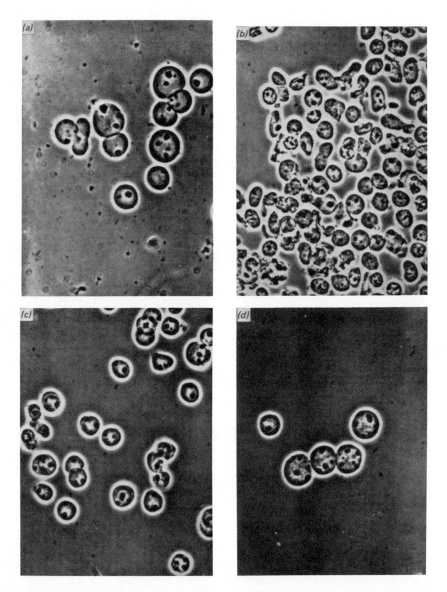

Fig. 9.7. Photomicrographs of unstained rat nuclei (Johnston *et al.*, 1968). Nuclei are from the experiment shown in Fig. 9.6; (a) unfractionated nuclei; (b) diploid zone (195–245 ml); (c) diploid zone (245–315 ml); and (d) tetraploid zone (360–510 ml).

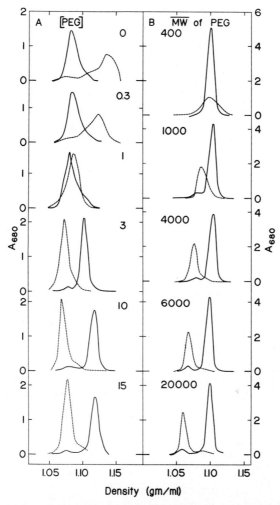

Fig. 9.8. Isopycnic sedimentation of spinach chloroplasts in silica sol gradients with different concentrations and kinds of poly(ethylene glycol) (Morgenthaler *et al.*, 1975). In each frame the solid line represents the absorbancy profile of intact chloroplasts and the dotted line the profile of stripped chloroplast membranes. The frame for 3% PEG 6000 on the left reflects the standard conditions described in the text. The two kinds of particles respond differently to different concentrations of PEG 6000 (left column) and to other mean molecular weights of PEG (right column).

For reasons that are not at all clear, the positions of the two zones of chloroplasts are strongly affected by the concentration of PEG and may even be reversed (Morgenthaler et al., 1975).

Percoll may be substituted for Ludox AM in the gradient solutions (Price and Reardon, 1982). The general procedure may also be used for the purification of chloroplasts from kilogram-quantities of spinach in continuous-flow zonal rotors (Morgenthaler et al., 1975; Price and Reardon, 1982). Functional chloroplasts can also be recovered from the alga Euglena gracilis, but the composition of the gradient is considerably altered from that for chloroplasts from higher plants (Ortiz et al., 1980; Price and Reardon, 1982).

9.3.3   Sequential Product Recovery of Mitochondria, Lysosomes, and Peroxisomes of Rat Liver (Brown et al., 1973)

Frequently the object in fractionations is to determine the quantitative distribution of some component among the various subcellular compartments rather than the qualitative purification of any one component. Brown et al. (1973) point out that a single rate separation can hardly resolve the wide range of particle sizes normally encountered in cells. A field–time integral which moves mitochondria near to their isopycnic point scarcely moves lysosomes and peroxisomes from the sample zone. In a study preparatory to analyzing the target organelles of the tumor-seeking metal gallium, Brown and co-workers exploited edge-loading zonal rotors in a procedure which permits one to collect discrete cuts from the end of a gradient following progressively larger values of $\omega^2\Delta t$. The three particles examined here through marker enzymes belong to the classical mitochondrial fraction of Hogeboom et al. (1948), whose subsequent resolution into lysosomes and peroxisomes earned de Duve a Nobel prize.

Rotor.   B-XXIX.

Solution.   Prepare sucrose solutions at concentrations of 6% w/w, 8.5% w/w, 20% w/w, 30% w/w, and 45% w/w.

Sample.   Rat livers are disrupted in 8.5% w/w sucrose with five vertical strokes of a Potter–Elvehjem homogenizer driven at 1000 rpm. The brei is clarified by centrifugation at 1300 rpm for 10 min.

Gradient.   One liter of a linear 20–30% w/w sucrose followed by a cushion of 45% w/w sucrose to fill rotor is used.

Temperature.   4°C.

Procedure.   At a rotor speed of 2500 rpm, 100 cm³ of sample is loaded at the center and displaced to a starting radius of 3.3 cm with 6% w/w sucrose. The rotor is then accelerated to 10,000 rpm, returned to 2500 rpm over an elapsed $\int\omega^2 dt$ of 0.25 rad²/μsec. and the distal 280 ml (cushion + 40 cm³ of the heavy end of the gradient) collected at the edge by pumping water to the center. The displaced volume was then replaced with fresh 45% w/w sucrose and the cycle repeated at a larger value of $\int \omega^2 dt$.

Results. The distribution of cytochrome oxidase, acid phosphatase, and catalase marks the occurrence of mitochondria, lysosomes, and peroxisomes in the several fractions (Fig. 9.9).

It is evident that the mitochondria are nicely separated from the other particles. Although lysosomes and peroxisomes largely overlap in this rate separation, they would be readily separable in a subsequent isopycnic centrifugation.

Comments. Sequential product recovery is a useful adjunct to rate–zonal separation. As noted elsewhere, several particles can only be resolved by inclusion of a rate–zonal step (cf. Canonico and Bird, 1970). All of these particles can be highly purified by alternate procedures (cf. Fleischer and Packer, 1974), but few of the conventional methods are suitable for quantitative distribution.

The procedure of Brown *et al.* (1973) is easily extended to nuclei by using a cushion of silica or Metrizamide and to ribosomes by higher centrifugal fields.

Percoll is probably a better gradient material than sucrose for the isolation of mitochondria. Mitochondria from skeletal and heart muscle, for example, can be resolved from sarcoplasmic reticulum in Percoll, but not in sucrose gradients (Mickelson *et al.*, 1980) and mitochondria from leaves can be resolved from chloroplast fragments better in Percoll than in sucrose gradients (Jackson *et al.*, 1979).

9.3.4 Synaptosomes (Whittaker and Barker, 1971)

Background and principles. When brain tissue is broken under conditions of moderate shear, the cell enlargements at the sites of presynaptic terminals are detached and the plasma membranes reseal forming enscapulations that retain most of the morphology of the intact terminal. These bodies, which are essentially enucleated neuronal cells are called *synaptosomes* (Whittaker *et al.*, 1964). In addition to mitochondria, ribosomes, and other typical cytoplasmic constituents, synaptosomes contain *synaptic vesicles*, tiny membrane-bound packets of acetylcholine.

Synaptosomes are prepared from breis in sucrose or Ficoll preferably and separated by isopycnic sedimentation in sucrose gradients either in swinging-bucket or zonal rotors (Cotman *et al.*, 1968). The latter method often yields synaptosomes with a rather ragged morphology, probably because of shear in crossing the fluid seal.

Rotors. Both a Sorvall SS-1 and a Spinco SW 25 rotor are used.

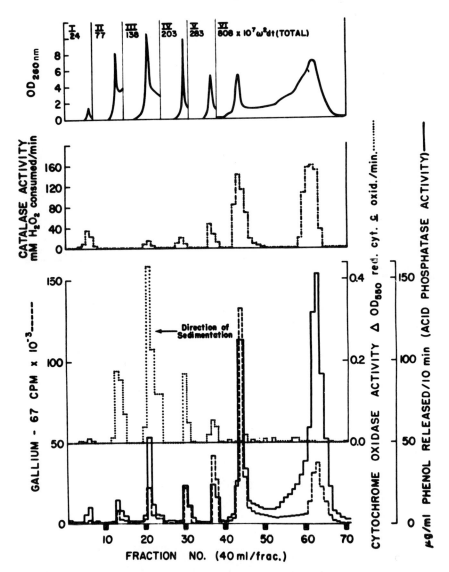

Fig. 9.9. Fractionation of rat liver by multi-stage rate-zonal centrifugation (Brown *et al.*, 1973). A rat liver homogenate was loaded onto a sucrose gradient in a zonal rotor and fractions collected after selected intervals by unloading from the edge. The upper curve shows the absorbancy profile of the portions of the gradient removed after indicated values of rad²/sec. The next curve shows the recovery of cytochrome oxidase, a marker for mitochondria, which is centered in fraction III. The bottom curve shows the recovery of acid phosphatase, which is a marker for lysosomes. Injected gallium-67 is also seen to distribute with the lysosomes.

Solutions.   Sucrose solutions of 0.32 *M*, 0.8 *M*, and 1.2 *M*, sucrose are all adjusted to pH 6.5–7.0 with Tris base.

Sample.   One guinea pig brain is scraped free of caudate nuclei, hippocampus, and white matter, and quickly weighed. Carry out all subsequent operations in ice water. Prepare a 10% w/v brei in 0.32 *M* sucrose. A Plexiglas–glass homogenizer should be used at about 800 rpm with 6 complete up and down strokes.* Cool in ice for 30 sec and repeat. The brei is centrifuged for 11 min at 3000 rpm in a Sorvall SS-1 and the supernatant collected. Resuspend the pellet in 0.32 *M* sucrose and recentrifuge. The combined supernatants are centrifuged at 12,000 rpm for 60 min, and the pellet resuspended in 2–3 ml 0.32 *M* sucrose for every gram of original tissue. This suspension is then layered over a gradient in a Spinco SW-25 rotor.

Gradient (Linear)

Starting solution: 10 cm³ 0.8 *M* sucrose.

Limiting solution: 10 cm³ 1.6 *M* sucrose.

Sample: 2–3 cm³ of crude suspension.

Temperature.   4°C.

Centrifugation.   Spin at 25,000 rpm for 2 hr.

Results.   Myelin floats as a layer over the gradient, mitochondria layer at approximately 1.4 *M*, and synaptosomes band broadly in between (Fig. 9.10).

Synaptosomes prepared in this way are contaminated principally with plasma membranes containing cytoplasm but without synaptic vesicles (Fig. 9.11) (cf. detailed criticisms of Cotman, 1974). An alternative gradient

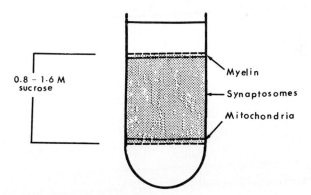

Fig. 9.10.   Isopycnic sedimentation of synaptosomes in a sucrose gradient (redrawn from Whittaker and Barker, 1971). A partially purified suspension of particles from guinea pig brain is sedimented into a linear gradient of sucrose. Synaptosomes are broadly distributed between a layer of myelin on the surface and a layer of mitochondria at approximately 1.4 *M* sucrose.

* Anderson (1956) pointed out that most of the shear in a Potter–Elvehjem type homogenizer is produced by vertical movement of fluid past the cylindrical pestle.

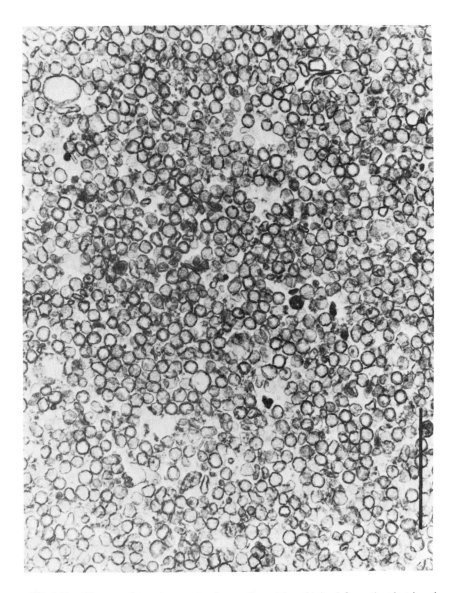

Fig. 9.11. Electron photomicrograph of synaptic vesicles obtained from the electric eel (V. P. Whittaker). Cholinergic synaptic vesicles were obtained by isopycnic sedimentations of extracts of electric organ of *Torpedo*. Bar = 1 μm.

procedure employing Ficoll (Cotman, 1974), minimizes contamination with mitochondria (but, see Hernandez, 1974).

9.4 MULTIMOLECULAR SYSTEMS

The smaller and simpler a particle, the more closely its behavior corresponds to theory. Ribosomes have been a favorite in the testing of theoretical models because they approximate closely the notion of a sedimenting particle as a hard, noninteracting sphere. By the same token investigators have been able to achieve near theoretical resolution and capacity in the centrifugation of ribosomes in density gradients.

Viruses behave almost as agreeably in density gradients as ribosomes. Indeed the sensitivity of many viruses to pelleting made density gradient centrifugation virtually *de rigeur* almost from the start of serious purification of animal viruses.

9.4.1 Polysomes from Rat Liver (Noll, 1969a)

The protocol described is a procedure for the analytical separation of polysomes. Noll and co-workers have used this procedure with particular success in the dissection of the mechanism of protein synthesis.

Prepare a crude suspension of polysomes by differential centrifugation as follows:

Male Wistar rats are starved for 16–18 h and then killed by decapitation. The livers (weighing about 10 g per 300 g animal) are removed as quickly as possible, blotted, trimmed of connective tissues and placed in tared 50-cm^3 breakers containing 10 cm^3 of ice-cold homogenizing buffer (0.25 M sucrose; 20 mM Tris, pH 7.5; 4 mM MgCl$_2$; 10 mM KCl; 1 mM 2-mercaptoethanol). After weighing, buffer is added to give a final ratio of 2.5 cm^3/g liver. The livers are minced with scissors in the cold room and homogenized in a Potter–Elvehjem glass vessel with a motor-driven Teflon pestle (0.25 mm clearance), slowly at first to avoid heating, 6–8 up and down strokes after all large pieces have been disintegrated.

The homogenate is spun in 40-cm^3 plastic tubes at 13,000 rev/min for 10 min. Under these conditions cell debris, nuclei, mitochondria and lysosomes are sedimented into the pellet. Approximately half of the opaque, red-brown supernatant above the multilayered pellet is removed with a syringe from the middle of the tube. Care should be taken not to contaminate the post-mitochondrial supernatant (PMS) with material from the pellet or from the white lipid layer floating on the top. The needle on the syringe should be made of stainless steel.

Addition of sodium deoxycholate (1.5 ml of a 10% w/v solution per 10 ml PMS) to a final concentration of 1.3% in the post-mitochondrial supernatant dissolves the membranes of the endoplasmic reticulum and produces a clear, dark red fluid.

The PMS may be examined directly for the polysome distribution pattern by centrifugation through a sucrose gradient, or it may be processed for the preparative isolation of purified polysomes by centrifugation through a sucrose double layer as follows. Two-ml portions of ice-cold 2 M sucrose in buffer (50 mM KCl, 20 mM Tris–HCl, pH 7.5, 5 mM MgCl$_2$) are dispensed into 10-ml polycarbonate screw-cap centrifuge tubes. An equal volume of buffered 0.5 M sucrose is carefully layered over the bottom 2 M sucrose layer. The tubes are then filled with the PMS and centrifuged for 1 h at 60,000 rev/min and 2°C. The whitish particular matter that has sedimented at the interface of the sucrose double layer is probably DOC. The ferritin forms an intense yellow band below the interface. The pellets should be nearly colorless and completely transparent.

The supernatant is removed by aspiration with a capillary pipette and the sides of the tube are wiped clean with tissue paper. The pellets are then rinsed once again with several milliliters of cold buffer and dissolved by gentle agitation in 0.5 ml of distilled water or buffer. Dissolution is facilitated if the pellets are allowed to swell in water for about 30 min. If necessary, the solutions are clarified by low speed centrifugation. Good polysome preparations are opalescent; the light scattering disappears, however, if the polysomes are converted into single ribosomes with RNase. The purity of the polysomes is checked by measuring the absorbancy of a 1:200 dilution at 240, 260 and 280 mμ. The 260/280 ratio should approach 1.7.

The polysomes may be stored in convenient portions (to prevent repeated freezing and thawing) at -60°C without loss of activity.

Gradient. A 12-cm^3 exponential gradient is generated in a tube of the IEC SB-283 rotor with the parameters chosen for $\rho_p = 1.4$, gm/cm^3 T = 2° and C$_s = 15\%$ w/v sucrose (Appendix Table D1) with the following salts throughout: 50 mM KCl, 20 mM Tris–HCl, pH 7.5, and 5 mM MgCl$_2$.

Sample. Use 0.2 cm^3 containing 4 A$_{260}$ · cm^3 of crude polysomes.

Centrifugation. Spin for 1 hr at 60,000 rpm.

Results. The gradient can be analyzed by puncturing the bottom of the tube, passing the gradient through a photometric flow cell, and collecting fractions. In one such analysis (Fig. 9.12) (Noll, 1969b), the ribosomes resolve into a number of zones. The largest zone contains 80 S ribosomes; more rapidly sedimenting zones corresponding to polysomes of up to 7 ribosomes can be discerned.

Comment. Isokinetic gradients have become the standard for the isolation of ribosomes. They are also valuable, but less commonly used for the separation of RNA and DNA (cf. Coulter-Mackie *et al.*, 1980; Korba *et al.*, 1981).

9.4.2 Ribosomal subunits from *E. coli* (Eikenberry *et al.*, 1970)

The characterization of ribosomal proteins requires prodigious quantities of ribosomes in a high state of purity. In the study of *E. coli* ribosomal proteins a limiting step was the resolution of the ribosomes into the 30 S and 50 S subunits. To this end we investigated the theoretical and practical limits of gradient capacity in the B-XV zonal rotor and found that up to 2 gm of crude ribosomes could be resolved into subunits in a single run.

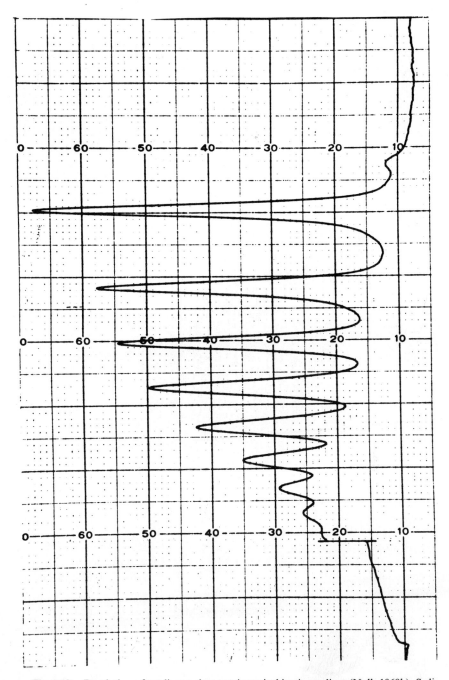

Fig. 9.12. Resolution of rat liver polysomes in an isokinetic gradient (Noll, 1969b). Sedimentation was for 2 hr at 37,000 rpm. Gradient was collected from the bottom of the tube; sedimentation is right to left. The largest peak corresponds to 80 S monosomes; polysomes of up to 7 monosomes can be discerned. From *Anal. Biochem.* with permission.

A suspension of about 40 mg of crude ribosomes per cm^3 is prepared from
E. coli harvested in exponential growth by the method of Tissières *et al.*
(1959). The ribosomes are dialyzed against 10 mM Tris–HCl pH 7.4, 1 mM
$MgCl_2$, and 100 mM KCl to dissociate the ribosomes into subunits and
clarified by low speed centrifugation.

Rotor.   A titanium B-XV (IEC) is used in the experiments. Identical
results can be expected in the B-15, B-29, and other rotors of similar
geometry.

Gradient.   A 6-cm hyperbolic gradient shape (Appendix D6) is employed.
The actual gradient extends from 7.4% w/w sucrose at 808 cm^3 to 38% w/w
at 1600 cm^3 with a cushion of 45% w/w sucrose. All of the solutions contain
a buffer of 10 mM Tris–HCl pH 7.4, 1 mM $MgCl_2$, and 100 mM KCl
throughout.

Sample.   The sample, containing up to 2 gm of ribosomes, is introduced
in a linear inverse gradient by means of a two-cylinder generator with 50 cm^3
of buffered 7.4% w/w sucrose in the mixing chamber and 50 cm^3 or ribosomes
in the other chamber.

Overlay.   The sample was followed by 708 cm^3 of buffer.

Temperature.   5°C.

Centrifugation.   Centrifugation is continued for 3.8×10^{11} rad^2/sec or
nearly 8 hr at 35,000 rpm (cf. Appendix A4).

Results.   The absorbancy profile (Fig. 9.13) of the recovered gradient
shows two trapezoidal zones of particles, corresponding to 30 S and 50 S
ribosomal subunits. The yield was 75–85% of the starting material. The
insets in the figure show the absorbancy profiles of samples taken from the
two zones and recentrifuged separately on analytical gradients. This and
other evidence indicated less than 1% cross contamination.

Comment.   Chaires and Kegeles (1978) have analyzed the sedimentation
behavior of ribosomes and ribosomal subunits by computer simulation. Their
model, which includes the pressure-induced, reversible dissociation of 70 S
ribosomes, predicts zone broadening dependent on rotor speed.

Although ribosomes and ribosomal subunits are too dense to be banded
isopycnically in sucrose gradients and lose some of their constituent proteins
in CsCl gradients, they can be separated isopycnically in gradients of metrizamide, in which they have ρ_{eq} values of only 1.2 to 1.3 gm/cm^3 (Buckingham
and Gros, 1975). The resolution does not look good enough for the preparation of pure ribosomal subunits, but may be very useful in the separation
of other ribonucleoprotein particles from ribosomes.

9.4.3   Influenza Virus (Sorrentino *et al.*, 1973)

A persuasive argument for the development of zonal rotors was the need
for an instrument for the large-scale isolation of viruses. Reimer *et al.* (1967)

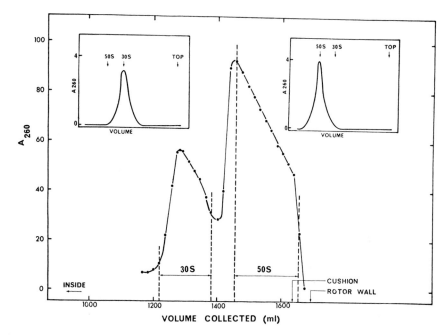

Fig. 9.13. Rate–zonal separation of 2.0 gm of *E. coli* ribosomes into subunits (Eikenberry *et al.*, 1970). Fractions between the vertical dashed lines were pooled and the ribosomes recovered by centrifugation. The yield was 450 mg of 30 S and 1050 mg of 50 S subunits. The insets show analytical sucrose density gradient analyses of the final products, showing negligible cross-contamination.

in fact demonstrated that commercially useful quantities of influenza virus could be collected and purified in the B-XVI rotor by continuous-flow centrifugation with isopycnic banding (Fig. 9.14). The procedure outlined here is an adaptation of that of Reimer *et al.* to the larger and more sophisticated K-III rotor.

Virus. Influenza virus is produced by standard techniques in the allantoic cavity of 11-day-old embryonated hens eggs.

Sharples Centrifugation (Clarification). Prior to the concentration of virus containing allantoic fluid, the crude allantoic fluid is clarified through an SS-16 model Sharples centrifuge at a flow rate of 360 liters/hr at 13,200 *g*. Formaldehyde solution is added to the clarified allantoic fluids to give a final dilution of 1:5000.

Sharples Centrifugation (Concentration). Allantoic fluids containing virus inactivated with formaldehyde are centrifuged in a laboratory model Sharples centrifuge at 62,000 *g* and a flow rate of 1200 cm^3/hr. After centrifugation the resultant viral sediment is resuspended to 1/20 of the original volume in 0.01 *M* phosphate buffered saline, pH 7.2.

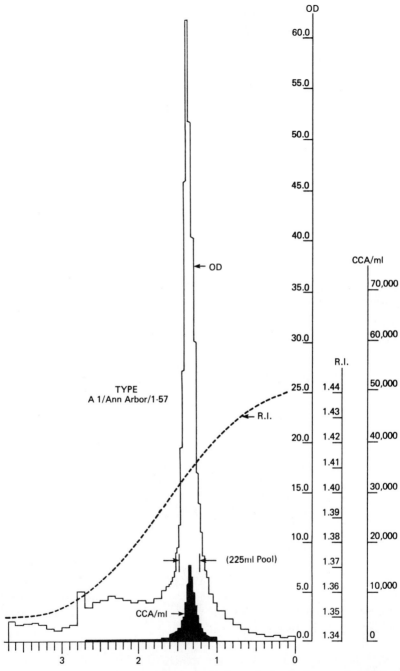

Fig. 9.14. Harvest of influenza virus in the K-II zonal rotor (Reimer *et al.*, 1967). Absorbancy profile (solid line) and hemaglutinin titers of influenza virus (solid blocks) were measured on gradient (dotted lines) recovered from K-II rotor.

Zonal Centrifugation. The reorienting gradient technique of isopycnic sucrose density gradient zonal centrifugation used is essentially that described by Reimer *et al.* (1967). The model K series zonal centrifuge with a K-III rotor is used.

Clarified allantoic fluids used for the preparation of manufactured lots of bivalent vaccine are centrifuged at a flow rate of 22 liters/hr in a K-III titanium rotor at approximately 90,000 *g*. Sucrose solution (60% w/w) and phosphate buffer (0.01 *M*, pH 7.2) are added separately to the rotor in the volumes required and the gradient is formed dynamically.

Results. In a series of runs the yield of virus in the centrifugation step averages about 60% of the clarified allantoic fluid (Table 9.3). The virus particles are exceptionally pure, as shown by electron microscopy (Fig. 9.15) and by high CCA chicken cell agglutinin activities. In addition, influenza vaccine prepared from these viruses produces negligible adverse reactions in human volunteers. It should be noted that previously a major problem with influenza vaccines was low potency and serious side reactions, especially in geriatric patients.

Comment. Centrifugation in sucrose gradients has been used in the isolation of nearly all viruses. Other gradient materials include iodinated aromatics (cf. Rickwood, 1976; Coulter-Mackie *et al.*, 1980) and silica sols (cf. Pertoft and Laurent, 1977).

Table 9.3. Yield and Purity of Different Preparations of Influenza Virus Vaccine[a]

Lot No.	Starting material		Final vaccine		
	Volume (liters)	CCA[d] (per mg protein)	CCA (per mg protein)	Purification index	% Recovery
7114Z[b]	48	150	11,980	79.86	48
7114S[c]	48	150	5,891	39.00	82
7115Z	48	209	9,500	45.45	42
7115S	48	209	3,410	16.00	41
7116Z	48	206	10,081	48.93	49
7116S	48	206	4,349	21.00	55
7145Z	48	226	13,472	59.61	35
7145S	48	226	2,447	10.80	60
7146Z	49	143	7,866	55.00	45
7146S	49	143	2,176	15.20	60

[a] Sorentino *et al.*, 1973.
[b] Z is zonal density gradient.
[c] S is Sharples.
[d] Chicken cell agglutin.

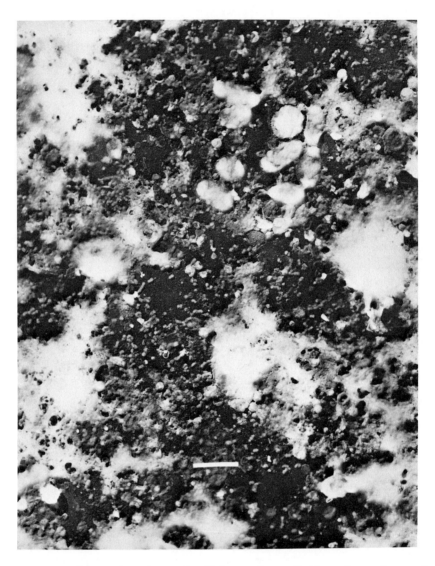

Fig. 9.15. Electron photomicrographs of influenza virus purified by continuous-flow zonal centrifugation in the K-II rotor (Peck, 1968; Electro-Nucleonics, Inc.). (a) The crude virus prepared by a conventional method. Bar = 1 μm. (b) Virus after recovery from the gradient. Bar = 1 μm.

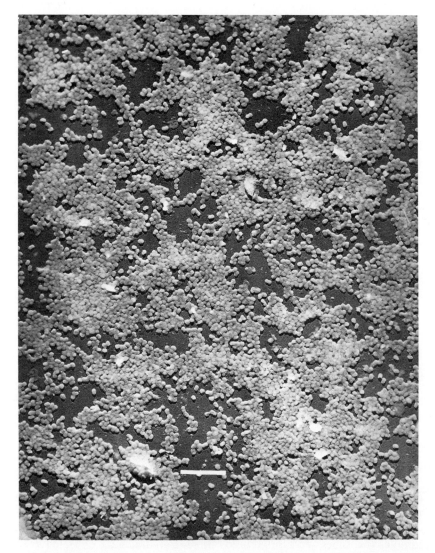

Fig. 9.15. *Continued*

9.5 MACROMOLECULES

Density gradient centrifugation becomes progressively more difficult as the particle weight falls toward 500,000 u and below. Fortunately, alternative methods, such as gel permeation and electrophoresis, become progressively more rewarding in this same region. Despite the welcome advances with gels related to agarose and controlled-pore glass, there are still a number of separations of macromolecules where the advantages lie with density gradient centrifugation.

9.5.1 Separation of DNA by Reograd Centrifugation in Angle Rotors (Flamm *et al.*, 1966)

The equilibrium density of species of DNA in CsCl increases regularly with the GC content of the DNA (cf. Szybalski, 1968). Moreover, gradients of DNA are readily formed by sedimentation equilibrium provided that the radial distances are kept modest. In this method of Flamm *et al.* the small radial distance in the Spinco Model 40 angle rotor is more advantageous than the much longer path of the SW-39 rotor. In addition, the reorientation of the gradient at the end of the run facilitates collection of the particle zones by amplifying the thickness of the particle zones and the distances between them.

Sample.   High-molecular-weight DNA from any source can be used. In this experiment amounts of rat liver DNA ranging from 23 to 135 μg were mixed with 2.7 μg of [^{14}C]DNA from *E. coli.*

Rotor.   Use a Spinco 40 or vertical rotors of 33,000 rpm or more.

Gradients.   A solution of 4.3750 gm of optical grade CsCl dissolved in 3.4 ml 0.01 M Tris pH 8.2 which also contains the DNA is prepared. The final volume is 4.5 ml with the remaining volume in the tube filled with paraffin oil.

Centrifugation. The suspension is spun at 33,000 rpm at 25°C for 60–65 hr. The sedimentation–equilibrium gradients generated in the 40 compared with the SW-39 rotors are shown in Figure 9.16. Although the gradients with respect to radius must be identical, the gradient as a function of rotor volume is clearly steeper in the swinging-bucket rotor. Considerably shorter intervals are required for the establishment of the gradient in vertical rotors.

At the end of the centrifugation, the rotor is allowed to decelerate to rest. The gradient reorients and in doing so, the separation of isodense lines in the rotor is magnified (drawing at right of Fig. 9.17).

Analysis.   The gradient can be analyzed as in any tube system. In the example, the tubes were punctured, three-drop fractions collected from the bottom, and the fractions analyzed for absorption at 260 nm and radioactivity.

Results.   The DNA from *E. coli,* $\rho_{eq} = 1.712$ gm/cm^3 was clearly separated from the rat liver DNA, $\rho_{eq} = 1.702$ gm/cm^3, almost independently of the amount of DNA added (Fig. 9.18). In contrast, similar experiments with the SW-39 rotors produced much poorer resolution (Fig. 9.19).

Comment.   Vertical rotors offer still better resolution in isopycnic sepa-

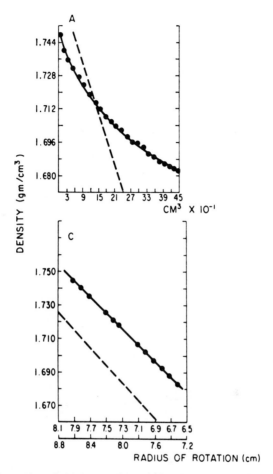

Fig. 9.16. Properties of density gradients self-generated in angle and swinging-bucket rotors (Flamm *et al.*, 1966). Gradients were prepared by centrifuging solutions of CsCl initially of 1.720 gm/cm^3 at 33,000 rpm for 60–65 hr. The solid lines represent the gradients obtained with a Spinco 40 angle rotor, the dashed lines with a Spinco SW-39 rotor. The upper curve is a plot of the density as a function of rotor volume and the lower curve a plot of the density as function of rotor radius.

rations than angle rotors (cf. Section 7.3), but the range of density in a given tube is less than in angle or swinging bucket rotors.

Creeth and Horton (1977) have computed the relative advantages of a variety of alkali salts with respect to resolution, preparative separations, and situations where a species bands outside or near the ends of the gradient.

Resolution of different DNAs can be enhanced by adding materials to the gradient which bind differentially to different conformers (e.g., ethidium

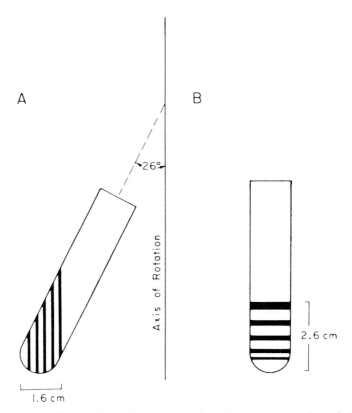

Fig. 9.17. Amplification in band separation obtained upon reorientation of the angle rotor (Flamm *et al.*, 1966). (A) shows a Spinco 40 angle rotor containing imaginary bands of particles in a density gradient with the rotor spinning. (B) shows that the bands are more widely separated from one another when the gradient has reoriented in the tube that has come to rest.

bromide, Radloff *et al.*, 1967), to (dG + dC)-rich sequences (silver ion, Jensen and Davidson, 1966), or to (dA + dT)-rich sequences (e.g., netropsin, Matthews *et al.*, 1978; bisbenzimide, Hudspeth *et al.*, 1980). Ethidium bromide and bisbenzimide have the further advantages of rendering the DNA fluorescent.

Szafarz (1977) claims that sodium iodide is superior to sucrose in the rate sedimentation of DNA, because the viscosity of the iodide is less. The consequence is that the capacity of the gradient is higher and the anomalous sedimentation behavior of very high molecular weight DNA is avoided. Iodide gradients are also suitable for the banding of RNA (Gonzalez *et al.*, 1978). The one, very large disadvantage of iodide is its strong absorption in the ultraviolet range. This makes it difficult to detect the DNA by its absorp-

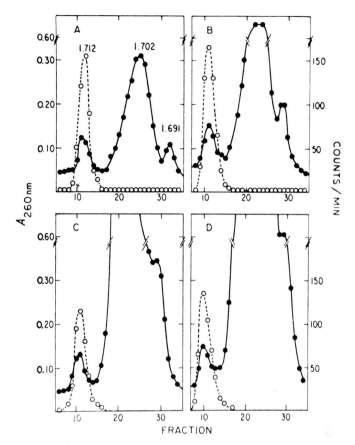

Fig. 9.18.   Resolution of different species of DNA by isopycnic sedimentation in an angle rotor (Flamm *et al.*, 1966). Mixtures of labeled *E. coli* DNA (dotted lines) and different amounts of mouse liver DNA (solid lines) were centrifuged to equilibrium in a Spinco 40 angle rotor as described in the text. The amounts of mouse liver DNA were (A) 23 μg; (B) 45 μg; (C) 90 μg; and (D) 135 μg. Even at the largest loading, the satellite band at 1.712 gm/cm^3 was resolved from the main band.

tion at 260 nm and decreases the fluorescence excitation of DNA–ethidium bromide complexes.

9.5.2   Rate–Zonal Separation of DNA in Gradients of Alkaline Sucrose (McGrath and Williams, 1966; Peterson *et al.*, 1974)

Background and Principles

The analysis of DNA according to size is important both for the preparation of homogeneous samples and the examination of chromosome breaks,

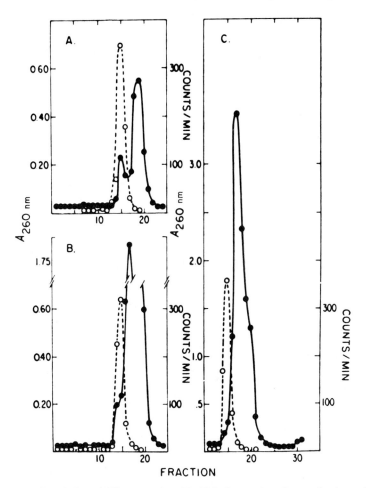

Fig. 9.19. Resolution of different species of DNA by isopycnic sedimentation in a swinging-bucket rotor (Flamm *et al.*, 1966). The experiment was similar to that of Fig. 9.18, except that the sedimentation was carried out in a Spinco SW 39 rotor. The amounts of mouse liver DNA were A, 15 μg; B, 45 μg; C, 90 μg. Note that the satellite band at 1.712 gm/cm^3 was unresolved at all but the lowest amount of DNA.

such as can be caused indirectly by radiation and various other mutagens. A major problem is that almost any manipulation of DNA species as they occur in bacterial and eukaryotic chromosomes will result in breakage. McGrath and Williams (1966) found that cells could be gently lysed in a layer of strong alkali overlying sucrose gradients and the DNA subsequently sedimented into the gradient with little, if any, breakage resulting from shear. The resulting sedimentation profiles have been widely exploited in the investigation of radiation- and alkylation-induced breaks in chromosomes.

Unfortunately, the interpretation of these profiles has been the subject of great controversy. Ormerod and Lehmann (1971) and Levin and Hutchinson (1973) warn that the apparent sedimentation coefficients of very large DNAs may decrease at high rotor speeds and that this speed dependence increases with size and concentration in such a way that random collections of DNA may appear to be less heterogeneous and to possess a smaller average particle weight than they actually do. Other workers have reported anomalously high sedimentation rates, that could result from aggregation, association with other cell components, etc. Anomalous sedimentation of DNA may be due in some cases to wall effects. It was first observed in tubes of cellulose nitrate (Levin and Hutchinson, 1973), but not in polyallomer tubes (Clark and Lange, 1976) nor in polycarbonate tubes whose geometry was modified to eliminate wall effects (Rosenbloom and Cox, 1974). In addition, Ehmann and Lett (1973) warn against simplistic estimates of the ratio of number-average to weight-average particle weights, M_n/M_a, which is a common measure of the number of chromosome breaks.

Peterson et al. (1974), whose protocol is followed here, have conducted their measurements with an eye toward the various possible artifacts.

Rotors. Use an SW-25 or any similar swinging-bucket rotor.

Solutions

Gradient: 5% w/v and 25% w/v nuclease-free sucrose* containing 1.0 M NaCl, 1 mM EDTA, 60 mM Na p-aminosalicylate, and NaOH to pH 12.5.

Lysing layer: 0.005 M EDTA, 0.5 M NaOH, 0.005 M NaKHPO$_4$, and 0.05 M NaCl.

Cell resuspension mix: 0.01 M EDTA, 0.01 M NaKHPO$_4$, and 0.1 M NaCl. Also Eagle's Basal Medium and DNA from bacteriophage T4.

Sample. Cells of mouse C3H/10T1/2CL8 embryo fibroblasts between Passages 5 and 16 are harvested from cultures growing exponentially in 75-cm plastic flasks by scraping with a rubber policeman into 0.2 ml of cold phosphate-buffered saline containing 0.01 M EDTA. After centrifugation, the cells are resuspended in Eagle's basal medium supplemented with 10% serum and diluted to 10^4 cells/ml in the same medium. Aliquants (5 ml) of cell suspensions are then seeded in 60-mm plastic petri dishes and incubated at 37°C in an atmosphere of 5% CO$_2$ in air.

At 24 hr after seeding, cultures are given 0.2 μCi of [2-^{14}C]thymidine (TdR-^{14}C) per ml for 24 hr in order to prelabel the cellular DNA. After the 24-hr period, the radioactive medium is replaced with complete medium and the cells are incubated for a further 90 min.

---

* Nuclease-free sucrose may be obtained commercially or by running stock solutions through a sulfonic acid-type of ion-exchange column followed by heat sterilization (cf. Section 5.1.1), or by treatment with activated charcoal.

Cultures are also treated with N-methyl-N'-nitro-N-nitrosoguanidine (MNNG), an alkylating agent in order to produce chromosome breaks. The details of this treatment are irrevelant to the immediate objectives. At the time of harvest, cells are detached from the dish with a rubber policeman and added to 0.2 cm^3 of the cell resuspension mix. This suspension, containing about 5×10^4 cells, is introduced into the lysing layer of the gradients.

Gradient. Polyallomer tubes are loaded with 30 cm^3 each of linear gradients made from the 5% w/v and 25% w/v sucrose solutions described above. Each gradient is overlayed with 0.2 cm^3 1.0 N NaOH immediately prior to the addition of the cells.

Addition of sample. The 0.2 cm^3 of cells are mixed in the lysing layer and held for 30 min.

Temperature. $20°$C.

Centrifugation. Spin at 24,500 rpm for 3 hr. Peterson *et al.* (1974) report that "a major source of error is the lack of precision that attends measurements of the centrifugation speed and time." In the absence of direct measurement of the $\int \omega^2 dt$, it is especially important to determine the maximum speed and the acceleration and deceleration intervals as precisely as possible.

Results. The gradient is collected from the bottom of the tubes, fractions are collected, and the radioactivity is determined. The radioactivity of each fraction is then plotted against the fraction number in order to obtain profiles of the DNA. An example is shown in Fig. 9.20. One sees that the DNA from the untreated cells bands in an approximately Gaussian distribution near the middle of the tube. The DNA from cells which had been treated with MNNG band at higher levels in the tube, indicating slower sedimentation.

Discussion and interpretation. The gradient used in these experiments is approximately isokinetic over the middle half of the tube; so that values of $s_{20,w}$ can be estimated from the distance sedimented. Specifically,

$$s_{20,w} = \frac{kr}{\int \omega^2 dt}$$

d is of course determined from the fraction number in which the radioactivity is measured and k, the calibration constant, is determined by the behavior of DNA of known length, in this case the DNA of T4 phage.

Molecular weights can be calculated in turn from the empirical equation of Studier (1965)

$$M = 1.561 \times 10^3 (s_{20,w})^{2.5} \tag{9.1}$$

In these and similar experiments one frequently wants to determine the heterogeneity of the DNA. That rationale for such determinations is as follows: an absolutely homogeneous species of DNA will sediment in an

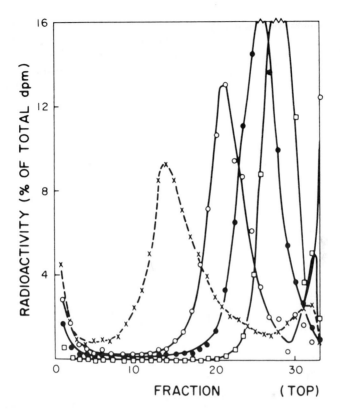

Fig. 9.20. Sedimentation of DNA from mouse fibroblast cells in alkaline sucrose gradients (Peterson *et al.*, 1974). Cells were labeled with [^{14}C]-TdR and lysed on top of gradient. Separation on the 5–25% w/v sucrose gradients was by rate zonal sedimentation. Several of the samples of cells were treated with an alkylating agent, MNNG, to induce chromosome breaks: (○), 0.5 μg MNNG/ml; (●), 1.0 μg MNNG/ml; (□), 2.0 μg/ml: (X), control.

approximately Gaussian distribution with a small but finite band width; the same species of DNA, partially degraded, will migrate as a wider band with a more slowly moving mean. There is, moreover, a quantitative treatment of the data involving the number-average and the weight-average molecular sights. However, Ehmann and Lett (1973) point out that this treatment is valid only in certain cases, namely, when the distribution of molecular weights is approximately random.

A simplistic application of Eq. (9.1), from which the molecular weight distributions are obtained, already leads to erroneous interpretations. Specifically, if one calculates the molecular weight of the fraction at the center of a zone of homogeneous particles, the number obtained is presumably valid. However, since the zone has finite width, larger and smaller molecular weights can similarly be calculated for fractions on either side of the center, yielding values which are patently wrong. A complete analysis of the sedimentation profiles must take into account the zone spreading of homogeneous particles and compute from the shape of a sedimenting zone the probabilities that particles of a given molecular weight will be found within a given fraction.

The separation of different size classes of DNA by agarose–gel electro-phoresis is far easier than rate sedimentation, particularly for multiple samples. If there is any advantage to rate sedimentation, it must be in terms of capacity. Rate sedimentation is applicable (with the caveats noted above) to DNA molecules as large as can be obtained (ca. 10^9 dalton). On the small end of the scale, one can separate restriction fragments down to about 350 base pairs (ca. 230,000 dalton) (El-Gewely and Helling, 1980); on the high side, resolution becomes poor above about 30×10^6 dalton (McDonell et al., 1977).

If ethidium bromide is added to the sample, the sedimenting bands can be detected by fluorescence and different conformers can be resolved (El-Gewely and Helling, 1980).

Linear gradients were employed in the protocol of Peterson et al. (1974) described here, but isokinetic gradients offer the advantage of easier inter-polation of molecular weights (cf. Coulter-Mackie et al., 1980; Korba et al., 1981). Isokinetic gradients are only slightly more difficult to construct than linear gradients.

9.5.3 Separation of mRNA from Calf Lens by Rate–Zonal Sedimentation in an Equivolumetric Gradient (Berns et al., 1971)

The isolation of single species of mRNA is dependent on finding or in-ducing cells to produce a single kind of protein. Examples include reticu-locytes, which produce only hemoglobin, and certain instances of virus-infected cells, which may produce principally viral coat proteins. Another example, described here, is the lens of the mammalian eye, which produces a specific class of proteins, called crystallins.

Different sizes of RNA can be separated by rate–zonal sedimentation. The description of this preparative separation is from Berns et al. (1971) and A. J. M. Berns and H. Bloemendal, personal communication.

Preparation of sample.   Polysomes are prepared from 2- to 3-month-old calf lenses as described by Schoenmakers et al. (1967). "The polysomes were suspended in 0.05 M Tris–HCl, pH 7.4, to a final concentration of about 6 mg/ml, 1/10 volume at 10% w/v SDS added, and the solution kept at 37°C for 5 min. One volume of the buffer in 12% w/w sucrose was added before pumping the sample into the rotor."

Rotor. A B30a or other B-XIV types of rotors may be used.

Gradient. The gradient is an exponential approximation of equivolumetric gradient shape for $\rho = 1.60$ gm/cm^3 (cf. Appendix D3). Specifically, 37% w/w buffered sucrose is pumped into a mixing chamber containing 300 cm^3 of buffer (Fig. 5.6b). The first 50 cm^3 of gradient is stored for use as an overlay.

Sample. Use 15–30 cm^3 of diluted polysome suspension containing approximately 45–90 mg of RNA.

Overlay. After balancing, the stored portion of the gradient is pumped in following the sample. This is followed by buffer for a total volume of 150 cm^3 of overlay.

Centrifugation. Spin at 1.48 rad^2/psec, which corresponds to 50,000 rpm for 15 hr, at 2°C.

Analysis. The gradient is analyzed by flow photometry at 260 nm.

Results. The absorbancy profile (Fig. 9.21) shows a 14 S RNA, subsequently identified as the mRNA for α crystalline A$_2$, between another putative mRNA at 10 S and the massive zone of rRNA at 18 S. Both the

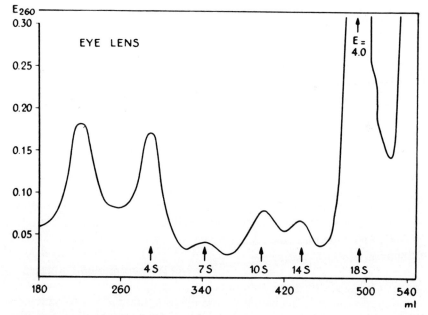

Fig. 9.21. Rate sedimentation of polysomal RNA from calf lens in an equivolumetric gradient (Berns *et al.*, 1971). RNA was extracted from calf lens polysomes and sedimented into an equivolumetric gradient. Note that the method resolves RNAs of 4 S, 7 S, 10 S, and 14 S, in addition to the larger ribosomal RNAs. The 10 S fraction probably contained the mRNA for len; protein.

10 S and 14 S mRNAs were then purified to apparent homogeneity by rate–zonal sedimentation in isokinetic gradients in tubes.

The separations by Berns *et al.* have a double significance quite apart from the study of the synthesis of lens proteins. Small amounts of mRNAs can be resolved in the presence of massive amounts of rRNAs. The RNAs can be successfully separated down to at least 4 S.

9.5.4 Separation of Plasma Lipoproteins by Flotation in Mixed Gradients of Sucrose and Sodium Bromide (Mallinson and Hinton, 1973)

Four kinds of lipoproteins in human blood plasma are routinely distinguished on the basis of their densities: high-density lipoproteins (HDL), low-density lipoproteins (LDL), very low density lipoproteins (VLDL), and chylomicrons. Wilcox and Heimberg (1968) showed that the conventional method of differential flotation through solutions of different densities could be greatly improved by subjecting the plasma to density gradient flotation through gradients of potassium bromide stabilized with sucrose in zonal rotors. In a single run the HDL and LDL components were cleanly separated while the VLDL and chylomicrons collected at the top of the gradient.

Mallinson and Hinton (1973) improved on the procedure of Wilcox and Heimberg by providing two successive gradients: a lower gradient NaBr is surmounted by a gradient of plain sucrose with the result that VLDL and chylomicrons are separately resolved.

Preparation of samples. The method is suitable for 10–20 cm^3 of serum to which 1 mg/cm^3 EDTA has been added immediately after separation from the clot, EDTA–plasma, or concentrated lipoproteins prepared by centrifuging serum or plasma to a density of 1.23 gm/cm^3 and centrifuging 18 hr at 100,000 *g*.

Rotor. Use a B-XIV zonal rotor. A narrower initial sample zone is expected with an edge-loading B-XXX. The method can be easily scaled up for use with B-XV or B-XXIX rotors.

Gradient. A double, linear gradient is employed. A 0–45% w/v sucrose gradient of 300 cm^3 is followed by a 300 cm^3 gradient of NaBr from $\rho = 1.2$ gm/cm^3 to 1.4 gm/cm^3. EDTA is present throughout at a concentration of 0.35 mM.

Sample. The serum, plasma, or concentrated lipoprotein, adjusted to $\rho = 1.4$ gm/cm^3 with solid sodium bromide, are pumped to the edge of the rotor and followed by an underlay of sodium bromide at $\rho = 1.50$ gm/cm^3 to fill the rotor (i.e., until the top of the sucrose gradient begins to emerge from the center line).

Centrifugation. The rotor is accelerated to 42,000 rpm and continued for 30 min at 15°C. After deceleration the gradient is displaced from the center by pumping a solution of sodium bromide of $\rho = 1.50$ gm/cm^3 (or, in the case of edge-unloading rotors, displaced from the edge by pumping water to the center). The absorbancy of the gradient is monitored at 280 nm and 10-cm^3 fractions collected.

Results. As shown in Fig. 9.22, the lipoproteins resolve into a large zone between 400 cm^3 and the edge, which consists of HDL; the asymmetric zone in the center of the gradient is LDL; a sharp zone of VLDL near the top of the gradient; and finally the chylomicron fraction, which hangs on the top. Some minor components are also visible between 100 and 200 cm^3.

Mallinson and Hinton also demonstrated that the general method can be employed on an analytical scale in swinging-bucket rotors. They point out that such a procedure could be useful in clinical analyses of serum. There has been further progress along these lines. Clinical samples can be analyzed in less than 1 hr of flotation in vertical rotors (Chung *et al.*, 1980), although at some loss of resolution over that obtainable in swinging buckets Nilsson *et al.*, 1981). The lipoprotein may be prestained with Sudan black for easier detection (Terpstra *et al.*, 1981).

9.5.5 Separation of Serum Globulins by Rate Sedimentation in an Isometric Gradient (Spragg *et al.*, 1969)

Although there are certainly a number of published accounts of the separation of soluble enzymes by density gradient sedimentation, starting with the famous paper of Martin and Ames (1961), there has not been a concerted effort to determine the limit of resolution of proteins as there has been, for example, with ribosomes.

Spragg *et al.* (1969) designed an isometric gradient shape to move particles across a gradient as rapidly as possible and still preserve a narrow zone width. Indeed, they hoped for one that would be constant.

Rotor. The protocol is described for a B-XIV; however, any of the B-XIV-type of rotors, such as the B-14 Ti and B-30a can be substituted.

Gradient. An isometric sucrose gradient is generated with a programmable generator according to Appendix D8. Exponential approximations have not been described. As with any nonlinear gradient shape, it is important that changes in the size or location of the sample zone not result in any shift of the gradient shape up or down. Changes in sample volumes can be compensated by adjustments in the volume of the overlay.

Sample. Human serum, 20 cm^3, containing Bence–Jones macroglobulin.

Temperature. 22°C.

Centrifugation. Spin at 1.5 radians^2/psec, which corresponds to about 15 hr at 50,000 rpm.

Results. The absorbance profile is shown in Fig. 9.23. There are two

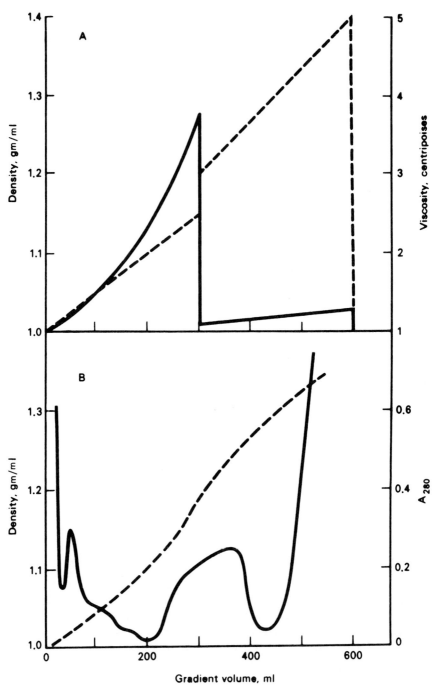

Fig. 9.22. Separation of serum lipoproteins by density gradient flotation (Mallinson and Hinton, 1973). (A) shows the viscosity (solid line) and density (dotted line) of the complex gradient of sucrose and NaBr has loaded into the B-XIV zonal rotor. (B) shows the sedimentation profile of the serum lipoproteins after centrifugation as described in the text. The solid line is the absorbance at 280 nm and the dotted line the density at 15°.

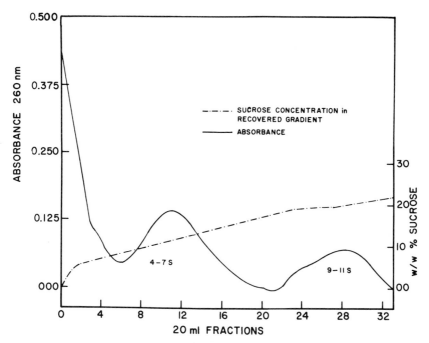

Fig. 9.23. Separation of serum globulins in an isometric gradient (C. T. Rankin, Jr., J. P. Breillatt, and N. G. Anderson, unpublished). The isometric gradient is designed to minimize the time required to separate small particles; this was an overnight run. Human serum containing Bence–Jones macroglobulin was centrifuged in a B-XIV rotor and spun for 1.5×10^{12} radians^2/sec^1. Note that 4–7 S albumins are resolved from 9–11 S globulins.

zones of proteins, one corresponding to 9–11 S with distinct asymmetry and a more symmetrical one at 4–7 S.

Although the experiment establishes an upper limit for the resolution of soluble proteins, one cannot be sure that the gradient shape is necessarily optimal for small particles. Specifically, a steeper gradient might counteract anomalous zone broadening. Note that better resolution was apparently achieved in experiments with steeper gradients described in Figs. 3.22 and 9.21. Although this latter separation concerns RNAs of a size similar to the proteins analyzed here, the comparison is indirect.

REFERENCES

Anderson, N. G. (1956). Techniques for the mass isolation of cellular components. *Phys. Tech. Biol. Res.* **3,** 299–352.
Berns, A. J. M., de Abreu, R. A., van Kraaikamp, M., Benedetti, E. L., and Bloemendal, H.

(1971). Synthesis of lens protein *in vitro*. V. Isolation of messenger-like RNA from lens by high resolution zonal centrifugation. *FEBS Lett.* **18**, 159–163.

Birnie, G. D. (1972). "Subcellular Components," 2nd ed. Butterworth, London.

Birnie, G. D., and Rickwood, D. (eds.) (1978). "Centrifugal Separations in Molecular and Cell Biology." Butterworths, London.

Boone, C. W., Harell, G. S., and Bond, H. E. (1968). The resolution of mixtures of viable mammalian cells into homogeneous fractions by zonal centrifugation. *J. Cell Biol.* **36**, 369–378.

Bowen, R. A., St. Onge, J. M., Colton, J. B., and Price, C. A. (1972). Density gradient centrifugation as an aid to sorting planktonic organisms. I. Gradient materials. *Mar. Biol.* **14**, 242–247.

Brown, D. H., Carlton, E., Byrd, B., Harrell, B., and Hayes, R. L. (1973). A rate-zonal centrifugation procedure for screening particle populations by sequential product recovery utilizing edge-unloading zonal rotors. *Arch. Biochem. Biophys.* **155**, 9–18.

Buckingham, M. E., and Gros, F. (1975). The use of Metrizamide to separate cytoplasmic ribonucleoprotein particles in muscle cell cultures: A method for the isolation of messenger RNA, independent of its poly (A) content. *FEBS Lett.* **53**, 355–359.

Buckner, D., Eisel, R., and Perry, S. (1968). Blood cell separation in the dog by continuous-flow centrifugation. *Blood* **31**(5), 653–672.

Canonico, P. G., and Bird, J. W. C. (1970). Lysosomes in skeletal muscle tissue. Zonal centrifugation evidence for multiple cellular sources. *J. Cell Biol.* **45**, 321–333.

Ca.simpoolas, N. (ed.) (1977). "Methods in Cell Separation," Vol. 1. Plenum, New York.

Chaires, J. B., and Kegeles, G. (1977). Sucrose density gradient sedimentation of *Escherichia coli* ribosomes. *Biophys. Chem.* **7**, 173–178.

Cheng, T. C., Huang, J.-W., Karadogan, H. Renwrantz, L. R., and Yoshino, T. P. (1980). Separation of oyster hemocytes by density gradient centrifugation and identification of their surface receptors. *J. Invertebr. Pathol.* **36**, 35–40.

Chermann, J.-C., and Lavergne, M., eds. (1973). "European Symposium of Zonal Centrifugation in Density Gradients," Spectra 2000, No. 4. Editions Cité Nouvelle.

Chevrenka, C. H., and Elrod, L. H. (1972). "A Manual of Methods for Large-Scale Zonal Centrifugation." Beckman Instruments, Palo Alto, Calif.

Chevrenka, C. H., and McEwen, C. R. (1971). "A Manual of Methods for Large-Scale Zonal Centrifugation." Beckman Instruments, Spinco Division, Palo Alto, California.

Chung, B.-H., Wilkinson, T., Geer, J. C., and Segrest, J. P. (1980). Preparative and quantitative isolation of plasma lipoproteins: Rapid, single discontinuous density gradient ultracentrifugation in a vertical rotor. *J. Lipid Res.* **21**, 284–291.

Clark, R. W., and Lange, C. S. (1976). The sucrose gradient and native DNA $s_{20,w}$, an examination of measurement problems. *Biochim. Biophys. Acta* **454**, 567–577.

Cline, G. B., and Dagg, M. K. (1973). Particle separations in the J- and RK-types of Flo-Band zonal rotors. *In* "Advances With Zonal Rotors" (E. Reid, ed.), Vol. 3, pp. 261–273. Longmans, Green, New York.

Cline, G. B., snd Ryel, R. B. (1971). Zonal centrifugation. *In* "Methods in Enzymology" (W. B. Jakoby, ed.), Vol. 22, pp. 168–204. Academic Press, New York.

Conn, P. M., Tsuruhara, T., Dafau, M., and Catt, K. J. (1977). Isolation of highly purified Leydig cells by density gradient centrifugation. *Endocrinology* **101**, 639–642.

Cotman, C., Mahler, H. R., and Anderson, N. G. (1968). Isolation of a membrane fraction in nerve-end membranes from rat brain by zonal centrifugation. *Biochim. Biophys. Acta* **163**, 272–275.

Coulter-Mackie, M. B., Bradbury, W. C., and Dales, S. (1980). *In vivo* and *in vitro* models of demyelinating diseases. IV. Isolation of Halle measles virus-specific RNA from BGMK cells and preparation of complementary DNA. *Virology* **102**, 327–338.

Creeth, J. M., and Horton, J. R. (1977). Macromolecular distribution near the limits of density-gradient columns. Some applications to the separation and fractionation of glycoproteins. *Biochem. J.* **161**, 449–463.

Cutts, J. H. (1970). "Cell Separation: Methods Used in Hematology." Academic Press, New York.

Eagle, H. (1959). Amino acid metabolism in mammalian cell cultures. *Science* **130**, 432–437.

Ehmann, U. K., and Lett, J. T. (1973). Review and evaluation of molecular weight calculations from the sedimentation profiles of irradiated DNA. *Radiat. Res.* **54**, 152–162.

Eikenberry, E. F., Bickle, T. A., Traut, R. R., and Price, C. A. (1970). Separation of large quantities of ribosomal sub-units by zonal ultracentrifugation. *Eur. J. Biochem.* **12**, 113–116.

Flamm, W. G., Bond, H. E., and Burr, H. E. (1966). Density-gradient centrifugation of DNA in a fixed angle rotor. A higher order of resolution. *Biochim. Biophys. Acta* **129**, 310–317.

Fleischer, S., and Packer, L. (eds.) (1974). "Biomembranes" Part A. Methods in Enzymology XXXI, Academic Press, New York.

Fleischer, S., and Packer, L., eds. (1979a). "Biomembranes" Part F. Methods in Enzymology LV, Academic Press, New York.

Fleischer, S., and Packer, L., eds. (1979b). "Biomembranes" Part G. Methods in Enzymology LVI, Academic Press, New York.

Gonzalez, F. J., Garrett, C. T., Wiener, D., and Caine, M. D. (1978). The use of potassium iodide equilibrium density gradient centrifugation in the purification of RNA for hybridization with nonreiterated DNA sequences. *Anal. Biochem.* **85**, 146–156.

Gorczynski, P. M., Miller, R. G., and Phillips, R. A. (1970). Homogeneity of antibody producing cells as analysed by their buoyant density in gradients of Ficoll. *Immunology* **19**, 817–829.

Granick, S. (1938). Quantitative isolation of chloroplasts from higher plants. *Am. J. Bot.* **25**, 558–561.

Haley, N. J., Shio, H., and Fowler, S. (1977). Characterization of lipid-laden aortic cells from cholesterol-fed rabbits. I. Resolution of aortic cell populations by Metrizamide density gradient centrifugation. *Lab. Invest.* **37**, 287–296.

Halvorson, H. O., Carter, B. L. A., and Tauro, P. (1971). Use of synchronous cultures of yeast to study gene position. *In* "Methods in Enzymology" (L. Grossman and K. Moldave, eds.), Vol. 21, Part D, pp. 462–470. Academic Press, New York.

Hendricks, A. W. (1972). Purification of plant nuclei using colloidal silica. *FEBS Lett.* **24**, 101–105.

Hernandez, A. G. (1974). Protein synthesis by synaptosomes from rat brain. *Biochem. J.* **142**, 7–17.

Hinton, R. H., Dobrota, M., Fitzsimons, J. T. R., and Reid, E. (1970). Preparation of a plasma membrane fraction from rat liver by zonal centrifugation. *Eur. J. Biochem.* **12**, 349–361.

Hogeboom, G. H., Schneider, W. C., and Palade, G. E. (1948). Cytochemical studies of mammalian tissues. I. Isolation of intact mitochondria from rat liver; some biochemical properties of mitochondria and submicroscopic particulate material. *J. Biol. Chem.* **172**, 619–636.

Hudspeth, M. E. S., Shumard, D. S., and Tatti, K. M. (1980). Rapid purification of yeast mitochondrial DNA in high yield. *Biochim. Biophys. Acta* **610**, 221–228.

Jackson, C., Dench, J. E., Hall, D. O., and Moore, A. L. (1979). Separation of mitochondria from contaminating subcellular structures utilizing silica sol gradient centrifugation. *Plant Physiol.* **64**, 150–153.

Jensen, R. H., and Davidson, N. (1966). Spectrophotometic, potentiometric, and density gradient ultracentrifugation studies of the binding of silver by DNA. *Biopolymers* **4**, 17–32.

Johnston, I. R., Mathias, A. P., Pennington, E., and Ridge, D. (1968). The fractionation of nuclei from mammalian cells by zonal centrifugation. *Biochem. J.* **109**, 127–135.

Juhos, E. (1966). Density gradient centrifugation of bacteria and nonspecific bacteriophage in silica sols. *J. Bacteriol.* **91**, 1376–1377.

Korba, B. E., Hays, J. B., and Boehmer, S. (1981). Sedimentation velocity of DNA in isokinetic sucrose gradients: Calibration against molecular weight using fragments of defined length. *Nucleic Acids Res.* **9**, 4403–4412.

Lammers, W. T. (1971). Insoluble material in natural water. *In* "Water and Water Pollution Handbook" (L. L. Ciaccio, ed.), Vol. 2, pp. 593–638. Dekker, New York.

Leech, R. M. (1964). The isolation of structurally intact chloroplasts. *Biochim. Biophys. Acta* **79**, 637–639.

Levin, D., and Hutchinson, F. (1973). Natural sucrose sedimentation of very large DNA from *Bacillus subtilis*. *J. Mol. Biol.* **75**, 455–478.

Lieblová, J., Beran, K., and Streiblová, E. (1964). Fractionation of a population of *Saccharomyces cerevisiae* yeasts by centrifugation in a dextran gradient. *Folia Microbiol.* (*Prague*) **9**, 205–213.

Lipsich, L. A., Lucas, J. J., and Kates, J. R. (1979). Separation of cytoplasts and whole cells using density gradients of Renografin. *J. Cell. Physiol.* **98**, 637–642.

McDonnell, M. W., Simon, M. N., and Studier, F. W. (1977). Analysis of restriction fragments of T7 DNA and determination of molecular weights by electrophoresis in neutral and alkaline gels. *J. Mol. Biol.* **110**, 119–146.

McGrath, R. A., and Williams, R. W. (1966). Reconstruction *in vivo* of irradiated *Escherichia coli* deoxyribonucleic acid; the rejoining of broken pieces. *Nature* (*London*) **212**, 534–535.

Mallinson, A., and Hinton, R. H. (1973). The use of sucrose-sodium bromide gradients in the separation of plasma lipoproteins. *In* "Advances with Zonal Rotors" (E. Reid, ed.), "Methods in Developmental Biochemistry," Vol. 3, pp. 113–119. Longman, Guildford, 275 pp.

Martin, R. G., and Ames, B. N. (1961). A method for determining the sedimentation behavior of enzymes: Application to protein mixtures. *J. Biol. Chem.* **236**, 1372–1379.

Maruyama, Y., and Yanagita, T. (1956). Physical methods for obtaining synchronous cultures *E. coli*. *J. Bacteriol.* **71**, 542–546.

Mateyko, G. M., and Kopac, M. J. (1963). Cytophysical studies on living normal and neoplastic cells. II. Isopyknotic cushioning during high-speed centrifugation. *Ann. N. Y. Acad. Sci.* **105**, 219–285.

Mathias, A. P. (1973). The properties of nuclei from rat brain and liver fractionated by zonal centrifugation. *Spectra 2000* **4**, 151–160.

Mathias, A. P., and Wynther, C. V. A. (1973). The use of Metrizamide in the fractionation of nuclei from brain and liver tissue by zonal centrifugation. *FEBS Lett.* **33**, 18–22.

Matthews, H. R., Johnson, E. M., Steer, W. M., Bradbury, E. M., and Allfrey, V. G. (1978). The use of netropsin with CsCl gradients for the analysis of DNA and its application to restriction nuclease fragments of ribosomal DNA from *Physarum polycephalum*. *Eur. J. Biochem.* **82**, 569–576.

Mayer, D., Stoehr, S., and Lange, L. (1977). Quantitative analysis of DNA, RNA, protein and glycogen in isolated rat hepatocytes separated by Metrizamide density gradients. *Cytobiologie* **15**, 321–334.

Mickelson, J. R., Greaser, M. L., and Bruce, M. B. (1980). Purification of skeletal-muscle mitochondria by density-gradient centrifugation with Percoll. *Anal. Biochem.* **109**, 255–260.

Moore, D. H. (1969). Gradient centrifugation. *In* "Physical Techniques in Biological Research" (D. H. Moore, ed.), 2nd ed., Vol. 2, Part B, pp. 285–314. Academic Press, New York.

Morgenthaler, J.-J., Price, C. A., Robinson, J. M., and Gibbs, M. (1974). Photosynthetic activity of spinach chloroplasts after isopycnic centrifugation in gradients of silica. *Plant Physiol.* **54**, 532–534.

Morgenthaler, J.-J., Marsden, M. P. F., and Price, C. A. (1975). Factors affecting the separation of photosynthetically competent chloroplasts in gradients of silica sols. *Arch. Biochem. Biophys.* **168**, 289–301.

Nanni, G., Baldini, I., and Ferro, M. (1969). Separation of different lymphocyte populations by Ficoll linear density gradient centrifugation. *Boll. Soc. Ital. Biol. Sper.* **45**, 935–939.

Nilsson, J., Mannickarottu, V., and Edelstein, C. (1981). An improved detection system applied to the study of serum lipoproteins after single-step density gradient ultracentrifugation. *Anal. Biochem.* **110**, 342–348.

Noll, H. (1969a). Polysomes: Analysis of structure and function. *In* "Techniques in Protein Biosynthesis" (P. N. Cambell and J. R. Sargent, eds.), Vol. 2, pp. 101–179. Academic Press, New York.

Noll, H. (1969b). An automatic high-resolution gradient analyzing system. *Anal. Biochem.* **27**, 130–149.

Novick, P., Field, C., and Schekman, R. (1980). The identification of 23 complementation groups required for post-translational events in the yeast secretory pathway. *Cell* **21**, 205–215.

Ormerod, M. G., and Lehmann, A. R. (1971). Artifacts arising from the sedimentation of high molecular weight DNA on sucrose gradients. *Biochim. Biophys. Acta* **247**, 369–372.

Ortiz, W., Reardon, E. M., and Price, C. A. (1980). Preparation of chloroplasts from *Euglena* highly active in protein synthesis. *Plant Physiol.* **66**, 291–294.

Peake, P. W. (1979). Isolation and characterization of the hemocytes of *Calliphora vicina* on density gradients of Ficoll. *J. Insect Physiol.* **25**, 795–803.

Peck, F. B. (1968). Purified influenza virus vaccine. *J. Am. Med. Assoc.* **206**, 2277–2282.

Peeters, H. (ed.) (1979). "Separation of Cells and Subcellular Elements." Pergamon, Oxford.

Pertoft, H. (1966). Gradient centrifugation in colloidal silica-polysaccharide media. *Biochim. Biophys. Acta* **126**, 594–596.

Pertoft, H. (1969). The separation of rat liver cells in colloidal silica-polyethylene glycol gradients. *Exp. Cell Res.* **57**, 338–350.

Pertoft, H. (1970). Separation of cells from a mast cell tumor in density gradients of colloidal silica. *JNCI, J. Natl. Cancer Inst.* **44**, 1251–1256.

Pertoft, H., and Laurent, T. C. (1977). Isopycnic separation of cells and cell organelles by centrifugation in modified colloidal silica gradients. *Methods Cell Sep.* **1**, 25–65.

Pertoft, H., Bäck, O., and Lindahl-Kiessline, K. (1968). Separation of various blood cells in colloidal silica-polyvinylpyrrolidone gradients. *Exp. Cell Res.* **50**, 355–368.

Pertoft, H., Rubin, K., Kjellen, L., Laurent, T. C., and Klingeborn, B. (1977). The viability of cells grown or centrifuged in a new density gradient medium, Percoll *Exp. Cell Res.* **110**, 449–457.

Pertoft, H., Hirtenstein, M., and Kagedal, L. (1979). Cell separations in a new density gradient

Medium, Percoll. *In* "Cell Populations" (E. Reid, ed.), "Meth. Surveys (B): Biochemistry," Vol. 8, pp. 67–80. Ellis Horwood, Chichester.

Peterson, A. R., Bertram, J. S., and Heidelberger, C. (1974). DNA damage and its repair in transformable mouse fibroblasts treated with N-methyl-N'nitro-N-nitrosoguanidine. *Cancer Res.* **34,** 1592–1599.

Phillips, R. A., and Miller, R. G. (1970). Antibody producing cells: Analysis and purification by velocity sedimentation. *Cell Tissue Kinet.* **3,** 263–274.

Pretlow, T. G., II, and Boone, C. W. (1969). Separation of mammalian cells using programmed gradient sedimentation. *Exp. Mol. Pathol.* **11,** 139–152.

Pretlow, T. G. II, and Pretlow, T. P. (1977). Separation of viable cells by velocity sedimentation in an isokinetic gradient of Ficoll in tissue culture medium. *In* "Methods in Cell Separation" (N. Catsimpoolas, ed.), Vol. 1, pp. 171–191. Plenum, New York, 361 pp.

Price, C. A. (1970). Plant cell fractionation: An overview. *In* "Microsymposium on Particle Separation from Plant Materials" (C. A. Price, ed.), Oak Ridge Natl. Lab. CONF-700119, pp. 1–13. Natl. Tech. Inf. Serv., Springfield, Virginia.

Price, C. A., Mendiola-Morgenthaler, L. R., Goldstein, M., Breden, E. N., and Guillard, R. R. L. (1974). Harvest of planktonic marine algae by centrifugation into gradients of silica in the CF-6 continuous-flow zonal rotor. *Biol. Bull.* (*Woods Hole, Mass.*) **147,** 136–145.

Price, C. A., St. Onge-Burns, J. M., Colton, J. B., and Joyce, J. E. (1977). Automatic sorting of zooplankton by isopycnic sedimentation in gradients of silica: Performance of a "rho spectrometer." *Mar. Biol.* **42,** 225–231.

Price, C. A., Reardon, E. M., and Guillard, R. R. L. (1978). Collection of dinoflagellates and other marine microalgae by centrifugation in density gradients of a modified silica sol. *Limnol. Oceanogr.* **23,** 548–553.

Price, C. A., and Reardon, E. M. (1982). Isolation of chloroplasts for protein synthesis from spinach and *Euglena gracilis* by centrifugation in silica sols. *In* "Methods in Chloroplast Molecular Biology" (M. Edelman, R. Hallick, and N. Chua, eds.), Elsevier-North Holland, in press.

Price, C. A., Reardon, E. M., and Guillard, R. R. L. (1982). Collection and analysis of marine phytoplankton by density gradient centrifugation in Percoll gradients. Commun. Woods Hole Oceanographic Institution, Woods Hole, Mass., U.S.A., in press.

Probst, H., and Maisenbacher, J. (1975). Selection of synchronous cell populations from Ehrlich ascites tumor cells by zonal centrifugation. *Methods Cell Biol.* **10,** 173–184.

Reid, E., ed. (1970). "Separations with Zonal Rotors." University of Surrey, Guildford, Surrey, U. K.

Reid, E., ed. (1973). "Advances with Zonal Rotors," Vol. 3. Longmans, Green, New York.

Reid, E., ed. (1979a). "Cell Populations" Methods Dev. Biochem. Vol. 8, Ellis Horwood, Chichester.

Reid, E., ed. (1979b). "Plant Organelles" Methods Dev. Biochem. Vol. 9, Ellis Horwood, Chichester.

Reimer, C. B., Baker, R. S., van Frank, R. M., Newlin, T. E., Cline, G. B., and Anderson, N. G. (1967). Purification of large quantities of influenza virus by density gradient centrifugation. *J. Virol.* **1,** 1207–1216.

Rickwood, H., ed. (1976). "Biological Separations in Iodinated Density-Gradient Media." Information Retrieval, London.

Rosenbloom, J., and Cox, E. C. (1966). Sedimentation coefficient of T-even bacteriophage DNA. *Biopolymers* **4,** 747–757.

Russell, H., Thomas, M. L., Clark, V. W., Jr., Cline, G. B., and Anderson, N. G. (1967).

Purification of *Treponema pallidum* by zonal centrifugation. *Oak Ridge Natl. Lab.* [*Spec. Rep.*] **ORNL-SP-4171**, 48–57.

Schoenmakers, J. G. G., Zweers, A., and Bloemendal, H. (1967). Synthesis of lens protein *in vitro*. I. Properties of polyribosomes. *Biochim. Biophys. Acta* **145**, 120–126.

Schumacher, M., Schaefer, G., Holstein, A. F., and Hilz, H. (1978). Rapid isolation of mouse Leydig cells by centrifugation in Percoll density gradients with complete retention of morphological and biochemical integrity. *FEBS Lett.* **91**, 333–338.

Scott, W. N., Yoder, M. J., and Gennaro, J. F. (1978). Isolation of highly enriched preparations of two types of mucosal cells of the turtle's urinary bladder. *Proc. Soc. Exp. Biol. Med.* **1158**, 565–571.

Sebastian, J., Carter, B. L. A., and Halvorson, H. O. (1971). Use of yeast populations fractionated by zonal centrifugation to study the cell cycle. *J. Bacteriol.* **108**, 1045–1050.

Shortman, K. (1968). The separation of different cell classes from lymphoid organs. II. The purification and analysis of lymphocyte populations by equilibrium density gradient centrifugation. *Aust. J. Exp. Biol. Med. Sci.* **46**, 375–396.

Sitz, T. O., Kent, A. B., Hopkins, H. A., and Schmidt, R. R. (1970). Equilibrium density-gradient procedure for selection of synchronous cells from asynchronous cultures. *Science* **168**, 1231–1232.

Sorrentino, J., Metzgar, D. P., and Bolyn, A. E. (1973). Purification of influenza vaccine on a commercial scale using density gradient centrifugation. *Spectra 2000* **4**, 205–210.

Sorokin, C. (1963). Characteristics of the process of aging in algal cells. *Science* **140**, 385.

Spragg, S. P., Morrod, R. S., and Rankin, C. T., Jr. (1969). The optimization of density gradients for zonal centrifugation. *Sep. Sci.* **4**, 467–481.

Studier, F. W. (1965). Sedimentation studies of the size and shape of DNA. *J. Mol. Biol.* **11**, 373–390.

Szafarz, D. (1977). An improved method for DNA alkaline gradient analysis and its application to the effect of carcinogens on mouse liver DNA. *Biochimie* **59**, 775–778.

Szybalski, W. (1968). Use of cesium sulfate for equilibrium density gradient centrifugation. *In* "Methods in Enzymology" (S. P. Colowick and N. O. Kaplan, eds.), Vol. 12, Part B, pp. 330–360. Academic Press, New York.

Tamir, H., and Gilvarg, C. (1966). Density gradient centrifugation for the separation of sporulating forms of bacteria. *J. Biol. Chem.* **241**, 1085–1090.

Terpstra, A. H. M., Woodward, C. J. M., and Sanchez-Muniz, F. J. (1981). Improved techniques for the separation of serum lipoproteins by density gradient ultracentrifugation: Visualization by prestraining and rapid separation of serum lipoproteins from small volumes of serum. *Anal. Biochem.* **111**, 149–157.

Thomas, M. L., Clark, J. W., Jr., Cline, G. B., Anderson, N. G., and Russell, H. (1972). Separation of *Treponema pallidum* from tissue substances by continuous-flow zonal centrifugation. *Appl. Microbiol.* **23**, 714–720.

Tissières, A., Watson, J. D., Schlessinger, D., and Hollingworth, B. R. (1959). Ribonucleoprotein particles from *Escherichia coli*. *J. Mol. Biol.* **1**, 221–233.

Vallee, B. L., Hughes, W. L., Jr., and Gibson, J. G., 2nd (1947). A method for the separation of leukocytes from whole blood by flotation on serum albumin. *Blood* **1**, Spec. Issue, 82–87.

Vasconcelos, A., Pollack, M., Mendiola, L. R., Hoffmann, H.-P., Brown, D. H., and Price, C. A. (1971). Isolation of intact chloroplasts from *Euglena gracilis* by zonal centrifugation. *Plant Physiol.* **47**, 217–221.

Warmsley, A. M. H., and Pasternak, C. A. (1970). Use of conventional and zonal centrifugation to study the life cycle of mammalian cells. Phospholipid and macromolecular synthesis in neoplastic mast cells. *Biochem. J.* **119**, 493–499.

Whittaker, V. P., and Barker, L. A. (1971). The subcellular fractionation of brain tissue with
     special reference to the preparation of synaptosomes and their component organelles.
     Methods Neurochem. **2,** 1–52.
Whittaker, V. P., Michaelson, I. A., and Kirkland, R. J. A. (1964). The separation of synaptic
     vesicles from disrupted nerve-ending particles ('synaptosomes'). *Biochem. J.* **90,** 293–303.
Wilcox, H. G., and Heimberg, M. (1968). The isolation of human serum lipoproteins by zonal
     ultracentrifugation. *Biochim. Biophys. Acta* **152,** 424–426.
Wolff, D. A. (1975). The separation of cells and subcellular particles by colloidal silica density
     gradient centrifugation. *Methods Cell Biol.* **10,** 85–104.

Appendix A

Some Useful Units, Values, and Conversions

A1. MATHEMATICAL VALUES AND RELATIONS

Symbol or expression	Value	
pi (π)	3.1415	927
e	2.71828	18285
$\log_{10}x$	0.43429	44819 $\log_e x$
$\log_e x$	2.30258	50930 $\log_{10}x$
$\log_{10}2$	0.30102	99957
$\log_e 2$	0.09314	71806
$e^{-1/2}$	0.606531	
e^{-1}	0.367879	
e^{-2}	0.13533	52832
$e^{1/2}$	1.648721	
e^2	7.38905	60991

Gaussian Distributions

Since narrow particle zones are typically recovered as Gaussian distributions, it is useful to assemble some of the properties of these distributions.

The concentration of particles $c(v)$ in Fig. A.1 is in a Gaussian distribution with respect to volume V. The highest concentration of particle $\bar{c}$ is at the origin $V = 0$. The distribution can be written as

$$c(v) = \bar{c}\epsilon^{\frac{-V^2}{2\sigma^2}}$$

315

where σ is the *dispersion, first moment,* or *standard deviation* (cf. Fig. A.1). The total amount of particles is evidently

$$m_t = \int_{-\infty}^{+\infty} c(v)dV$$

The value of this integral is

$$m_t = \int_{-\infty}^{+\infty} c(v)dV = \int_{-\infty}^{+\infty} \bar{c}\epsilon^{\frac{-V^2}{2\sigma^2}}dV = \sqrt{2\pi}\,\bar{c}\sigma = 2.50663\bar{c}\sigma$$

A normalized Gaussian distribution in which $m = 1$ can also be considered. In this case

$$c(V) = \frac{\epsilon^{\frac{-V^2}{2\sigma^2}}}{\sqrt{2\pi}\,\sigma}$$

whence,

$$\bar{c} = 1/\sqrt{2\pi}\,\sigma$$

At $V = \pm\sigma$

$$c(\sigma) = \bar{c}\,\epsilon^{-1/2} \qquad c(\sigma) = 0.6065\bar{c}$$

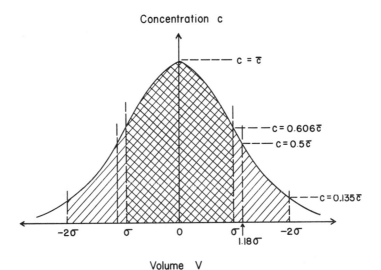

Fig. A.1.   Gaussian distribution function. The curve represents the concentration $c(V)$ with respect to volume of a Gaussian distribution of particles. The cross-hatched area represents the fraction (0.683) of particles contained between $+\sigma$ and $-\sigma$. The diagonal shading represents the fraction (0.955) between $+2\sigma$ and -2σ.

Thus the concentration at the first moment is 0.6065 of the peak height. One can similarly compute the values of c at different points along the abcissa and the fraction of particles included.

	Distance from the center of the zone		
	$\pm\sigma$	$\pm1.17741\sigma$	$\pm2\sigma$
$c/\bar{c}$ (fraction of peak height)	0.6065	0.5	0.135
m/m_t (fraction of total mass of particles)	0.683	0.754	0.955

A2. PHYSICAL AND CHEMICAL VALUES AND CONVERSIONS
OBSOLETE TERMS ARE ITALICIZED

Term	Abbreviations	Value
Multipliers		
milli-	m-	10^{-3}
micro-	μ-	10^{-6}
nano- (formerly "*millimicro*"-)	n- (mμ-)	10^{-9}
pico (formerly "*micromicro*"-)	p- ($\mu\mu$-)	10^{-12}
Centrifugal fields and forces		
Svedberg	S	10^{-13} sec
		0.1 psec
gravity	G	980.655 dyn/cm^2
relative centrifugal field	RCF	$1.118 \times 10^{-5}r$(cm) $\times$ (rpm)^2 gravities
(also, relative centrifugal *force*)		1.019727×10^{-3} cm rad^2/sec^2
dyn/sec^2	dyn/sec^2	1.0197×10^{-3} G
revolutions per minute	rpm	0.10472 rad/sec
(revolutions per minute)^2	(rpm)^2	1.09662×10^{-2} rad^2/sec
radians	rad	57.29578 degrees
		0.15916 revolutions
radians per second	ω	9.5493
(radians per second)^2	ω^2	91.189
Interconversion of American and metric units		
pound	lb	453.5924 277 gm
kilogram	kg	2.2046 22341 lb
gallon (American)	gal	3.78533 liter
Units of pressure		
pascal	Pa	1 N/m^2
		9.869×10^{-6} atm
		10 dyn/cm^2
atmosphere	atm	1.013×10^5 Pa
		1.0332 kg/cm^2

A2.   Continued

Term	Abbreviations	Value
		1.0133 bars
		1.01325×10^6 dyn/cm^2
		14.6960 psi
		760 mm Hg (pressure of at 0°C)
Torr	(none)	133.3 Pa
		1 mm of Hg (pressure of, at 0°C)
mm of Hg (pressure of, at 0°C)	mm	1333.22 dyn/cm^2
		0.00131579 atm
micron (of vacuum)	μ	10^{-3} mm of Hg
kilogram per square centimeter	kg/cm^2	0.96777 atm
		14.223 psi
pounds per square inch	psi	0.070307 kg/cm^2
		0.068046 atm
Time		
second	sec	
minute	min	60 sec
hour	hr	60 min; 3600 sec
day	day	24 hr
		1.44×10^3 min
		8.64×10^4 sec
Chemical units		
Avogadro constant	N$_A$	6.02252×10^{23}
dalton	d	1.66024×10^{-24} gm
or		
atomic mass unit	u	(e.g., 1 molecule of 10^5 molecular weight weighs 10^5 d or 10^5 u
molar gas constant	R	82.06 cm^3/atom deg·mole
		8.3144×10^7 erg/deg·mole
		8.3144 joule/deg·mole
		1.013×10^6 dyn/cm^2·deg·mole
		1.987 cal/gm·deg·mole
		0.08206 liter atm/deg·mole
		22.4 atm/mole·liter (at 0°C)
curie	Ci	3.7×10^{10} disintegration/sec
Dynamic viscosity		
poise	(none)	1.0 dyn·sec/cm^2 (unit of viscosity)
		0.1 Pa·sec
pascal second	Pa·sec	10 *poise*
Diffusion coefficients		
(no name)	m^2/sec	
fick		10^{-7} cm^2/sec
Length		
Angstrom	Å	0.1 nm

A3. VALUES OF $\omega^2 t$ FOR DIFFERENT SPEEDS AND TIMES (COMPUTED BY E. F. EIKENBERRY)[a]

		Time			
rpm	ω^2	360 sec 6 min 0.1 hr	600 sec 10 min 0.1667 hr	1200 sec 20 min 0.3333 hr	1800 sec 30 min 0.5 hr
500	2.742 E 3	9.870 E 5	1.645 E 6	3.290 E 6	4.935 E 6
1000	1.097 E 4	3.948 E 6	6.580 E 6	1.316 E 7	1.974 E 7
1500	2.467 E 4	8.883 E 6	1.480 E 7	2.961 E 7	4.441 E 7
2000	4.387 E 4	1.579 E 7	2.632 E 7	5.264 E 7	7.896 E 7
2500	6.854 E 4	2.467 E 7	4.112 E 7	8.225 E 7	1.234 E 8
3000	9.870 E 4	3.553 E 7	5.922 E 7	1.184 E 8	1.777 E 8
4000	1.755 E 5	6.317 E 7	1.053 E 8	2.106 E 8	3.158 E 8
5000	2.742 E 5	9.870 E 7	1.645 E 8	3.290 E 8	4.935 E 8
6000	3.948 E 5	1.421 E 8	2.369 E 8	4.737 E 8	7.106 E 8
8000	7.018 E 5	2.527 E 8	4.211 E 8	8.422 E 8	1.263 E 9
10000	1.097 E 6	3.948 E 8	6.580 E 8	1.316 E 9	1.974 E 9
15000	2.467 E 6	8.883 E 8	1.480 E 9	2.961 E 9	4.441 E 9
20000	4.387 E 6	1.579 E 9	2.632 E 9	5.264 E 9	7.896 E 9
25000	6.854 E 6	2.467 E 9	4.112 E 9	8.225 E 9	1.234 E 10
30000	9.870 E 6	3.553 E 9	5.922 E 9	1.184 E 10	1.777 E 10
35000	1.343 E 7	4.836 E 9	8.060 E 9	1.612 E 10	2.418 E 10
40000	1.755 E 7	6.317 E 9	1.053 E 10	2.106 E 10	3.158 E 10
45000	2.221 E 7	7.994 E 9	1.332 E 10	2.665 E 10	3.997 E 10
50000	2.742 E 7	9.870 E 9	1.645 E 10	3.290 E 10	4.935 E 10
55000	3.317 E 7	1.194 E 10	1.990 E 10	3.981 E 10	5.971 E 10
60000	3.948 E 7	1.421 E 10	2.369 E 10	4.737 E 10	7.106 E 10
65000	4.633 E 7	1.668 E 10	2.780 E 10	5.560 E 10	8.340 E 10
70000	5.373 E 7	1.934 E 10	3.224 E 10	6.448 E 10	9.672 E 10
75000	6.169 E 7	2.221 E 10	3.701 E 10	7.402 E 10	1.110 E 11
rpm	3600 sec 60 min 1.0 hr	7200 sec 120 min 2.0 hr	1.44×10^4 sec 240 min 4.0 hr	2.16×10^4 sec 360 min 6.0 hr	2.88×10^4 sec 480 min 8.0 hr
500	9.870 E 6	1.974 E 7	3.948 E 7	5.922 E 7	7.896 E 7
1000	3.948 E 7	7.896 E 7	1.579 E 8	2.369 E 8	3.158 E 8
1500	8.883 E 7	1.777 E 8	3.553 E 8	5.330 E 8	7.106 E 8
2000	1.579 E 8	3.158 E 8	6.317 E 8	9.475 E 8	1.263 E 9
2500	2.467 E 8	4.935 E 8	9.870 E 8	1.480 E 9	1.974 E 9
3000	3.553 E 8	7.106 E 8	1.421 E 9	2.132 E 9	2.842 E 9
4000	6.317 E 8	1.263 E 9	2.527 E 9	3.790 E 9	5.053 E 9
5000	9.870 E 8	1.974 E 9	3.948 E 9	5.922 E 9	7.896 E 9
6000	1.421 E 9	2.842 E 9	5.685 E 9	8.527 E 9	1.137 E 10
8000	2.527 E 9	5.053 E 9	1.011 E 10	1.516 E 10	2.021 E 10
10000	3.948 E 9	7.896 E 9	1.579 E 10	2.369 E 10	3.158 E 10

Continued

A3.   Continued

	Time				
rpm	3600 sec 60 min 1.0 hr	7200 sec 120 min 2.0 hr	1.44×10^4 sec 240 min 4.0 hr	2.16×10^4 sec 360 min 6.0 hr	2.88×10^4 sec 480 min 8.0 hr
15000	8.883 E 9	1.777 E 10	3.553 E 10	5.330 E 10	7.106 E 10
20000	1.579 E 10	3.158 E 10	6.317 E 10	9.475 E 10	1.263 E 11
25000	2.467 E 10	4.935 E 10	9.870 E 10	1.480 E 11	1.974 E 11
30000	3.553 E 10	7.106 E 10	1.421 E 11	2.132 E 11	2.842 E 11
35000	4.836 E 10	9.672 E 10	1.934 E 11	2.902 E 11	3.869 E 11
40000	6.317 E 10	1.263 E 11	2.527 E 11	3.790 E 11	5.053 E 11
45000	7.994 E 10	1.599 E 11	3.198 E 11	4.797 E 11	6.396 E 11
50000	9.870 E 10	1.974 E 11	3.948 E 11	5.922 E 11	7.896 E 11
55000	1.194 E 11	2.388 E 11	4.777 E 11	7.165 E 11	9.554 E 11
60000	1.421 E 11	2.842 E 11	5.685 E 11	8.527 E 11	1.137 E 12
65000	1.668 E 11	3.336 E 11	6.672 E 11	1.001 E 12	1.334 E 12
70000	1.934 E 11	3.869 E 11	7.738 E 11	1.161 E 12	1.548 E 12
75000	2.221 E 11	4.441 E 11	8.883 E 11	1.332 E 12	1.777 E 12

rpm	4.32×10^4 sec 720 min 12.0 hr	5.4×10^4 sec 900 min 15.0 hr	5.55×10^4 sec 1280 min 18.0 hr	21.0 hr	24.0 hr
500	1.184 E 8	1.480 E 8	1.777 E 8	2.073 E 8	2.369 E 8
1000	4.737 E 8	5.922 E 8	7.106 E 8	8.291 E 8	9.475 E 8
1500	1.066 E 9	1.332 E 9	1.599 E 9	1.865 E 9	2.132 E 9
2000	1.895 E 9	2.369 E 9	2.842 E 9	3.316 E 9	3.790 E 9
2500	2.961 E 9	3.701 E 9	4.441 E 9	5.182 E 9	5.922 E 9
3000	4.264 E 9	5.330 E 9	6.396 E 9	7.461 E 9	8.527 E 9
4000	7.580 E 9	9.475 E 9	1.137 E 10	1.326 E 10	1.516 E 10
5000	1.184 E 10	1.480 E 10	1.777 E 10	2.073 E 10	2.369 E 10
6000	1.705 E 10	2.132 E 10	2.558 E 10	2.985 E 10	3.411 E 10
8000	3.032 E 10	3.790 E 10	4.548 E 10	5.306 E 10	6.064 E 10
10000	4.737 E 10	5.922 E 10	7.106 E 10	8.291 E 10	9.475 E 10
15000	1.066 E 11	1.332 E 11	1.599 E 11	1.865 E 11	2.132 E 11
20000	1.895 E 11	2.369 E 11	2.842 E 11	3.316 E 11	3.790 E 11
25000	2.961 E 11	3.701 E 11	4.441 E 11	5.182 E 11	5.922 E 11
30000	4.264 E 11	5.330 E 11	6.396 E 11	7.462 E 11	8.527 E 11
35000	5.803 E 11	7.254 E 11	8.705 E 11	1.016 E 12	1.161 E 12
40000	7.580 E 11	9.475 E 11	1.137 E 12	1.326 E 12	1.516 E 12
45000	9.593 E 11	1.199 E 12	1.439 E 12	1.679 E 12	1.919 E 12
50000	1.184 E 12	1.480 E 12	1.777 E 12	2.073 E 12	2.369 E 12
55000	1.433 E 12	1.791 E 12	2.150 E 12	2.508 E 12	2.866 E 12
60000	1.705 E 12	2.132 E 12	2.558 E 12	2.985 E 12	3.411 E 12
65000	2.002 E 12	2.502 E 12	3.002 E 12	3.503 E 12	4.003 E 12
70000	2.321 E 12	2.902 E 12	3.482 E 12	4.062 E 12	4.643 E 12
75000	2.665 E 12	3.331 E 12	3.997 E 12	4.663 E 12	5.330 E 12

[a] Values of $\omega^2 t$ are in radians^2/sec^{-1}.

A4.   RELATION OF $\omega^2 t$ TO RPM (FIG. A2)

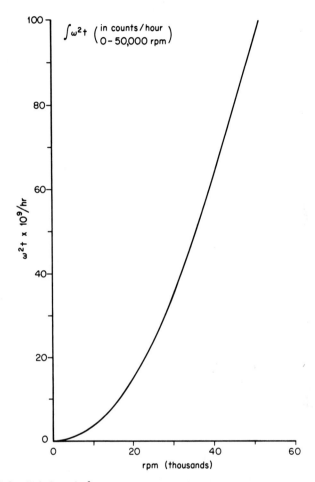

Fig. A.2.   Relation of $\omega^2 t$ to rpm. (Courtesy of N. G. Andrews, MAN Program.)

A5. NOMOGRAPH RELATING CENTRIFUGAL FIELD, IN RADIUS, AND SPEED (FIG. A3)

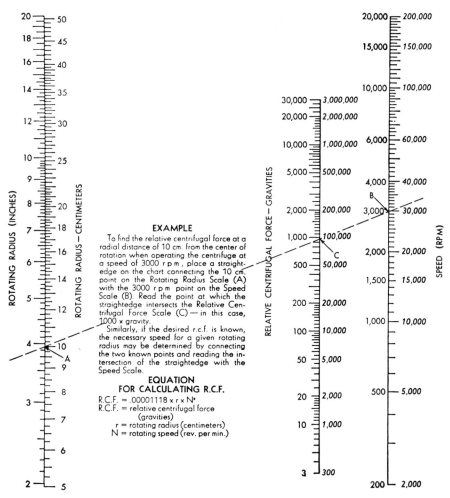

Fig. A.3. Nomograph for computing relative centrifugal field. (Courtesy of IEC/Damon.)

Appendix B

Properties of Particles

B1. NATURAL PARTICLES

Particle	Weight (d)	Sedimentation coefficient (Svedbergs)	Density (gm/cm^3)	Frictional coefficient (f/f_0)
Milk lipase[a]	6,669	1.14	1.30	1.190
Insulin[a]	24,430	1.95	1.36	1.516
Pig heart lactate dehydrogenase[a]	109,000	6.93	1.35	1.127
Human fibrinogen[a]	339,700	7.63	1.38	2.336
E. coli 16 S ribosomal RNA[b]	560,000	16.7	1.663[c]	—
Horse liver catalase[a]	221,600	11.2	1.40	1.246
Apoferritin[a]	466,900	17.60	1.34	1.141
E. coli 30 S ribosomal subunit	990,000	30.6	1.72	—
Bovine liver glutamate dehydrogenase[a]	1,015,000	26.60	1.33	1.250
E. coli 23 S ribosomal RNA	1,100,000	23	1.663[c]	—
E. coli 50 S ribosomal subunit[d]	1,700,000	50.0	1.72	
β- lipoprotein[a]	2,663,000	5.9	1.03	1.243
E. coli 70 S ribosome[d]	2,690,000	69.1	1.72	—
Turnip yellow mosaic virus[a]	4,970,000	106	1.50	1.255
Human adenovirus 2 DNA[b]	23,000,000	25	1.714	—
Tobacco mosaic virus[a]	31,340,000	185	1.37	1.927
Silkworm polyhedral virus[a]	916,200,000	1,871	1.30	1.515
Lysosomes	—	ca. 9,000	1.18	—
Peroxisomes	—	ca. 20,000	1.24	—
Mitochondria	—	ca. 30,000	1.18	—

Continued

B1.   Continued

Pollen grains	Diameter (μm)	Source
Paper mulberry	12–13	Coulter Electronics, Inc.
Ragweed	19–20	Coulter Electronics, Inc.
Pecan	45–50	Coulter Electronics, Inc.
Corn (maize)	85–90	Coulter Electronics, Inc.

[a] Compiled by M. H. Smith. (1968). Molecular weights of proteins and some other materials including sedimentation, diffusion and frictional coefficients and partial specific volumes. *In* "Handbook of Biochemistry and Biophysics" (H. A. Sober, ed.), 2nd ed. C3–C25. Chemical Rubber Company, Cleveland.

[b] Compiled by L. A.MacHattie, and C. A. Thomas. (1968). Viral DNA molecules. *In* "Handbook of Biochemistry and Biophysics" (H. A. Sober, ed.), 2nd ed. Section H. Chemical Rubber Company, Cleveland.

[c] Equilibrium density in Cs_2SO_4.

[d] Tissieres, A., Watson, J. D., Schlessinger, D., and Hollingworth, B. R. (1959). Ribonucleoprotein particles from *Escherichia coli. J. Mol. Biol.* **1**, 221–233.

B2.   FRICTIONAL COEFFICIENTS FOR DIFFERENT SHAPES

Frictional ratio θ for ellipsoids of revolution[a]

Prolate ($r_1 > r_2$)		Oblate ($r_2 > r_1$)	
r_1/r_2	$\theta = f/f_0$	r_2/r_1	$\theta = f/f_0$
1.0	1.000	1.0	1.000
2.0	1.044	2.0	1.042
3.0	1.112	3.0	1.105
4.0	1.182	4.0	1.165
5.0	1.255	5.0	1.224
6.0	1.314	6.0	1.277
7.0	1.375	7.0	1.326
8.0	1.433	8.0	1.374
9.0	1.490	9.0	1.416
10.0	1.543	10.0	1.458
20.0	1.996	20.0	1.782

[a] From T. Svedberg and K. O. Pedersen (1940). "The Ultracentrifuge." Oxford Univ. Press (Clarendon), London and New York.

B3. ARTIFICIAL PARTICLES

Particle	Density g/cm^3	Diameter	Source
Polystyrene latex beads	1.05	from 0.088 $\pm$ 0.008 μm to 0.557 $\pm$ 0.011 μm	Particle Information Service
Polystyrene latex beads	1.05	from 0.088 $\pm$ 0.008 μm to 1.1 $\pm$ 0.005 μm	Duke Standards Co.
		from 0.5 to 90 μm	Coulter Electronics Inc.
Poly(vinyl styrene) "latex" beads	1.05		Dow Chemical Co.
Poly(vinylstyrene)-poly(vinyltoluene) "latex" beads	1.05		Dow Chemical Co.
Polystyrene divinyl benzene beads		from 3.5 $\pm$ 0.2 μm to 100 $\pm$ 10 μm	Duke Standards Co.
Fluorescent polystyrene divinyl benzene beads		from 30 $\pm$ 3 μm to 100 $\pm$ 6 μm	Duke Standards Co.
Silica sols	see Appendix C11		
Density-gradient beads	1.10–1.60		Spinco Division/Beckman
Density marker beads	1.017–1.142 in saline 1.037–1.136 in sucrose		Pharmacia Fine Chemicals
Calibrated floats (glass)	0.8–3.0 $\pm$ 0.00002	6 mm	Techne
FC-78 (perfluoridated hydrocarbon)	1.7035[a]	liquid	Minnesota Mining & Manufacturing
Maxidens	1.9	liquid	Nygaard AS

Poly(vinyl chloride)	M_w	M_n	Pressure Chemical Co.
	68,600	25,500	
	118,200	41,000	
	132,000	54,000	

Polystyrene	Normal particle weight (d)	M_w/M_n (approx)	Pressure Chemical Co.
	200,000	1.10	
	498,000	1.20	
	670,000	1.15	
	1,800,000	1.20	
	2,000,000	1.25	

[a] Density is a known function of pressure and hence centrifugal speed; cf. A. J. Richard, J. Glick, and R. Burkat (1970). An inert liquid marker for density gradient ultracentrifugation in CsCl. *Anal. Biochem.* **37**, 378–384.

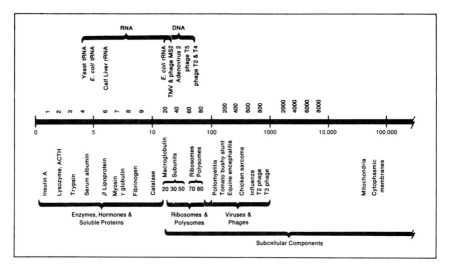

Fig. B.1. Partial spectrum of sedimentation coefficients of biological particles. (Courtesy of Spinco Division/Beckman Instruments.)

Appendix C

Properties of Gradient Materials

C1. DENSITY AND VISCOSITY OF AQUEOUS SOLUTIONS OF SUCROSE*

The polynomials comprising Barber's (1966) equations represent the best least-square fits to the data over the range of temperature and concentration used. Although the computed data may be more precise than the tabulated data, the two kinds of data may disagree for specific values. For example, the actual values of ρ and η of pure water differ strikingly from the computed value. The computed values for water reported here are internally consistent when used in calculations involving sucrose.

The first three columns represent the concentration of sucrose. Molarity represents here the moles of sucrose per 1000 cm^3 of solution at the indicated temperature rather than the conventional meaning of molarity.

Density and Viscosity of Aqueous Solutions of Sucrose at 0°C

%(w/w)	%(w/v)	Molarity	Density	Viscosity
0	0.00	0.000	1.0004	1.78
1	1.00	0.029	1.0043	1.831
2	2.01	0.058	1.0082	1.884
3	3.03	0.088	1.0122	1.941
4	4.06	0.118	1.0162	2.002
5	5.10	0.149	1.0203	2.067

Continued

* Computed by E. F. Eikenberry from empirical equations of Barber (1966), and Appendix C2. E. J. Barber (1966). Calculation of density and viscosity of sucrose solutions as a function of concentration and temperature. *Natl. Cancer Inst. Monog.* **21**, 219–239.

C1.   Continued

%(w/w)	%(w/v)	Molarity	Density	Viscosity
6	6.14	0.179	1.0244	2.135
7	7.19	0.210	1.0285	2.208
8	8.26	0.241	1.0326	2.286
9	9.33	0.272	1.0368	2.369
10	10.41	0.304	1.0411	2.458
11	11.49	0.335	1.0453	2.552
12	12.59	0.367	1.0496	2.653
13	13.70	0.400	1.0539	2.761
14	14.81	0.432	1.0583	2.877
15	15.94	0.465	1.0627	3.001
16	17.07	0.498	1.0671	3.134
17	18.21	0.532	1.0716	3.277
18	19.36	0.565	1.0761	3.430
19	20.53	0.599	1.0806	3.596
20	21.70	0.634	1.0852	3.774
21	22.88	0.668	1.0898	3.967
22	24.07	0.703	1.0944	4.175
23	25.27	0.738	1.0991	4.401
24	26.49	0.773	1.1038	4.646
25	27.71	0.809	1.1085	4.912
26	28.94	0.845	1.1133	5.202
27	30.18	0.881	1.1181	5.519
28	31.44	0.918	1.1229	5.866
29	32.70	0.955	1.1278	6.246
30	33.98	0.992	1.1327	6.665
31	35.26	1.030	1.1376	7.126
32	36.56	1.068	1.1426	7.636
33	37.87	1.106	1.1476	8.201
34	39.19	1.144	1.1527	9.829
35	40.52	1.183	1.1578	9.53
36	41.86	1.222	1.1629	10.31
37	43.21	1.262	1.1680	11.20
38	44.58	1.302	1.1732	12.19
39	45.95	1.342	1.1784	13.31
40	47.34	1.383	1.1837	14.58
41	48.74	1.424	1.1889	16.03
42	50.15	1.465	1.1943	17.69
43	51.58	1.506	1.1996	19.59
44	53.01	1.548	1.2050	21.78
45	54.46	1.591	1.2104	24.31
46	55.92	1.633	1.2159	27.24
47	57.40	1.676	1.2214	30.65
48	58.89	1.720	1.2269	34.64
49	60.38	1.764	1.2324	39.24
50	61.90	1.808	1.2380	44.74
51	63.42	1.852	1.2437	51.29

C1.   Continued

%(w/w)	%(w/v)	Molarity	Density	Viscosity
52	64.96	1.897	1.2493	59.11
53	66.51	1.943	1.2550	68.52
54	68.07	1.988	1.2607	79.93
55	69.65	2.034	1.2665	93.85
56	71.24	2.081	1.2723	111.0
57	72.85	2.128	1.2781	132.3
58	74.47	2.175	1.2840	158.9
59	76.10	2.223	1.2899	192.6
60	77.74	2.271	1.2958	235.7
61	79.40	2.319	1.3018	291.4
62	81.08	2.368	1.3078	364.2
63	82.77	2.418	1.3138	460.6
64	84.47	2.467	1.3199	589.9
65	86.18	2.517	1.3260	766.1
66	87.92	2.568	1.3321	1000
67	89.66	2.619	1.3383	1352
68	91.42	2.670	1.3445	1842
69	93.20	2.722	1.3507	2557
70	94.99	2.775	1.3570	3621

Density and Viscosity of Aqueous Solutions of Sucrose at 4°C

%(w/w)	%(w/v)	Molarity	Density	Viscosity
0	0.0	0.0	1.0004	1.564
1	1.00	0.029	1.0043	1.608
2	2.01	0.058	1.0082	1.654
3	3.03	0.088	1.0122	1.703
4	4.06	0.118	1.0161	1.755
5	5.10	0.149	1.0202	1.810
6	6.14	0.179	1.0242	1.868
7	7.19	0.210	1.0283	1.931
8	8.25	0.241	1.0324	1.997
9	9.32	0.272	1.0366	2.067
10	10.40	0.304	1.0407	2.142
11	11.49	0.335	1.045	2.222
12	12.59	0.367	1.0492	2.308
13	13.69	0.400	1.0535	2.399
14	14.80	0.432	1.0578	2.497
15	15.93	0.465	1.0622	2.601
16	17.06	0.498	1.0666	2.713
17	18.20	0.531	1.0710	2.833
18	19.35	0.565	1.0755	2.962
19	20.51	0.599	1.0800	3.101
20	21.69	0.633	1.0845	3.250

Continued

C1.   Continued

%(w/w)	%(w/v)	Molarity	Density	Viscosity
21	22.87	0.668	1.0891	3.411
22	24.06	0.702	1.0937	3.585
23	25.26	0.737	1.0983	3.773
24	26.47	0.773	1.1030	3.977
25	27.69	0.808	1.1077	4.198
26	28.92	0.844	1.1124	4.438
27	30.16	0.881	1.1172	4.700
28	31.41	0.917	1.1220	4.986
29	32.67	0.954	1.1268	5.299
30	33.95	0.991	1.1317	5.643
31	35.23	1.029	1.1366	6.02
32	36.53	1.067	1.1416	6.436
33	37.83	1.105	1.1466	6.895
34	39.15	1.143	1.1516	7.405
35	40.48	1.182	1.1566	7.971
36	41.82	1.221	1.1617	8.602
37	43.17	1.261	1.1668	9.308
38	44.53	1.301	1.1720	10.10
39	45.90	1.341	1.1772	10.99
40	47.29	1.381	1.1824	12.00
41	48.69	1.422	1.1876	13.14
42	50.10	1.463	1.1929	14.44
43	51.52	1.505	1.1983	15.93
44	52.95	1.547	1.2036	17.63
45	54.40	1.589	1.2090	19.59
46	55.86	1.632	1.2144	21.85
47	57.33	1.675	1.2199	24.26
48	58.81	1.718	1.2254	27.51
49	60.31	1.762	1.2309	30.99
50	61.82	1.806	1.2365	35.14
51	63.34	1.850	1.2421	40.04
52	64.88	1.895	1.2478	45.86
53	66.43	1.940	1.2534	52.82
54	67.99	1.986	1.2591	61.19
55	69.56	2.032	1.2649	71.33
56	71.15	2.078	1.2706	83.71
57	72.75	2.125	1.2765	98.95
58	74.37	2.172	1.2823	117.9
59	76.00	2.220	1.2882	141.6
60	77.64	2.268	1.2941	171.5
61	79.30	2.316	1.3000	209.8
62	80.97	2.365	1.3060	259.3
63	82.65	2.414	1.3120	324.0
64	84.35	2.464	1.3181	409.7
65	86.07	2.514	1.3242	524.7
66	87.79	2.564	1.3303	681.3

C1.   Continued

%(w/w)	%(w/v)	Molarity	Density	Viscosity
67	89.54	2.615	1.3365	897.8
68	91.29	2.667	1.3426	1202
69	93.07	2.719	1.3489	1638
70	94.85	2.771	1.3551	2273

Density and Viscosity of Aqueous Solutions of Sucrose at 5°C

%(w/w)	%(w/v)	Molarity	Density	Viscosity
0	0.0	0.0	1.0004	1.516
1	1.00	0.029	1.0043	1.558
2	2.01	0.058	1.0082	1.603
3	3.03	0.088	1.0121	1.650
4	4.06	0.118	1.0161	1.700
5	5.10	0.149	1.0201	1.753
6	6.14	0.179	1.0241	1.809
7	7.19	0.210	1.0282	1.869
8	8.25	0.241	1.0323	1.933
9	9.32	0.272	1.0365	2.001
10	10.40	0.304	1.0406	2.073
11	11.49	0.335	1.0448	2.150
12	12.58	0.367	1.0491	2.232
13	13.69	0.400	1.0534	2.319
14	14.80	0.432	1.0577	2.413
15	15.93	0.465	1.0620	2.513
16	17.06	0.498	1.0644	2.621
17	18.20	0.531	1.0708	2.736
18	19.35	0.565	1.0753	2.859
19	20.51	0.599	1.0798	2.992
20	21.68	0.633	1.0843	3.135
21	22.86	0.668	1.0889	3.290
22	24.05	0.702	1.0935	3.456
23	25.25	0.737	1.0981	3.636
24	26.46	0.773	1.1028	3.831
25	27.68	0.808	1.1075	4.043
26	28.91	0.844	1.1122	4.272
27	30.15	0.881	1.1170	4.523
28	31.40	0.917	1.1218	4.796
29	32.67	0.954	1.1266	5.094
30	33.94	0.991	1.1315	5.422
31	35.22	1.029	1.1364	5.781
32	36.52	1.066	1.1413	6.177
33	37.82	1.105	1.1463	6.614
34	39.14	1.143	1.1513	7.099
35	40.47	1.182	1.1563	7.636

Continued

C1.   Continued

%(w/w)	%(w/v)	Molarity	Density	Viscosity
36	41.81	1.221	1.1614	8.236
37	43.16	1.260	1.1665	8.905
38	44.52	1.300	1.1717	9.656
39	45.89	1.340	1.1768	10.50
40	47.28	1.381	1.1821	11.45
41	48.67	1.422	1.1873	12.53
42	50.08	1.463	1.1926	13.76
43	51.51	1.504	1.1979	15.16
44	52.94	1.546	1.2033	16.76
45	54.38	1.588	1.2087	18.60
46	55.84	1.631	1.2141	20.72
47	57.31	1.674	1.2195	23.18
48	58.80	1.717	1.2250	26.03
49	60.29	1.761	1.2306	29.28
50	61.80	1.805	1.2361	33.16
51	63.32	1.850	1.2417	37.73
52	64.86	1.894	1.2474	43.16
53	66.41	1.940	1.2530	49.63
54	67.97	1.985	1.2587	57.39
55	69.54	2.031	1.2645	66.79
56	71.13	2.078	1.2702	78.24
57	72.73	2.124	1.2760	92.31
58	74.34	2.172	1.2819	109.7
59	75.97	2.219	1.2877	131.5
60	77.61	2.267	1.2937	159.0
61	79.27	2.315	1.2996	194.0
62	80.94	2.364	1.3056	239.1
63	82.63	2.413	1.3116	297.9
64	84.32	2.463	1.3176	375.6
65	86.04	2.513	1.3237	479.4
66	87.76	2.564	1.3298	620.3
67	89.51	2.614	1.3360	814.3
68	91.26	2.666	1.3422	1086
69	93.03	2.718	1.3484	1473
70	94.82	2.770	1.3546	2034

Density and Viscosity of Aqueous Solutions of Sucrose at 10°C

%(w/w)	%(w/v)	Molarity	Density	Viscosity
0	0.0	0.0	1.0002	1.308
1	1.00	0.029	1.004	1.343
2	2.01	0.058	1.0079	1.380
3	3.03	0.088	1.0118	1.420
4	4.06	0.118	1.0157	1.462
5	5.09	0.148	1.0196	1.506

C1.   Continued

%(w/w)	%(w/v)	Molarity	Density	Viscosity
6	6.14	0.179	1.0236	1.553
7	7.19	0.210	1.0277	1.603
8	8.25	0.241	1.0317	1.655
9	9.32	0.272	1.0358	1.711
10	10.39	0.303	1.0400	1.771
11	11.48	0.335	1.0441	1.835
12	12.58	0.367	1.0484	1.902
13	13.68	0.399	1.0526	1.974
14	14.79	0.432	1.0569	2.051
15	15.91	0.465	1.0612	2.134
16	17.04	0.498	1.0655	2.222
17	18.18	0.531	1.0699	2.316
18	19.33	0.564	1.0743	2.417
19	20.49	0.598	1.0788	2.525
20	21.66	0.632	1.0833	2.642
21	22.84	0.667	1.0878	2.768
22	24.03	0.702	1.0923	2.903
23	25.22	0.737	1.0969	3.049
24	26.43	0.772	1.1016	3.206
25	27.65	0.807	1.1062	3.377
26	28.88	0.843	1.1109	3.562
27	30.12	0.880	1.1157	3.763
28	31.37	0.916	1.1204	3.982
29	32.63	0.953	1.1252	4.221
30	33.90	0.990	1.1301	4.481
31	35.18	1.027	1.1349	4.767
32	36.47	1.065	1.1398	5.080
33	37.77	1.103	1.1448	5.424
34	39.09	1.142	1.1498	5.805
35	40.41	1.180	1.1548	6.225
36	41.75	1.219	1.1598	6.692
37	43.10	1.259	1.1649	7.211
38	44.46	1.298	1.1700	7.790
39	45.83	1.338	1.1752	8.438
40	47.21	1.379	1.1803	9.166
41	48.60	1.420	1.1856	9.987
42	50.01	1.461	1.1908	10.92
43	51.43	1.502	1.1961	11.97
44	52.86	1.544	1.2014	13.17
45	54.30	1.586	1.2068	14.54
46	55.76	1.629	1.2122	16.11
47	57.22	1.671	1.2176	17.92
48	58.70	1.715	1.2231	20.00
49	60.20	1.758	1.2286	22.37
50	61.70	1.802	1.2341	25.17
51	63.22	1.847	1.2397	28.45
52	64.75	1.891	1.2453	32.32

Continued

C1. Continued

%(w/w)	%(w/v)	Molarity	Density	Viscosity
53	66.30	1.936	1.2509	36.89
54	67.85	1.982	1.2566	42.34
55	69.42	2.028	1.2623	48.87
56	71.01	2.074	1.2681	56.76
57	72.61	2.121	1.2739	66.35
58	74.22	2.168	1.2797	78.11
59	75.84	2.215	1.2855	92.65
60	77.48	2.263	1.2914	110.8
61	79.13	2.311	1.2973	133.6
62	80.80	2.360	1.3033	162.7
63	82.48	2.409	1.3093	200.0
64	84.17	2.459	1.3153	248.6
65	85.88	2.509	1.3214	312.5
66	87.61	2.559	1.3275	397.7
67	89.35	2.610	1.3336	513.0
68	91.10	2.661	1.3398	671.1
69	92.87	2.713	1.3460	891.7
70	94.65	2.765	1.3522	1205

Density and Viscosity of Aqueous Solutions of Sucrose at 15°C

%(w/w)	%(w/v)	Molarity	Density	Viscosity
0	0.0	0.0	0.9996	1.140
1	1.00	0.029	1.0034	1.170
2	2.01	0.058	1.0073	1.202
3	3.03	0.088	1.0111	1.235
4	4.05	0.118	1.0150	1.271
5	5.09	0.148	1.0189	1.308
6	6.13	0.179	1.0229	1.348
7	7.18	0.209	1.0269	1.390
8	8.24	0.240	1.0309	1.434
9	9.31	0.272	1.0350	1.481
10	10.39	0.303	1.0391	1.531
11	11.47	0.335	1.0432	1.584
12	12.56	0.367	1.0474	1.640
13	13.67	0.399	1.0516	1.701
14	14.78	0.431	1.0558	1.765
15	15.9	0.464	1.0601	1.833
16	17.03	0.497	1.0644	1.906
17	18.16	0.530	1.0688	1.985
18	19.31	0.564	1.0732	2.068
19	20.47	0.598	1.0776	2.158
20	21.64	0.632	1.0820	2.255
21	22.81	0.666	1.0865	2.358

C1. Continued

%(w/w)	%(w/v)	Molarity	Density	Viscosity
22	24.00	0.701	1.0911	2.470
23	25.19	0.736	1.0956	2.590
24	26.40	0.771	1.1002	2.719
25	27.62	0.806	1.1048	2.859
26	28.84	0.842	1.1095	3.010
27	30.08	0.878	1.1142	3.174
28	31.33	0.915	1.1189	3.352
29	32.58	0.952	1.1237	3.546
30	33.85	0.989	1.1285	3.757
31	35.13	1.026	1.1334	3.987
32	36.42	1.064	1.1382	4.239
33	37.72	1.102	1.1432	4.515
34	39.03	1.140	1.1481	4.818
35	40.35	1.179	1.1531	5.153
36	41.69	1.217	1.1581	5.522
37	43.03	1.257	1.1632	5.931
38	44.39	1.296	1.1682	6.386
39	45.76	1.336	1.1734	6.893
40	47.14	1.377	1.1785	7.460
41	48.53	1.417	1.1837	8.096
42	49.93	1.458	1.1889	8.812
43	51.35	1.500	1.1942	9.62
44	52.77	1.541	1.1995	10.54
45	54.21	1.583	1.2048	11.58
46	55.66	1.626	1.2102	12.77
47	57.13	1.669	1.2156	14.12
48	58.61	1.712	1.2211	15.68
49	60.10	1.755	1.2265	17.45
50	61.60	1.799	1.2320	19.52
51	63.11	1.843	1.2376	21.93
52	64.64	1.888	1.2432	24.75
53	66.18	1.933	1.2488	28.06
54	67.73	1.978	1.2544	31.98
55	69.30	2.024	1.2601	36.64
56	70.88	2.070	1.2658	42.22
57	72.48	2.117	1.2716	48.95
58	74.08	2.164	1.2774	57.12
59	75.71	2.211	1.2832	67.13
60	77.34	2.259	1.2891	79.48
61	78.99	2.307	1.2950	94.86
62	80.65	2.356	1.3009	114.2
63	82.33	2.405	1.3069	138.7
64	84.02	2.454	1.3129	170.2
65	85.73	2.504	1.3189	211.0
66	87.45	2.554	1.3250	264.7
67	89.18	2.605	1.3311	336.0

Continued

C1.   Continued

%(w/w)	%(w/v)	Molarity	Density	Viscosity
68	90.93	2.656	1.3373	432.2
69	92.69	2.708	1.3434	563.8
70	94.47	2.760	1.3497	746.8

Density and Viscosity of Aqueous Solutions of Sucrose at 20°C

%(w/w)	%(w/v)	Molarity	Density	Viscosity
0	0.0	0.0	0.9988	1.004
1	1.00	0.029	1.0026	1.030
2	2.01	0.058	1.0064	1.057
3	3.03	0.088	1.0102	1.086
4	4.05	0.118	1.0141	1.116
5	5.08	0.148	1.0179	1.148
6	6.13	0.179	1.0219	1.182
7	7.18	0.209	1.0258	1.217
8	8.23	0.240	1.0298	1.255
9	9.30	0.271	1.0339	1.295
10	10.37	0.303	1.0380	1.337
11	11.46	0.334	1.0421	1.382
12	12.55	0.366	1.0462	1.430
13	13.65	0.398	1.0504	1.481
14	14.76	0.431	1.0546	1.535
15	15.88	0.463	1.0588	1.592
16	17.01	0.496	1.0631	1.654
17	18.14	0.530	1.0675	1.720
18	19.29	0.563	1.0718	1.790
19	20.44	0.597	1.0762	1.865
20	21.61	0.631	1.0806	1.946
21	22.78	0.665	1.0851	2.032
22	23.97	0.700	1.0896	2.125
23	25.16	0.735	1.0941	2.226
24	26.36	0.770	1.0987	2.333
25	27.58	0.805	1.1033	2.449
26	28.80	0.841	1.1079	2.575
27	30.04	0.877	1.1126	2.710
28	31.28	0.913	1.1173	2.857
29	32.53	0.950	1.1221	3.016
30	33.80	0.987	1.1268	3.189
31	35.08	1.024	1.1316	3.378
32	36.36	1.062	1.1365	3.583
33	37.66	1.100	1.1414	3.808
34	38.97	1.138	1.1463	4.053
35	40.29	1.177	1.1513	4.323
36	41.62	1.216	1.1563	4.620
37	42.96	1.255	1.1613	4.948

C1. Continued

%(w/w)	%(w/v)	Molarity	Density	Viscosity
38	44.32	1.294	1.1663	5.311
39	45.68	1.334	1.1714	5.714
40	47.06	1.374	1.1766	6.163
41	48.45	1.415	1.1817	6.664
42	49.85	1.456	1.1870	7.225
43	51.26	1.497	1.1922	7.857
44	52.68	1.539	1.1975	8.569
45	54.12	1.581	1.2028	9.375
46	55.57	1.623	1.2081	10.29
47	57.03	1.666	1.2135	11.33
48	58.50	1.709	1.2189	12.52
49	59.99	1.752	1.2244	13.86
50	61.49	1.796	1.2299	15.42
51	63.00	1.840	1.2354	17.23
52	64.52	1.885	1.2409	19.33
53	66.06	1.930	1.2465	21.79
54	67.61	1.975	1.2522	24.67
55	69.18	2.021	1.2578	28.07
56	70.75	2.067	1.2635	32.12
57	72.34	2.113	1.2693	36.96
58	73.95	2.160	1.2750	42.79
59	75.56	2.207	1.2808	49.85
60	77.20	2.255	1.2867	58.50
61	78.84	2.303	1.2926	69.15
62	80.50	2.351	1.2985	82.39
63	82.17	2.400	1.3044	99.01
64	83.86	2.450	1.3104	120.1
65	85.56	2.499	1.3164	147.0
66	87.28	2.549	1.3225	182.0
67	89.01	2.600	1.3286	227.8
68	90.75	2.651	1.3347	288.5
69	92.51	2.702	1.3409	370.2
70	94.29	2.754	1.3470	481.8

Density and Viscosity of Aqueous Solutions of Sucrose at 25°C

%(w/w)	%(w/v)	Molarity	Density	Viscosity
0	0.0	0.0	0.9977	0.891
1	1.00	0.029	1.0014	0.914
2	2.01	0.058	1.0052	0.938
3	3.02	0.088	1.0090	0.962
4	4.05	0.118	1.0128	0.989
5	5.08	0.148	1.0167	1.016
6	6.12	0.178	1.0206	1.045
7	7.17	0.209	1.0246	1.076

Continued

C1.   Continued

%(w/w)	%(w/v)	Molarity	Density	Viscosity
8	8.22	0.240	1.0285	1.108
9	9.29	0.271	1.0325	1.142
10	10.36	0.302	1.0366	1.179
11	11.44	0.334	1.0407	1.217
12	12.53	0.366	1.0448	1.258
13	13.63	0.398	1.0489	1.301
14	14.74	0.430	1.0531	1.347
15	15.86	0.463	1.0574	1.396
16	16.98	0.496	1.0616	1.449
17	18.12	0.529	1.0659	1.505
18	19.26	0.562	1.0703	1.564
19	20.41	0.596	1.0746	1.628
20	21.58	0.630	1.0790	1.697
21	22.75	0.664	1.0835	1.770
22	23.93	0.699	1.0879	1.848
23	25.12	0.734	1.0924	1.933
24	26.32	0.769	1.0970	2.023
25	27.53	0.804	1.1016	2.121
26	28.76	0.840	1.1062	2.226
27	29.99	0.876	1.1108	2.340
28	31.23	0.912	1.1155	2.462
29	32.48	0.949	1.1202	2.595
30	33.74	0.985	1.1250	2.739
31	35.02	1.023	1.1298	2.895
32	36.30	1.060	1.1346	3.064
33	37.60	1.098	1.1395	3.249
34	38.90	1.136	1.1444	3.451
35	40.22	1.175	1.1493	3.672
36	41.55	1.213	1.1543	3.914
37	42.89	1.253	1.1593	4.181
38	44.24	1.292	1.1643	4.474
39	45.60	1.332	1.1694	4.799
40	46.98	1.372	1.1745	5.159
41	48.36	1.412	1.1797	5.560
42	49.76	1.453	1.1848	6.007
43	51.17	1.494	1.1901	6.508
44	52.59	1.536	1.1953	7.071
45	54.02	1.578	1.2006	7.705
46	55.47	1.620	1.2059	8.421
47	56.93	1.663	1.2113	9.234
48	58.40	1.706	1.2167	10.16
49	59.88	1.749	1.2221	11.19
50	61.37	1.793	1.2276	12.39
51	62.88	1.837	1.2331	13.77
52	64.40	1.881	1.2386	15.37
53	65.94	1.926	1.2442	17.23
54	67.48	1.971	1.2498	19.29

C1.   Continued

%(w/w)	%(w/v)	Molarity	Density	Viscosity
55	69.04	2.017	1.2554	21.93
56	70.62	2.063	1.2611	24.93
57	72.20	2.109	1.2668	28.48
58	73.81	2.156	1.2726	32.73
59	75.42	2.203	1.2784	37.85
60	77.05	2.251	1.2842	44.05
61	78.69	2.298	1.2901	51.61
62	80.34	2.347	1.2959	60.93
63	82.01	2.396	1.3019	72.50
64	83.70	2.445	1.3078	87.00
65	85.39	2.494	1.3138	105.3
66	87.11	2.544	1.3199	128.8
67	88.83	2.595	1.3259	159.1
68	90.57	2.646	1.3320	198.8
69	92.33	2.697	1.3382	251.4
70	94.10	2.749	1.3444	322.0

Density and Viscosity of Aqueous Solutions of Sucrose at 30°C

%(w/w)	%(w/v)	Molarity	Density	Viscosity
0	0.0	0.0	0.9963	0.798
1	1.00	0.029	1.0000	0.818
2	2.00	0.058	1.0037	0.838
3	3.02	0.088	1.0075	0.86
4	4.04	0.118	1.0113	0.883
5	5.07	0.148	1.0152	0.907
6	6.11	0.178	1.0191	0.932
7	7.16	0.209	1.0230	0.959
8	8.21	0.240	1.0270	0.987
9	9.27	0.271	1.0310	1.016
10	10.34	0.302	1.0350	1.048
11	11.42	0.333	1.0391	1.081
12	12.51	0.365	1.0432	1.116
13	13.61	0.397	1.0473	1.154
14	14.72	0.430	1.0515	1.193
15	15.83	0.462	1.0557	1.235
16	16.95	0.495	1.0599	1.280
17	18.09	0.528	1.0642	1.328
18	19.23	0.561	1.0685	1.380
19	20.38	0.595	1.0728	1.434
20	21.54	0.629	1.0772	1.493
21	22.71	0.663	1.0816	1.555
22	23.89	0.698	1.0861	1.622
23	25.08	0.732	1.0906	1.694
24	26.28	0.767	1.0951	1.771
25	27.49	0.803	1.0997	1.854

Continued

C1. Continued

%(w/w)	%(w/v)	Molarity	Density	Viscosity
26	28.71	0.838	1.1043	1.943
27	29.94	0.874	1.1089	2.039
28	31.18	0.910	1.1136	2.143
29	32.42	0.947	1.1183	2.255
30	33.69	0.984	1.1230	2.376
31	34.96	1.021	1.1278	2.506
32	36.24	1.058	1.1326	2.648
33	37.53	1.096	1.1374	2.802
34	38.83	1.134	1.1423	2.970
35	40.15	1.173	1.1472	3.153
36	41.47	1.211	1.1522	3.353
37	42.81	1.250	1.1572	3.572
38	44.16	1.290	1.1622	3.813
39	45.52	1.329	1.1672	4.078
40	46.89	1.369	1.1723	4.372
41	48.27	1.410	1.1775	4.696
42	49.67	1.451	1.1826	5.058
43	51.07	1.492	1.1878	5.460
44	52.49	1.533	1.1931	5.911
45	53.92	1.575	1.1983'	6.417
46	55.36	1.617	1.2036	6.987
47	56.82	1.660	1.2090	7.630
48	58.28	1.702	1.2144	8.358
49	59.76	1.746	1.2198	9.168
50	61.26	1.789	1.2252	10.11
51	62.76	1.833	1.2307	11.18
52	64.28	1.877	1.2362	12.42
53	65.81	1.922	1.2418	13.84
54	67.35	1.967	1.2474	15.50
55	68.91	2.013	1.2530	17.43
56	70.48	2.059	1.2586	19.69
57	72.06	2.105	1.2643	22.36
58	73.66	2.152	1.2701	25.52
59	75.27	2.199	1.2758	29.30
60	76.89	2.246	1.2816	33.84
61	78.53	2.294	1.2875	39.34
62	80.18	2.342	1.2933	46.05
63	81.85	2.391	1.2992	54.30
64	83.53	2.440	1.3052	64.54
65	85.22	2.489	1.3112	77.35
66	86.93	2.539	1.3172	93.54
67	88.65	2.590	1.3232	114.2
68	90.39	2.640	1.3293	140.9
69	92.14	2.691	1.3354	175.8
70	93.91	2.743	1.3416	222.0

C2.   DENSITY AND VISCOSITY OF SUCROSE AS FUNCTIONS OF CONCENTRATION (BARBER, 1966)[*]

A.   In the range of 0 to 30° the density of sucrose may be related to temperature T and weight fraction Y by the relation

$$\rho_{T,m} = (B_1 + B_2 T + B_3 T^2) + (B_4 + B_5 T + B_6 T^2)Y$$
$$+ (B_7 + B_8 T + B_9 T^2)Y^2$$

where $\rho_{T,m}$ is the density of a sucrose solution, T the temperature (°C), Y the weight fraction sucrose, and the B_n are constants.

Constant	Value[a]
B_1	1.0003698
B_2	3.9680504×10^{-5}
B_3	$-5.8513271 \times 10^{-6}$
B_4	0.38982371
B_5	$-1.0578919 \times 10^{-3}$
B_6	1.2392833×10^{-5}
B_7	0.17097594
B_8	4.7530081×10^{-4}
B_9	$-8.9239737 \times 10^{-6}$

[a] Values are given to 8 figures for machine calculations; use of the first 5 figures would be sufficient for hand calculations.

B.   The viscosity of sucrose η between 0°C and 80°C can be expressed as a fraction of temperature T and the mole fraction y.

$$\log \eta_{T,m} = A + \frac{B}{T + C}$$

The mole fraction y is related to the weight fraction Y and the molecular weights of sucrose S and water W by the relation

$$y = \frac{Y/S}{Y/S + (1 - Y)/W}$$

[*] Barber, E. J. (1966). Calculation of density and viscosity of sucrose solutions as a function of concentration and temperature. *Natl. Cancer Inst. Monog.* **21,** 219–239.

The constants A and B are calculated from y by the relation

$$A = D_0 + D_1 y + D_2 y^2 + D_3 y_7{}^3 \cdots D_n y^n$$

	Range of equation, (wt %)	
Coefficients[a]	0–48	48–75
D_0	-1.5018327	-1.0803314
D_1	9.4112153	-2.0003484×10^1
D_2	-1.1435741×10^3	4.6066898×10^2
D_3	1.0504137×10^5	-5.9517023×10^3
D_4	-4.6927102×10^6	3.5627216×10^4
D_5	1.0323349×10^8	-7.8542145×10^4
D_6	-1.1028981×10^9	
D_7	4.5921911×10^9	

[a] Coefficient subscript indicates the exponent of the composition by which the coefficient is to be multiplied.

$$B = E_0 + E_1 y + E_2 y^2 + E_3 y_7{}^3 \cdots E_n y^n$$

	Range of equation (wt %)	
Coefficients[a]	0–48	48–75
E_0	2.1169907×10^2	1.3975568×10^2
E_1	1.6077073×10^3	6.6747329×10^3
E_2	1.6911611×10^5	-7.8716105×10^4
E_3	-1.4184371×10^7	9.0967578×10^5
E_4	6.0654775×10^8	-5.5380830×10^6
E_5	$-1.2985834 \times 10^{10}$	1.2451219×10^7
E_6	1.3532907×10^{11}	
E_7	$-5.4970416 \times 10^{11}$	

[a] Coefficient subscript indicates the exponent of the composition by which the coefficient is to be multiplied.

The value of C is related to the weight fraction y plus three additional constants.

$$C = G_1 - G_2[1 + (y/G_3)^2]^{1/2}$$

where

$$G_1 = 146.06635, \quad G_2 = 25.251728, \quad G_3 = 0.070674842.$$

C3. REFRACTIVE INDEX OF SUCROSE SOLUTIONS[a,b]

Percentage sugar	0	Percentage sugar	0	Percentage sugar	0	Percentage sugar	0
00. 1.3	330	22. 1.3	672	44. 1.4	076	65. 1.4	532
1.	344	23.	689	45.	096	66.	558
2.	359	24.	706	46.	117	67.	581
3.	374	25.	723	47.	137	68.	605
4.	388	26.	740	48.	158	69.	628
5.	403	27.	758	49.	179	70.	651
6.	418	28.	775	50.	200	71.	676
7.	433	29.	793	51.	221	72.	700
8.	448	30.	811	52.	242	73.	725
9.	464	31.	829	53.	264	74.	749
10.	479	32.	847	54.	285	75.	774
11.	494	33.	865	55.	307	76.	799
12.	510	34.	883	56.	329	77.	825
13.	526	35.	902	57.	351	78.	850
14.	541	36.	920	58.	373	79.	876
15.	557	37.	939	59.	396	80.	901
16.	573	38.	958	60.	418	81.	927
17.	590	39.	978	61.	441	82.	954
18.	606	40.	997	62.	464	83.	980
19.	622	41. 1.4	016	63.	486	84. 1.5	007
20.	639	42.	036	64.	509	85.	033
21.	655	43.	056				

[a] From "Handbook of Chemistry and Physics," 32nd ed. Chem. Rubber Publ. Co., Cleveland, Ohio.

[b] Measurements are for refractive index of light ($\lambda = 589$ nm) of aqueous solutions at 20°C.

C4. RECIPES FOR PREPARING STOCK SOLUTIONS OF AQUEOUS SUCROSE[a]

Concentration[b]	Sucrose (gm)	Water (cm³ at 20°C)	Yield (cm³ at 4°C)
30% (W/W)	1000	2329.1	2945.4
30% (W/W)	429.3	1000	1264.6
30% (W/W)	339.5	790.8	1000
60% (W/W)	1000	665.5	1287.9
60% (W/W)	1502.7	1000	1935.3
60% (W/W)	776.5	516.7	1000
65% (W/W)	1000	537.5	1161.8
65% (W/W)	1860.5	1000	2161.6
65% (W/W)	860.7	462.6	1000

Continued

C4.   Continued

Concentration[b]	Sucrose (gm)	Water (cm³ at 20°C)	Yield (cm³ at 4°C)
66% (W/W)	1000	514.2	1139
66% (W/W)	1944.7	1000	2214.9
66% (W/W)	878.0	451.5	1000
70% W/V @4	1000	807.8	1428.6
70% W/V @4	1238.0	1000	1768.5
70% W/V @4	700	565.4	1000
75% W/V @4	1000	711.5	1333.4
75% W/V @4	1405.4	1000	1874.0
75% W/V @4	750	533.6	1000
80% W/V @4	1000	627.1	1250
80% W/V @4	1594.6	1000	1993.4
80% W/V @4	800	501.7	1000
85% W/V @4	1000	552.4	1176.5
85% W/V @4	1810.2	1000	2129.7
85% W/V @4	850	469.6	1000
90% W/V @4	1000	485.9	1111.2
90% W/V @4	2058.0	1000	2286.7
90% W/V @4	900	437.3	1000
1 M @4	1000	2305.2	2921.4
1 M @4	433.8	1000	1267.3
1 M @4	342.3	789.1	1000
2 M @4	1000	840.2	1460.7
2 M @4	1190.2	1000	1738.5
2 M @4	684.6	575.2	1000

[a] Computed by E. F. Eikenberry.
[b] w/w or w/v at the temperatures indicated.

C5.   DILUTION OF STOCK SOLUTIONS OF SUCROSE[a]

Desired concentration (% w/w)	cm³ of stock diluted to 1000 cm³ final solution at 4°C				Desired concentration (% w/w)	cm³ of stock diluted to 1000 cm³ final solution at 4°C			
	70% w/v at 4°C	75% w/v at 4°C	80% w/v at 4°C	85% w/v at 4°C		60% (w/w)	65% (w/w)	66% (w/w)	2 M at 4
0	0	0	0	0	0	0	0	0	0
1	14.3	13.4	12.6	11.8	1	12.9	11.7	11.4	14.7
2	28.8	26.9	25.2	23.7	2	26	23.4	23	29.5
3	43.4	40.5	38	35.7	3	39.1	35.3	34.6	44.4
4	58.1	54.2	50.8	47.8	4	52.3	47.2	46.3	59.4
5	72.9	68	63.8	60	5	65.7	59.3	58.1	74.5

C5. Continued

Desired concentration (% w/w)	cm³ of stock diluted to 1000 cm³ final solution at 4°C			
	70% w/v at 4°C	75% w/v at 4°C	80% w/v at 4°C	85% w/v at 4°C
6	87.8	81.9	76.8	72.3
7	102.8	96	90	84.7
8	118	110.1	103.2	97.2
9	133.3	124.4	116.6	109.8
10	148.7	138.8	130.1	122.4
11	164.2	153.3	143.7	135.2
12	179.9	167.9	157.4	148.1
13	195.7	182.6	171.2	161.1
14	211.6	197.5	185.1	174.2
15	227.6	212.4	199.2	187.4
16	243.8	227.5	213.3	200.8
17	260.1	242.8	227.6	214.2
18	276.6	258.1	242	227.7
19	293.1	273.6	256.5	241.4
20	309.9	289.2	271.1	255.2
21	326.7	304.9	285.9	269.1
22	343.7	320.8	300.8	283.1
23	360.9	336.8	315.8	297.2
24	378.2	353	330.9	311.4
25	395.6	369.2	346.1	325.8
26	413.2	385.6	361.5	340.3
27	430.9	402.2	377.1	354.9
28	448.8	418.9	392.7	369.6
29	466.8	435.7	408.5	384.5
30	485	452.7	424.4	399.4
31	503.4	469.8	440.4	414.5
32	521.9	487.1	456.6	429.8
33	540.5	504.5	473	445.1
34	559.3	522	489.4	460.6
35	578.3	539.8	506	476.3
36	597.4	557.6	522.8	492
37	616.7	575.6	539.7	507.9
38	636.2	593.8	556.7	523.9
39	655.8	612.1	573.9	540.1
40	675.7	630.6	591.2	556.4
41	695.6	649.2	608.7	572.9
42	715.8	668	626.3	589.5
43	736.1	687	644.1	606.2
44	756.6	706.1	662	623.1
45	777.2	725.4	680.1	640.1
46	798.1	744.9	698.3	657.2
47	819.1	764.5	716.7	674.5

Desired concentration (% w/w)	cm³ of stock diluted to 1000 cm³ final solution at 4°C			
	60% (w/w)	65% (w/w)	66% (w/w)	2 M at 4
6	79.1	71.4	70	89.8
7	92.7	83.6	82	105.1
8	106.4	96	94.1	120.6
9	120.1	108.4	106.3	136.3
10	134	120.9	118.5	152
11	148	133.5	130.9	167.9
12	162.2	146.3	143.4	183.9
13	176.4	159.1	156	200.1
14	190.7	172.1	168.7	216.3
15	205.2	185.1	181.5	232.7
16	219.8	198.3	194.4	249.3
17	234.5	211.5	207.4	266
18	249.3	224.9	220.5	282.8
19	264.3	238.4	233.7	299.7
20	279.3	252	247	316.8
21	294.5	265.7	260.5	334.1
22	309.9	279.5	274	351.5
23	325.3	293.5	287.7	369
24	340.9	307.6	301.5	386.7
25	356.6	321.7	315.4	404.5
26	372.5	336	329.4	422.5
27	388.5	350.5	343.6	440.6
28	404.6	365	357.8	458.9
29	420.9	379.7	372.2	477.3
30	437.3	394.5	386.7	495.9
31	453.8	409.4	401.3	514.7
32	470.5	424.4	416.1	533.6
33	487.3	439.6	430.9	552.7
34	504.3	454.9	445.9	571.9
35	521.4	470.3	461.1	591.3
36	538.6	485.9	476.3	610.9
37	556	501.6	491.7	630.6
38	573.6	517.4	507.2	650.5
39	591.3	533.4	522.9	670.6
40	609.1	549.5	538.7	690.8
41	627.1	565.7	554.6	711.3
42	645.3	582.1	570.7	731.9
43	663.6	598.6	586.9	752.6
44	682.1	615.3	603.2	773.6
45	700.7	632.1	619.7	794.7
46	719.5	649	636.3	816
47	738.4	666.1	653	837.5

Continued

C5.   Continued

Desired concen-tration ($\%$ w/w)	cm^3 of stock diluted to 1000 cm^3 final solution at 4°C				Desired concen-tration ($\%$ w/w)	cm^3 of stock diluted to 1000 cm^3 final solution at 4°C			
	70$\%$ w/v at 4°C	75$\%$ w/v at 4°C	80$\%$ w/v at 4°C	85$\%$ w/v at 4°C		60$\%$ (w/w)	65$\%$ (w/w)	66$\%$ (w/w)	2 M at 4
48	840.3	784.3	735.2	692	48	757.5	683.4	669.9	859.2
49	861.7	804.2	754	709.6	49	776.8	700.8	687	881
50	883.2	824.3	772.8	727.4	50	796.3	718.3	704.2	903.1
51	905	844.6	791.8	745.3	51	815.9	737	721.5	925.3
52	926.9	865.1	811	763.3	52	835.6	753.8	739	947.8
53	949	885.8	830.4	781.5	53	855.6	771.8	756.6	970.4
54	971.3	906.6	849.9	799.9	54	875.7	790	774.4	993.2
55	993.8	927.6	869.6	818.4	55	896	808.3	792.3	
56		948.7	889.5	837.1	56	916.4	826.7	810.4	
57		970.1	909.5	856	57	937.1	845.3	828.7	
58		991.6	929.7	875	58	957.9	864.1	847.1	
59			950	894.1	59	978.8	883	865.6	
60			970.6	913.5	60	1000	902.1	884.3	

[a] Computed by E. F. Eikenberry.

C6.   COEFFICIENTS FOR DENSITY AND REFRACTIVE INDEX OF ALKALI SALTS*

Calculation of Density from Refractive Indices of
Solutions of Alkali Salts at 25°C[a]

Solute	Coefficients		Density range (gm/cm^3)
	a	b	
Cs$_2$SO$_4$	12.1200	15.1662	1.15–1.40
	13.6986	17.3233	1.40–1.70
CsBr	9.9667	12.2876	1.25–1.35
CsCl	10.8601	13.4974	1.25–1.90
Cs acetate	10.7527	13.4247	1.80–2.05
Cs formate	13.7363	17.4286	1.72–1.82
KBr	6.4786	7.6431	1.10–1.35
RbBr	9.1750	11.2410	1.15–1.65

[a] J. Vinograd and J. E. Hearst (1962). Equilibrium sedimentation of macromolecules and viruses in a density gradient. *Fortschr. Chem. Org. Naturst.* **20**, 372–422.

* D. B. Ludlum and R. C. Warner (1965). Equilibrium centrifugation in cesium sulfate solutions. *J. Biol. Chem.* **240**, 2961–2965.

Ludlum and Warner (1965) give following formula for density, $\rho_{25°}$, of Cs_2SO_4: $\rho_{25°} = 0.9954 + 11.1066\,(\eta - \eta_0) + 26.4460\,(\eta - \eta_0)^2$, where η is the refractive index of the solution and η_0 that of water.

The empirical relation is

$$\rho = a\eta_0 - b$$

where all measurements are made at 25°C.

C7. ADDITIVE MIXING RELATIONS FOR DILUTIONS OF CsCl SOLUTIONS*

$$v_{1,w} = (\rho_c - \rho°)/(\rho_c - 0.997) \qquad (C.1)$$

$$v_w = v_c(\rho_c - \rho°)/(\rho° - 0.997) \qquad (C.2)$$

where v is volume and the subscripts w and c refer to water and the concentrated salt solution. The quantity $\rho°$ is the desired density. The subscript 1 in Eq. (C.1) indicates the volume required to prepare 1 ml of solution.

C8. DENSITY AT 25°C OF CsCl SOLUTIONS AS A FUNCTION OF REFRACTIVE INDEX[a]

Refractive index (sodium D line, 25°C)	Density (gm/cm³)	Refractive index (sodium D line, 25°C)	Density (gm/cm³)	Refractive index (sodium D line, 25°C)	Density (gm/cm³)
1.34400	1.09857	1.35020	1.16591	1.35640	1.23324
1.34410	1.09966	1.35030	1.16699	1.35650	1.23433
1.34420	1.10075	1.35040	1.16808	1.35660	1.23541
1.34430	1.10183	1.35050	1.16917	1.35670	1.23650
1.34440	1.10292	1.35060	1.17025	1.35680	1.23758
1.34450	1.10400	1.35070	1.17134	1.35690	1.23867
1.34460	1.10509	1.35080	1.17242	1.35700	1.23976
1.34470	1.10618	1.35090	1.17351	1.35710	1.24084
1.34480	1.10726	1.35100	1.17460	1.35720	1.24193
1.34490	1.10835	1.35110	1.17568	1.35730	1.24301
1.34500	1.10943	1.35120	1.17677	1.35740	1.24410
1.34510	1.11052	1.35130	1.17785	1.35750	1.24519
1.34520	1.11161	1.35140	1.17894	1.35760	1.24627

Continued

* J. Vinograd (1963). Sedimentation equilibrium in a buoyant density gradient. *In* "Methods in Enzymology" (S. P. Colowick and N. O. Kaplan, eds.), Vol. 6, pp. 854–870. Academic Press, New York.

C8.   Continued

Refractive index (sodium D line, 25°C)	Density (gm/cm³)	Refractive index (sodium D line, 25°C)	Density (gm/cm³)	Refractive index (sodium D line, 25°C)	Density (gm/cm³)
1.34530	1.11269	1.35150	1.18003	1.35770	1.24736
1.34540	1.11378	1.35160	1.18111	1.35780	1.24844
1.34550	1.11486	1.35170	1.18220	1.35790	1.24953
1.34560	1.11595	1.35180	1.18328	1.35800	1.25062
1.34570	1.11704	1.35190	1.18437	1.35810	1.25170
1.34580	1.11812	1.35200	1.18546	1.35820	1.25279
1.34590	1.11921	1.35210	1.18654	1.35830	1.25387
1.34600	1.12029	1.35220	1.18763	1.35840	1.25496
1.34610	1.12138	1.35230	1.18871	1.35850	1.25605
1.34620	1.12247	1.35240	1.18980	1.35860	1.25713
1.34630	1.12355	1.35250	1.19089	1.35870	1.25822
1.34640	1.12464	1.35260	1.19197	1.35880	1.25930
1.34650	1.12572	1.35270	1.19306	1.35890	1.26039
1.34660	1.12681	1.35280	1.19414	1.35900	1.26148
1.34670	1.12790	1.35290	1.19523	1.35910	1.26256
1.34680	1.12898	1.35300	1.19632	1.35920	1.26365
1.34690	1.13007	1.35310	1.19740	1.35930	1.26473
1.34700	1.13115	1.35320	1.19849	1.35940	1.26582
1.34710	1.13224	1.35330	1.19957	1.35950	1.26691
1.34720	1.13333	1.35340	1.20066	1.35960	1.26799
1.34730	1.13441	1.35350	1.20175	1.35970	1.26908
1.34740	1.13550	1.35360	1.20283	1.35980	1.27016
1.34750	1.13658	1.35370	1.20392	1.35990	1.27125
1.34760	1.13767	1.35380	1.20500	1.36000	1.27234
1.34770	1.13876	1.35390	1.20609	1.36010	1.27342
1.34780	1.13984	1.35400	1.20718	1.36020	1.27451
1.34790	1.14093	1.35410	1.20826	1.36030	1.27559
1.34800	1.14201	1.35420	1.20935	1.36040	1.27668
1.34810	1.14310	1.35430	1.21043	1.36050	1.27777
1.34820	1.14419	1.35440	1.21152	1.36060	1.27885
1.34830	1.14527	1.35450	1.21261	1.36070	1.27994
1.34840	1.14636	1.35460	1.21369	1.36080	1.28102
1.34850	1.14744	1.35470	1.21478	1.36090	1.28211
1.34860	1.14853	1.35480	1.21586	1.36100	1.28320
1.34870	1.14962	1.35490	1.21695	1.36110	1.28428
1.34880	1.15070	1.35500	1.21804	1.36120	1.28537
1.34890	1.15179	1.35510	1.21912	1.36130	1.28645
1.34900	1.15287	1.35520	1.22021	1.36140	1.28754
1.34910	1.15396	1.35530	1.22129	1.36150	1.28863
1.34920	1.15505	1.35540	1.22238	1.36160	1.28971
1.34930	1.15613	1.35550	1.22347	1.36170	1.29080
1.34940	1.15722	1.35560	1.22455	1.36180	1.29188

C8. Continued

Refractive index (sodium D line, 25°C)	Density (gm/cm^3)	Refractive index (sodium D line, 25°C)	Density (gm/cm^3)	Refractive index (sodium D line, 25°C)	Density (gm/cm^3)
1.34950	1.15830	1.35570	1.22564	1.36190	1.29297
1.34960	1.15939	1.35580	1.22672	1.36200	1.29406
1.34970	1.16048	1.35590	1.22781	1.36210	1.29514
1.34980	1.16156	1.35600	1.22890	1.36220	1.29623
1.34990	1.16265	1.35610	1.22998	1.36230	1.29731
1.35000	1.16373	1.35620	1.23107	1.36240	1.29840
1.35010	1.16482	1.35630	1.23215	1.36250	1.29949
1.36260	1.30057	1.36900	1.37008	1.37550	1.44067
1.36270	1.30166	1.36910	1.37116	1.37560	1.44175
1.36280	1.30274	1.36920	1.37225	1.37570	1.44284
1.36290	1.30383	1.36930	1.37333	1.37580	1.44393
1.36300	1.30492	1.36940	1.37442	1.37590	1.44501
1.36310	1.30600	1.36950	1.37551	1.37600	1.44610
1.36320	1.30709	1.36960	1.37659	1.37610	1.44718
1.36330	1.30817	1.36970	1.37768	1.37620	1.44827
1.36340	1.30926	1.36980	1.37876	1.37630	1.44936
1.36350	1.31035	1.36990	1.37985	1.37640	1.45044
1.36360	1.31143	1.37000	1.38094	1.37650	1.45153
1.36370	1.31252	1.37010	1.38202	1.37660	1.45261
1.36380	1.31360	1.37020	1.38311	1.37670	1.45370
1.36390	1.31469	1.37030	1.38420	1.37680	1.45479
1.36400	1.31578	1.37040	1.38528	1.37690	1.45587
1.36410	1.31686	1.37050	1.38637	1.37700	1.45696
1.36420	1.31795	1.37060	1.38745	1.37710	1.45804
1.36430	1.31903	1.37070	1.38854	1.37720	1.45913
1.36440	1.32012	1.37080	1.38963	1.37730	1.46022
1.36450	1.32121	1.37090	1.39071	1.37740	1.46130
1.36460	1.32229	1.37100	1.39180	1.37750	1.46239
1.36470	1.32338	1.37110	1.39288	1.37760	1.46347
1.36480	1.32446	1.37120	1.39397	1,37770	1.46456
1.36490	1.32555	1.37130	1.39506	1.37780	1.46565
1.36500	1.32664	1.37140	1.39614	1.37790	1.46673
1.36510	1.32772	1.37150	1.39723	1.37800	1.46782
1.36520	1.32881	1.37160	1.39831	1.37810	1.46890
1.36530	1.32989	1.37170	1.39940	1.37820	1.46999
1.36540	1.33098	1.37180	1.40049	1.37830	1.47108
1.36550	1.33207	1.37190	1.40157	1.37840	1.47216
1.36560	1.33315	1.37200	1.40266	1.37850	1.47325
1.36570	1.33424	1.37210	1.40374	1.37860	1.47433
1.36580	1.33532	1.37220	1.40483	1.37870	1.47542
1.36590	1.33641	1.37230	1.40592	1.37880	1.47651
1.36600	1.33750	1.37240	1.40700	1.37890	1.47759

Continued

C8. Continued

Refractive index (sodium D line, 25°C)	Density (gm/cm^3)	Refractive index (sodium D line, 25°C)	Density (gm/cm^3)	Refractive index (sodium D line, 25°C)	Density (gm/cm^3)
1.36610	1.33858	1.37250	1.40809	1.37900	1.47868
1.36620	1.33967	1.37260	1.40917	1.37910	1.47976
1.36630	1.34075	1.37270	1.41026	1.37920	1.48085
1.36640	1.34184	1.37280	1.41135	1.37930	1.48194
1.36650	1.34293	1.37290	1.41243	1.37940	1.48302
1.36660	1.34401	1.37300	1.41352	1.37950	1.48411
1.36670	1.34510	1.37310	1.41460	1.37960	1.48519
1.36680	1.34618	1.37320	1.41569	1.37970	1.48628
1.36690	1.34727	1.37330	1.41678	1.37980	1.48737
1.36700	1.34836	1.37340	1.41786	1.37990	1.48845
1.36710	1.34944	1.37350	1.41895	1.38000	1.48954
1.36720	1.35053	1.37360	1.42003	1.38010	1.49062
1.36730	1.35161	1.37370	1.42112	1.38020	1.49171
1.36740	1.35270	1.37380	1.42221	1.38030	1.49280
1.36750	1.35379	1.37390	1.42329	1.38040	1.49388
1.36760	1.35487	1.37400	1.42438	1.38050	1.49497
1.36770	1.35596	1.37410	1.42546	1.38060	1.49605
1.36780	1.35704	1.37420	1.42655	1.38070	1.49714
1.36790	1.35813	1.37430	1.42764	1.38080	1.49823
1.36800	1.35922	1.37440	1.42872	1.38090	1.49931
1.36810	1.36030	1.37450	1.42981	1.38100	1.50040
1.36820	1.36139	1.37460	1.43089	1.38110	1.50148
1.36830	1.36247	1.37470	1.43198	1.38120	1.50257
1.36840	1.36356	1.37480	1.43307	1.38130	1.50366
1.36850	1.36465	1.37490	1.43415	1.38140	1.50474
1.36860	1.36573	1.37500	1.43524	1.38150	1.50583
1.36870	1.36682	1.37510	1.43632	1.38169	1.50691
1.36880	1.36790	1.37520	1.43741	1.38170	1.50800
1.36890	1.36899	1.37530	1.43850	1.38180	1.50909
		1.37540	1.43958	1.38190	1.51017
1.38200	1.51126	1.38850	1.58185	1.39500	1.65244
1.38210	1.51234	1.38860	1.58293	1.39510	1.65353
1.38220	1.51343	1.38870	1.58402	1.39520	1.65461
1.38230	1.51452	1.38880	1.58511	1.39530	1.65570
1.38240	1.51560	1.38890	1.58619	1.39540	1.65678
1.38250	1.51669	1.38900	1.58728	1.39550	1.65787
1.38260	1.51777	1.38910	1.58836	1.39560	1.65896
1.38270	1.51886	1.38920	1.58945	1.39570	1.66004
1.38280	1.51995	1.38930	1.59054	1.39580	1.66113
1.38290	1.52103	1.38940	1.59162	1.39590	1.66221
1.38300	1.52212	1.38950	1.59271	1.39600	1.66330
1.38310	1.52320	1.38960	1.59379	1.39610	1.66439

C8. Continued

Refractive index (sodium D line, 25°C)	Density (gm/cm³)	Refractive index (sodium D line, 25°C)	Density (gm/cm³)	Refractive index (sodium D line, 25°C)	Density (gm/cm³)
1.38320	1.52429	1.38970	1.59488	1.39620	1.66547
1.38330	1.52538	1.38980	1.59597	1.39630	1.66656
1.38340	1.52646	1.38990	1.59705	1.39640	1.66764
1.38350	1.52755	1.39000	1.59814	1.39650	1.66873
1.38360	1.52863	1.39010	1.59923	1.39660	1.66982
1.38370	1.52972	1.39020	1.60031	1.39670	1.67090
1.38380	1.53081	1.39030	1.60140	1.39680	1.67199
1.38390	1.53189	1.39040	1.60248	1.39690	1.67307
1.38400	1.53298	1.39050	1.60357	1.39700	1.67416
1.38410	1.53406	1.39060	1.60466	1.39710	1.67525
1.38420	1.53515	1.39070	1.60574	1.39720	1.67633
1.38430	1.53624	1.39080	1.60683	1.39730	1.67742
1.38440	1.53732	1.39090	1.60791	1.39740	1.67850
1.38450	1.53841	1.39100	1.60900	1.39750	1.67959
1.38460	1.53949	1.39110	1.61009	1.39760	1.68068
1.38470	1.54058	1.39120	1.61117	1.39770	1.68176
1.38480	1.54167	1.39130	1.61226	1.39780	1.68285
1.38490	1.54275	1.39140	1.61334	1.39790	1.68393
1.38500	1.54384	1.39150	1.61443	1.39800	1.68502
1.38510	1.54492	1.39160	1.61552	1.39810	1.68611
1.38520	1.54601	1.39170	1.61660	1.39820	1.68719
1.38530	1.54710	1.39180	1.61769	1.39830	1.68828
1.38540	1.54818	1.39190	1.61877	1.39840	1.68936
1.38550	1.54927	1.39200	1.61986	1.39850	1.69045
1.38560	1.55035	1.39210	1.62095	1.39860	1.69154
1.38570	1.55144	1.39220	1.62203	1.39870	1.69262
1.38580	1.55253	1.39230	1.62312	1.39880	1.69371
1.38590	1.55361	1.39240	1.62420	1.39890	1.69479
1.38600	1.55470	1.39250	1.62529	1.39900	1.69588
1.38610	1.55578	1.39260	1.62638	1.39910	1.69697
1.38620	1.55687	1.39270	1.62746	1.39920	1.69805
1.38630	1.55796	1.39280	1.62855	1.39930	1.69914
1.38640	1.55904	1.39290	1.62963	1.39940	1.70022
1.38650	1.56013	1.39300	1.63072	1.39950	1.70131
1.38660	1.56121	1.39310	1.63181	1.39960	1.70240
1.38670	1.56230	1.39320	1.63289	1.39970	1.70348
1.38680	1.56339	1.39330	1.63398	1.39980	1.70457
1.38690	1.56447	1.39340	1.63506	1.39990	1.70565
1.38700	1.56556	1.39350	1.63615	1.40000	1.70674
1.38710	1.56664	1.39360	1.63724	1.40010	1.70783
1.38720	1.56773	1.39370	1.63832	1.40020	1.70891
1.38730	1.56882	1.39380	1.63941	1.40030	1.71000

Continued

C8.   Continued

Refractive index (sodium D line, 25°C)	Density (gm/cm³)	Refractive index (sodium D line, 25°C)	Density (gm/cm³)	Refractive index (sodium D line, 25°C)	Density (gm/cm³)
1.38740	1.56990	1.39390	1.64049	1.40040	1.71108
1.38750	1.57099	1.39400	1.64158	1.40050	1.71217
1.38760	1.57207	1.39410	1.64267	1.40060	1.71326
1.38770	1.57316	1.39420	1.64375	1.40070	1.71434
1.38780	1.57425	1.39430	1.64484	1.40080	1.71543
1.38790	1.57533	1.39440	1.64592	1.40090	1.71651
1.38800	1.57642	1.39450	1.64701	1.40100	1.71760
1.38810	1.57750	1.39460	1.64810	1.40110	1.71869
1.38820	1.57859	1.39470	1.64918	1.40120	1.71977
1.38830	1.57968	1.39480	1.65027	1.40130	1.72086
1.38840	1.58076	1.39490	1.65135	1.40140	1.72194
1.40150	1.72303	1.40800	1.79362	1.41450	1.86421
1.40160	1.72412	1.40810	1.79471	1.41460	1.86530
1.40170	1.72520	1.40820	1.79579	1.41470	1.86638
1.40180	1.72629	1.40830	1.79688	1.41480	1.86747
1.40190	1.72737	1.40840	1.79796	1.41490	1.86856
1.40200	1.72846	1.40850	1.79905	1.41500	1.86964
1.40210	1.72955	1.40860	1.80014	1.41510	1.87073
1.40220	1.73063	1.40870	1.80122	1.41520	1.87181
1.40230	1.73172	1.40880	1.80231	1.41530	1.87290
1.40240	1.73280	1.40890	1.80339	1.41540	1.87399
1.40250	1.73389	1.40900	1.80448	1.41550	1.87507
1.40260	1.73498	1.40910	1.80557	1.41560	1.87616
1.40270	1.73606	1.40920	1.80665	1.41570	1.87724
1.40280	1.73715	1.40930	1.80774	1.41580	1.87833
1.40290	1.73823	1.40940	1.80882	1.41590	1.87942
1.40300	1.73932	1.40950	1.80991	1.41600	1.88050
1.40310	1.74041	1.40960	1.81100	1.41610	1.88159
1.40320	1.74149	1.40970	1.81208	1.41620	1.88267
1.40330	1.74258	1.40980	1.81317	1.41630	1.88376
1.40340	1.74366	1.40990	1.81425	1.41640	1.88485
1.40350	1.74475	1.41000	1.81534	1.41650	1.88593
1.40360	1.74584	1.41010	1.81643	1.41660	1.88602
1.40370	1.74692	1.41020	1.81751	1.41670	1.88810
1.40380	1.74801	1.41030	1.81860	1.41680	1.88919
1.40390	1.74909	1.41040	1.81969	1.41690	1.89028
1.40400	1.75018	1.41050	1.82077	1.41700	1.89136
1.40410	1.75127	1.41060	1.82186	1.41710	1.89245
1.40420	1.75235	1.41070	1.82294	1.41720	1.89353
1.40430	1.75344	1.41080	1.82403	1.41730	1.89462
1.40440	1.75452	1.41090	1.82512	1.41740	1.89571
1.40450	1.75561	1.41100	1.82620	1.41750	1.89679
1.40460	1.75670	1.41110	1.82729	1.41760	1.89788

C8.   Continued

Refractive index (sodium D line, 25°C)	Density (gm/cm³)	Refractive index (sodium D line, 25°C)	Density (gm/cm³)	Refractive index (sodium D line, 25°C)	Density (gm/cm³)
1.40470	1.75778	1.41120	1.82837	1.41770	1.89896
1.40480	1.75887	1.41130	1.82946	1.41780	1.90005
1.40490	1.75995	1.41140	1.83055	1.41790	1.90114
1.40500	1.76104	1.41150	1.83163	1.41800	1.90222
1.40510	1.76213	1.41160	1.83272	1.41810	1.90331
1.40520	1.76321	1.41170	1.83380	1.41820	1.90439
1.40530	1.76430	1.41180	1.83489	1.41830	1.90548
1.40540	1.76538	1.41190	1.83598	1.41840	1.90657
1.40550	1.76647	1.41200	1.83706	1.41850	1.90765
1.40560	1.76756	1.41210	1.83815	1.41860	1.90874
1.40570	1.76864	1.41220	1.83923	1.41870	1.90982
1.40580	1.76973	1.41230	1.84032	1.41880	1.91091
1.40590	1.77081	1.41240	1.84141	1.41890	1.91200
1.40600	1.77190	1.41250	1.84249	1.41900	1.91308
1.40610	1.77299	1.41260	1.84358	1.41910	1.91417
1.40620	1.77407	1.41270	1.84466	1.41920	1.91525
1.40630	1.77516	1.41280	1.84575	1.41930	1.91634
1.40640	1.77624	1.41290	1.84684	1.41940	1.91743
1.40650	1.77733	1.41300	1.84792	1.41950	1.91851
1.40660	1.77842	1.41310	1.81901	1.41960	1.91960
1.40670	1.77950	1.41320	1.85009	1.41970	1.92068
1.40680	1.78059	1.41330	1.85118	1.41980	1.92177
1.40690	1.78167	1.41340	1.85227	1.41990	1.92286
1.40700	1.78276	1.41350	1.85335	1.42000	1.92394
1.40710	1.78385	1.41360	1.85444	1.42010	1.92503
1.40720	1.78493	1.41370	1.85552	1.42020	1.92611
1.40730	1.78602	1.41380	1.85661	1.42030	1.92720
1.40740	1.78710	1.41390	1.85770	1.42040	1.92829
1.40750	1.78819	1.41400	1.85878	1.42050	1.92937
1.40760	1.78928	1.41410	1.85987	1.42060	1.93046
1.40770	1.79036	1.41420	1.86095	1.42070	1.93154
1.40780	1.79145	1.41430	1.86204	1.42080	1.93263
1.40790	1.79253	1.41440	1.86313	1.42090	1.93372
1.42100	1.93480	1.42120	1.93697	1.42140	1.93915
1.42110	1.93589	1.42130	1.93806		

ᵃ Compiled by N. G. Anderson and N. L. Anderson from the empirical relations of Ifft *et al.* (1961) $\rho\, 25° = 10.8601\, \overline{RI} \div 13.4974$ where $\overline{RI}$ is the refractive index at 25°C measured with the sodium D line.

J. B. Ifft, D. H. Voet, and J. Vinograd (1961). The determination of density distributions and density gradients in binary solutions at equilibrium in the ultracentrifuge. *J. Phys. Chem.* **65,** 1138–1145.

C9.   PROPERTIES OF SORBITOL[a]

Sorbitol (% w/w)	Density (gm/cm³)	Viscosity centipoise	Refractive index (4°C)	Refractive index (20°C)
1	1.0022	1.8	1.3350	1.3358
5	1.0170	2.0	1.3405	1.3420
10	1.0358	2.4	1.3482	1.3495
15	1.0546	—	1.3560	1.3577
20	1.0752	3.6	1.3640	1.3656
25	1.0964	—	1.3725	1.3741
30	1.1160	6.0	1.3812	1.3834
35	1.1388	7.3	1.3897	1.3920
40	1.1610	10.7	1.3993	1.4011
45	1.1850	15.7	1.4087	1.4060
50	1.2084	25.7	1.4195	1.4210
55	1.2330	46.2	1.4309	1.4312
60	1.2584	102.9	1.4402	1.4425

[a] C. Suerth, unpublished.

C10.   DENSITY, REFRACTIVE INDEX, AND VISCOSITY OF FICOLL

Density, viscosity, and partial specific volume of various concentrations at 25° [a]

C (gm solute/cm³)	η (centipoise)	ρ (gm soln./cm³)	$\overline{\gamma_0}$ (cm³/gm solution)
0.050	11.8	1.013	1.010
0.075	12.6	1.021	1.010
0.100	13.2	1.028	1.010
0.220	18.0	1.059	1.010
0.310	23.0	1.077	1.010
0.400	28.0	1.096	1.010
0.550	41.0	1.119	1.010
0.700	60.0	1.139	1.010

Densities in gm/cm³ at various concentrations and temperatures[b]

wt. %	$\rho_{2°}$	$\rho_{4°}$	$\rho_{10°}$	$\rho_{20°}$	Refractive index at 20°
0.68	1.000	1.003	1.002	0.998	1.3350
2.09	1.004	1.009	1.006	1.002	1.3360
4.92	1.012	1.019	1.105	1.011	1.3400
8.23	1.021	1.029	1.024	1.022	1.3433
11.75	1.030	1.039	1.033	1.032	1.3484

C10.   Continued

wt. %	$\rho_{2°}$	$\rho_{4°}$	$\rho_{10°}$	$\rho_{20°}$	Refractive index at 20°
18.74	1.048	1.059	1.052	1.051	1.3555
29.06	1.064	1.075	1.065	1.067	1.3622
31.22	1.080	1.091	1.083	1.082	1.3688
38.69	1.090	1.107	1.100	1.099	1.3764
43.09	1.113	1.125	1.121	1.227	1.3837

Viscosity in centipoise at various concentrations and temperatures[b]

wt. %	$\eta_{2°}$	$\eta_{4°}$	$\eta_{10°}$	$\eta_{20°}$
0.68	13'	14	12	10
2.09	16	16	14	13
4.92	16	16	15	16
8.23	23	20	19	17
11.75	22	20	20	20
18.74	39	34	30	24
25.06	60	51	49	35
31.22	91	90	79	58
38.69	159	151	122	90
48.09	295	273	212	157

The relation between the refractive index $\eta_D^{20°}$ and the concentration C in gm of Ficoll per 100 cm^3 is

$$\eta_D^{20°} = 1.330 + 0.00146C$$

[a] L. R. Bell and H. W. Hsu (1974). Transport phenomena in zonal centrifuge rotors. IX. Gradient properties of Ficoll and methyl cellulose (M-278). *Sep. Sci.* **9**, 401–410.

[b] Courtesy of Pharmacia Fine Chemicals.

C11.   PROPERTIES OF COLLOIDAL SILICAS[a]

A.   Properties of Commercial Preparations

Gradient material	Silica content (% w/w)	Approximate particle diameter (nm)	Density (gm/cm^3)	pH	Viscosity at 25°C (centipoise)
Ludox HS 40%	40.1	13–14	1.295	9.6	27
Ludox HS 30%	30.1	13–14	1.211	9.8	5.1
Ludox LS	30.1	15–16	1.209	8.3	10.4
Ludox AS[b]	30.1	13–14	1.206	9.4	16
Ludox AM[c]	30	13–14	1.209	9.1	10
Ludox SM	15	7–8	1.093	8.5	4
Ludox VS	16	5	1.11	10.4	2
Ludox	26	13–15	1.23	4.4	5–15
Nalcoag 1115)D-2195)	15	4	1.104	10.4	18
Nalcoag 1030	30	13	1.208	10.2	4
Nalcoag 1140	40	15	1.296	9.7	12
Nalcoag D-2149[b]	30	15	—	9.5	12
Nalcoag 1050	50	20	1.390	9.0	40
Nalcoa8 1034	34	20	1.23	3.2	10
Nalcoag 40 D04[d]	50	20	—	—	15
Nalcoag 41 D01[b]	40	20	1.292	9.3	30
Nalcoag 1060	50	60	1.39	8.5	10
E-119[c]	30	20	1.20	3.8	—
Percoll[e]	—	21–22	1.13	8.8	10

[a] Information on Ludox is through the courtesy of E. I. du Pont de Nemours & Co. (Inc.), Industrial and Biochemicals Department. Information on "Nalcoag" products is through the courtesy of the Nalco Chemical Company. Information on Percoll is from Pharmacia Fine Chemicals.

[b] Ammonium stabilized.

[c] Partially substituted with Al.

[d] Dispersed in cellosolve.

[e] Silica coated with polyvinylpyrrolidone.

B.   Comparison of Properties of Percoll and Other Gradient Materials

Gradient material	Concentration (% w/v)	Density (gm/cm^3)	Viscosity (cps at 20°C)	Osmolality (mOsm/kg H$_2$O)	Conductivity (mS/cm)
Percoll	26	1.13	10	10	0.60
Ludox HS	36	1.21	4.5	85	3.12
PVP-K15	10	1.02	3.1	195	0.62
Sodium Metrizoate	10	1.06	1.0	290	3.92
Metrizamide	30	1.16	2.0	260	0.12
Ficoll	30	1.10	49	130	0.08

C12.   DENSITY, REFRACTIVE INDEX, AND VISCOSITY OF METRIZAMIDE[a]

Concentration % (w/v)	Molarity (mol/liter)	Density (gm/cm^3)[b]		Ref. index[b]		Viscosity (cP)[b]	
		5°C	15°C	5°C	15°C	5°C	15°C
20	0.254	1.1102	1.1084	1.3657	1.3651	2.9	2.1
40	0.507	1.2207	1.2181	1.3981	1.3973	6.7	4.5
60	0.760	1.3321	1.3285	1.4310	1.4300	24.7	14.5
70	0.887	1.3860	1.3820	1.4470	1.4460	58.8	31.2
80	1.014	1.4408	1.4364	1.4635	1.4623	149	70.3
85	1.077	1.4663	1.4613	1.4712	1.4700	246	110

[a] Courtesy of Nyegaard & Co., AS, Oslo, Norway.
[b] The viscosities were measured with a Brookfield viscosimeter with a spindle U.L. adaptor. Pycnometers were used for measuring the densities. Refractive indices were measured on an Abbé refractometer (Zeiss).

C13.   RADIOOPAQUE AGENTS[a]

Name	Concen-tration (% w/v)	Density at 25°C (gm/cm^3)	Viscosity at 25°C (centipoise)	Osmolarity
Hypaque M 90	90	1.499	32.56	1.43
Renografin 76 NMG[b]	76	1.412	15.52	—
Renografin 76 NMG-Sodium[c]	76	1.419	14.39	1.27
Cardiografin	85	1.462	29.34	1.39
Angio-Conray	80	1.502	12.66	2.17
Conray 400	66.8	1.416	6.87	1.66
Metrizamide	85	1.466^d	246^d	0.67

[a] Information courtesy of Winthrop Laboratories and Nyegaard & Co.
[b] N-Methylglutamine salt.
[c] 66% N-Methylglutamine and 10% sodium salts.
[d] At 5°C.

C14.   DENSITY AND VISCOSITY OF DEUTERIUM OXIDE (HEAVY WATER)[a]

Temper-ature (°C)	Density (gm/cm^3)		Viscosity (cP)	
	Run 1[b]	Run 2[c]	Run 1	Run 2
5	1.103909	1.105531	1.9745	1.9812
10	1.104218	1.105849	1.6675	1.6725
15	1.104113	1.105751	1.4306	1.4343
20	1.103580	1.105215	1.2431	1.2468
25	1.102714	1.104362	1.0928	1.0963
30	1.101491	1.103142	0.9700	0.9730
35	1.099978	1.101631	0.8683	0.8708
40	1.098213	1.099867	0.7828	0.7852
45	1.096210	1.097864	0.7106	0.7126
50	1.093966	1.095618	0.6487	0.6503
55	1.091500	1.093151	0.5953	0.5965
60	1.088852	1.090500	0.5488	0.5502
65	1.086042	1.087688	0.5080	0.5094
70	1.083177	1.084822	0.4720	0.4731

[a] F. J. Millero, R. Dexter, and E. Hoff (1971). Density and viscosity of deuterium oxide solutions from 5-70-DEG. *J. Chem. Eng. Data* **16**, 85–87.
[b] 98.35 mole % deuterium oxide.
[c] 99.88 mole % deuterium oxide.

C15.   DENSITIES AND SPECIFIC VISCOSITIES OF MIXTURES OF CESIUM CHLORIDE IN H$_2$O AND D$_2$O[c] AT 0.0°C[a]

Density (gm/cm^3)	Specific viscosity[b]	
	CsCl/H$_2$O (η/ηH$_2$O)	CsCl/D$_2$O (η/ηH$_2$O)
1.000	1.000	
1.050	0.961	
1.095		1.300
1.100	0.914	1.288
1.125		1.241
1.150	0.871	1.197
1.175		1.155
1.200	0.836	1.117
1.250	0.808	1.060
1.300	0.787	1.015
1.350	0.772	0.979
1.400	0.762	0.951
1.450	0.757	0.929
1.500	0.756	0.914
1.550	0.758	0.904
1.600	0.766	0.899
1.650	0.780	0.899
1.700		0.907
1.750		0.926
1.800		0.951
1.850		0.984

[a] Provided by Dr. Raymond Kaempfer.
[b] Values obtained by interpolation of the curves of Fig. 1 in R. Kaempfer and M. Meselson (1971). In "Methods in Enzymology," (K. Moldave and L. Grossman, eds.), Vol. 20, Part C, Chapter 56. Academic Press, New York.
[c] 90% enriched for deuterium.

C16.   VALUES OF β° FOR SEVERAL GRADIENT-FORMING SALTS

A.   Variation of $\beta^\circ \times 10^{-9}$ with Solution Density[a]

$\rho^{\circ b}$	Sucrose	KBr	RbBr	RbCl	CsCl
1.02	8.091				
1.03	6.789				
1.04	5.605				
1.05	4.643		6.729	9.817	
1.06	4.019				
1.075		7.496			
1.08	3.449				
1.10	3.237	6.121	3.643	5.532	
1.12	3.121				
1.125		5.229			
1.14	3.091				
1.15		4.594	2.536	4.109	2.491
1.175		4.151			
1.20		3.848	2.122	3.445	1.984
1.225		3.637			
1.250		3.469	1.772	3.172	1.715
1.275		3.330			
1.30		3.213	1.635	3.083	1.546
1.325		3.112			
1.35			1.528	2.777	1.430
1.40			1.434	2.334	1.346
1.45			1.372		1.286
1.50					1.245
1.55					1.216
1.60					1.197
1.65					1.190
1.70					1.190
1.75					1.199
1.80					1.215
1.85					1.236

[a] J. Vinograd and J. E. Hearst (1962). Equilibrium sedimentation of macromolecules and viruses in a density gradient. *Fortschr. Chem. Org. Naturst.* **20**, 372–422.

[b] Density of the solution at 25°C.

B. Some Values of $\beta°$ for Several Solutes in Water and D_2O^a

Solute	Concentration (% w/w)	Solvent	Density (20°C)	$\beta° \times 10^{-9\,b}$	Remarks
CsCl	63	D_2O	1.98	1.25	saturated
Cs_2SO_4	64.1	H_2O	2.01	(0.33)	$\eta_r = 1.5$
Cs formate	70	H_2O	2.1	1.4	$\eta_r = 2$
Cs acetate	70	H_2O	2.0	(3)	$\eta_r = 3$
Rb formate	—	H_2O	1.85	(3)	
K acetate	72	H_2O	1.41	14.1	$\eta_r = 3$, satd
K acetate	50	D_2O	1.35	20	$\eta_r = 2$
K formate	77	H_2O	1.57	(6.7)	satd
K formate	74	D_2O	1.63	(6.7)	satd
K_2 tartrate	60	H_2O	1.49	?	$\eta_r = 11$
Na formate	49	H_2O	1.32	(10)	satd
Na formate	45	D_2O	1.40	(10)	satd
LiBr	63	H_2O	1.83	12.5	satd, absorbs UV
LiCl	30	D_2O	1.33	2.5	satd, $\eta_r = 3$

^{a} A. S. L. Hu, R. M. Bock, and H. O. Halvorson (1962). Separation of labeled from unlabeled proteins by equilibrium density gradient sedimentation. *Anal. Biochem.* **4,** 489–504.

^{b} The values in parentheses are estimates which may be in error by as much as 50%.

Other calculations and compilations of values of $\beta°$ are given by J. B. Ifft, W. R. Martin, and K. Kinzie. (1970). *Biopolymers* **9,** 597.

C17. INTEGRALS FOR COMPUTING SEDIMENTATION TIMES THROUGH LINEAR SUCROSE GRADIENTS

Computation from this table can be made for any rotor. The numbers in the body of the table are the values of $s_{20,w}\omega^2 t$ and can be used to compute the time required to migrate to a given position in the gradient, specifically to move to the concentration (% w/w) of sucrose indicated in the left-hand column. One needs only to know the z-intercept, as it were, of the gradient; that is the concentration of sucrose computed to the axis of rotation. This is normally a negative number.

McEwen gives the example of a 5–30% w/w sucrose gradient in an SW 39 rotor. From Table 6.1 one can determine that the radius at the top of the rotor is 6 cm and at the bottom it is 9 cm.

$z_0 = (5\%$ w/w $\times$ 9 cm$) - (20\%$ w/w $\times$ 6 cm$)/(9$ cm $- 6$ cm$) = -25\%$ w/w

For a particle of 1.10 at 0°C to move, say, 6% w/w to 12% w/w, one subtracts the integral under $z_0 = -25$ corresponding to 6% $(=0.4867)$ from that corresponding to 12% w/w ($=1.1759$). The difference is equal to $s_{20,w}\omega^2 t$

$$s_{20,w}\omega^2 t = 1.1759 - 0.4867 = 0.6892$$

If the $s_{20,w}$ of the particle should be 100 S and the centrifuge operates at 39,000 rpm, the time required would be

$$100 \times 10^{-13} \sec \frac{(39{,}000 \text{ rpm} \times 2\pi \text{ rad})^2}{60 \sec} t = 0.6892$$

$$t = 4.13 \times 10^3 \sec$$

McEwen, C. R. (1967). Tables for estimating sedimentation through linear concentration gradients of sucrose solution. *Anal. Biochem.* **20**, 114–149.

Values of Time Integral for Sucrose Gradient Centrifugation Temperature 0.0 Deg C Particle Density 1.10

WT.PCT. SUCROSE	ZO= 5	ZO= 0	ZO= -5	ZO= -10	ZO= -15	ZO= -20	ZO= -25	ZO= -30	ZO= -40	ZO= -60	ZO= -100
0	0.0	0.0	0.0	0.0	0.0	0.0	0.0	0.0	0.0	0.0	0.0
2	0.0	0.0	0.6517	0.3538	0.2430	0.1851	0.1495	0.1254	0.0949	0.0638	0.0385
4	0.0	1.5503	1.2161	0.7004	0.4933	0.3810	0.3104	0.2619	0.1996	0.1353	0.0823
6	0.0	2.6175	1.7457	1.0531	0.7578	0.5925	0.4867	0.4130	0.3172	0.2167	0.1327
8	3.4457	3.5221	2.2719	1.4244	1.0447	0.8263	0.6840	0.5837	0.4515	0.3109	0.1917
10	5.3925	4.3763	2.8205	1.8286	1.3647	1.0912	0.9099	0.7806	0.6083	0.4223	0.2622
12	6.9947	5.2471	3.4189	2.2846	1.7330	1.4001	1.1759	1.0142	0.7961	0.5572	0.3485
14	8.5374	6.1955	4.1039	2.8207	2.1734	1.7739	1.5006	1.3011	1.0289	0.7263	0.4577
16	10.1974	7.3020	4.9340	3.4849	2.7271	2.2485	1.9159	1.6704	1.3311	0.9479	0.6023
18	12.1917	8.7105	6.0229	4.3725	3.4762	2.8965	2.4869	2.1807	1.7519	1.2595	0.8075
20	14.9842	10.7703	7.6547	5.7237	4.6291	3.9019	3.3783	2.9813	2.4170	1.7564	1.1375
22	20.5157	14.9947	11.0720	8.5928	7.1017	6.0743	5.3154	4.7292	3.8793	2.8585	1.8758

Values of Time Integral for Sucrose Gradient Centrifugation Temperature 0.0 Deg C Particle Density 1.20

WT.PCT. SUCROSE	Z0= 5	Z0= 0	Z0= -5	Z0= -10	Z0= -15	Z0= -20	Z0= -25	Z0= -30	Z0= -40	Z0= -60	Z0= -100
0	0.0	0.0	0.0	0.0	0.0	0.0	0.0	0.0	0.0	0.0	0.0
2	0.0	0.0	0.6323	0.3430	0.2356	0.1795	0.1449	0.1216	0.0919	0.0618	0.0374
4	0.0	1.4383	1.1549	0.6638	0.4672	0.3607	0.2938	0.2478	0.1888	0.1280	0.0778
6	2.8537	2.3755	1.6195	0.9732	0.6991	0.5462	0.4484	0.3804	0.2919	0.1993	0.1220
8	4.3437	3.1209	2.0528	1.2789	0.9353	0.7386	0.6107	0.5208	0.4024	0.2768	0.1705
10	5.4606	3.7734	2.4716	1.5873	1.1794	0.9407	0.7831	0.6710	0.5220	0.3618	0.2243
12	6.4174	4.3796	2.8880	1.9045	1.4356	1.1555	0.9681	0.8335	0.6526	0.4556	0.2843
14	7.3012	4.9671	3.3121	2.2364	1.7082	1.3868	1.1690	1.0110	0.7967	0.5502	0.3519
16	8.1607	5.5557	3.7535	2.5895	2.0024	1.6390	1.3896	1.2072	0.9572	0.6779	0.4287
18	9.0304	6.1621	4.2220	2.9712	2.3246	1.9176	1.6351	1.4265	1.1380	0.8118	0.5168
20	9.9402	6.8028	4.7292	3.3910	2.6826	2.2298	1.9118	1.6750	1.3444	0.9659	0.6191
22	10.9206	7.4959	5.2891	3.8606	3.0870	2.5848	2.2283	1.9604	1.5831	1.1457	0.7395
24	12.0077	8.2632	5.9194	4.3954	3.5515	2.9953	2.5960	2.2935	1.8633	1.3584	0.8830
26	13.2481	9.1329	6.6442	5.0167	4.0952	3.4787	3.0310	2.6890	2.1980	1.6144	1.0571
28	14.7082	10.1437	7.4971	5.7545	4.7451	4.0595	3.5561	3.1680	2.6055	1.9282	1.2721
30	16.4873	11.3522	8.5280	6.6533	5.5419	4.7750	4.2053	3.7623	3.1137	2.3223	1.5440
32	18.7496	12.8446	9.8113	7.7820	6.5480	5.6825	5.0319	4.5211	3.7657	2.8311	1.8975
34	21.7937	14.7645	11.4808	9.2558	7.8684	6.8785	6.1248	5.5274	4.6342	3.5129	2.3744
36	26.2296	17.3743	13.7648	11.2862	9.6960	8.5401	7.6481	6.9336	5.8531	4.4753	3.0517
38	33.6444	21.2117	17.1461	14.3083	12.4279	11.0327	9.9399	9.0545	7.6988	5.9408	4.0896
40	51.3033	27.6782	22.8794	19.4578	17.1014	15.3108	13.8843	12.7136	10.8953	8.4922	5.9073
42		43.1941	36.7161	31.9434	28.4763	25.7565	23.5412	21.6923	18.7685	14.8096	10.4353

Values of Time Integral for Sucrose Gradient Centrifugation Temperature 0.0 Deg C Particle Density 1.30

WT.PCT. SUCROSE	Z0= 5	Z0= 0	Z0= -5	Z0= -10	Z0= -15	Z0= -20	Z0= -25	Z0= -30	Z0= -40	Z0= -60	Z0= -100
0	0.0	0.0	0.0	0.0	0.0	0.0	0.0	0.0	0.0	0.0	0.0
2	0.0	0.0	0.6252	0.3391	0.2329	0.1774	0.1433	0.1202	0.0909	0.0611	0.0369
4	0.0	1.4023	1.1344	0.6517	0.4585	0.3539	0.2883	0.2432	0.1853	0.1255	0.0763
6	2.6939	2.3013	1.5799	0.9483	0.6809	0.5318	0.4365	0.3702	0.2841	0.1939	0.1187
8	4.0728	3.0040	1.9884	1.2364	0.9035	0.7131	0.5895	0.5025	0.3882	0.2670	0.1644
10	5.0848	3.6075	2.3757	1.5217	1.1293	0.9000	0.7489	0.6415	0.4988	0.3455	0.2142
12	5.9318	4.1566	2.7529	1.8089	1.3613	1.0946	0.9164	0.7886	0.6171	0.4305	0.2685
14	6.6943	4.6767	3.1282	2.1027	1.6025	1.2993	1.0942	0.9457	0.7446	0.5231	0.3283
16	7.4147	5.1844	3.5089	2.4072	1.8563	1.5168	1.2845	1.1149	0.8830	0.6246	0.3945
18	8.1201	5.6926	3.9015	2.7271	2.1262	1.7502	1.4901	1.2987	1.0345	0.7367	0.4683
20	8.8311	6.2122	4.3129	3.0675	2.4165	2.0033	1.7145	1.5001	1.2019	0.8617	0.5513
22	9.5649	6.7538	4.7503	3.4343	2.7324	2.2807	1.9618	1.7231	1.3883	1.0022	0.6453
24	10.3388	7.3280	5.2220	3.8346	3.0800	2.5879	2.2370	1.9724	1.5980	1.1613	0.7527
26	11.1709	7.9471	5.7379	4.2768	3.4670	2.9319	2.5465	2.2538	1.8362	1.3435	0.8766
28	12.0827	8.6251	6.3100	4.7716	3.9029	3.3215	2.8987	2.5751	2.1095	1.5539	1.0208
30	13.1001	9.3797	6.9537	5.3328	4.4003	3.7681	3.3040	2.9461	2.4267	1.7999	1.1905
32	14.2569	10.2331	7.6885	5.9781	4.9755	4.2870	3.7765	3.3799	2.7994	2.0907	1.3926
34	15.6001	11.2147	8.5410	6.7315	5.6505	4.8983	4.3351	3.8942	3.2433	2.4392	1.6362
36	17.1917	12.3661	9.5486	7.6271	6.4566	5.6311	5.0070	4.5143	3.7808	2.8636	1.9349
38	19.1212	13.7428	10.7615	8.7111	7.4364	6.5250	5.8288	5.2749	4.4426	3.3890	2.3069
40	21.5265	15.4251	12.2527	10.0502	8.6516	7.6373	6.8542	6.2260	5.2735	4.0520	2.7792
42	24.6114	17.5372	14.1355	11.7485	10.1984	9.0574	8.1668	7.4462	6.3430	4.9099	3.3938
44	28.6879	20.2637	16.5781	13.9609	12.2202	10.9188	9.8914	9.0528	7.7562	6.0488	4.2142
46	34.2623	23.8877	19.8400	16.9265	14.9389	13.4285	12.2220	11.2281	9.6757	7.6028	5.3397
48	42.2094	28.8697	24.3435	21.0353	18.7165	16.9245	15.4754	14.2704	12.3685	9.7926	6.9339
50	54.1483	36.0068	30.8204	26.9639	24.1824	21.9946	20.2032	18.6992	16.3001	13.0032	9.2829
52	73.2918	46.7767	40.6299	35.9702	32.5071	29.7337	27.4336	25.4837	22.3396	17.9552	12.9238
54	107.3615	64.1169	56.4772	50.5614	45.0267	42.3283	39.2217	36.5624	32.2281	26.0948	18.9366
56	179.5187	95.0951	84.8785	76.7815	70.3767	65.0573	60.5320	56.6207	50.1774	40.9255	29.9427
58	179.5187	160.9384	145.4240	132.8183	122.5299	113.8302	106.3363	99.7970	88.9093	73.0449	53.8867
60	433.0125	393.0603	359.4978	331.4482	307.7947	287.4150	269.6265	253.9456	227.5360	188.4339	140.3039

Values of Time Integral for Sucrose Gradient Centrifugation Temperature 0.0 Deg C Particle Density 1.40

WT.PCT. SUCROSE	ZO= 5	ZO= 0	ZO= -5	ZO= -10	ZO= -15	ZO= -20	ZO= -25	ZO= -30	ZO= -40	ZO= -60	ZO=-100
0	0.0	0.0	0.0	0.0	0.0	0.0	0.0	0.0	0.0	0.0	0.0
2	0.0	0.0	0.6210	0.3368	0.2313	0.1762	0.1423	0.1194	0.0903	0.0607	0.0367
4	0.0	1.3835	1.1233	0.6451	0.4538	0.3503	0.2853	0.2407	0.1833	0.1242	0.0755
6	0.0	2.2635	1.5594	0.9354	0.6715	0.5244	0.4304	0.3650	0.2801	0.1912	0.1170
8	2.6174	2.9458	1.9559	1.2151	0.8876	0.7004	0.5789	0.4935	0.3812	0.2621	0.1614
10	3.9451	3.5269	2.3288	1.4897	1.1049	0.8803	0.7323	0.6272	0.4876	0.3377	0.2093
12	4.9104	4.0506	2.6885	1.7637	1.3262	1.0659	0.8921	0.7675	0.6004	0.4187	0.2611
14	5.7104	4.5417	3.0430	2.0411	1.5540	1.2592	1.0600	0.9159	0.7208	0.5061	0.3175
16	6.4229	5.0161	3.3987	2.3256	1.7911	1.4624	1.2378	1.0739	0.8501	0.6010	0.3794
18	7.0884	5.4856	3.7613	2.6211	2.0404	1.6780	1.4277	1.2437	0.9901	0.7046	0.4476
20	7.7319	5.9595	4.1365	2.9316	2.3052	1.9089	1.6324	1.4274	1.1427	0.8186	0.5233
22	8.3718	6.4469	4.5302	3.2617	2.5895	2.1585	1.8549	1.6281	1.3105	0.9449	0.6079
24	9.0225	6.9561	4.9484	3.6166	2.8977	2.4309	2.0989	1.8491	1.4964	1.0861	0.7031
26	9.6977	7.4962	5.3985	4.0024	3.2353	2.7310	2.3690	2.0946	1.7042	1.2450	0.8112
28	10.4108	8.0773	5.8888	4.4265	3.6089	3.0648	2.6707	2.3699	1.9384	1.4253	0.9347
30	11.1770	8.7113	6.4297	4.8980	4.0268	3.4401	3.0113	2.6817	2.2049	1.6320	1.0773
32	12.0132	9.4128	7.0337	5.4284	4.4996	3.8665	3.3996	3.0382	2.5113	1.8710	1.2434
34	12.9410	10.2000	7.7173	6.0326	5.0409	4.3568	3.8476	3.4506	2.8672	2.1504	1.4388
36	13.9886	11.0980	8.5031	6.7311	5.6696	4.9283	4.3716	3.9343	3.2864	2.4814	1.6717
38	15.1915	12.1383	9.4197	7.5502	6.4099	5.6038	4.9926	4.5090	3.7865	2.8784	1.9528
40	16.5978	13.3645	10.5066	8.5262	7.2957	6.4145	5.7400	5.2022	4.3920	3.3616	2.2970
42	18.2791	14.8408	11.8225	9.7132	8.3767	7.4070	6.6573	6.0550	5.1395	3.9612	2.7265
44	20.3318	16.6550	13.4478	11.1853	9.7220	8.6455	7.8048	7.1239	6.0798	4.7189	3.2724
46	22.8899	18.9291	15.4947	13.0462	11.4278	10.2202	9.2671	8.4888	7.2841	5.6940	3.9785
48	26.1482	21.8411	18.1268	15.4476	13.6357	12.2634	11.1685	10.2668	8.8579	6.9736	4.9101
50	30.4005	25.6597	21.5922	18.6195	16.5600	14.9759	13.6978	12.6361	10.9611	8.6912	6.1667
52	36.1044	30.8049	26.2784	22.9218	20.5366	18.6727	17.1516	15.8768	13.8459	11.0564	7.9056
54	43.9651	37.9247	32.7849	28.9124	25.0811	23.8433	21.9909	20.4248	17.9051	14.3975	10.3735
56	55.2143	48.1524	42.1611	37.5680	34.1249	31.3457	29.0248	27.0453	23.8292	19.2919	14.0054
58	71.9707	63.4405	56.2176	50.5766	45.2309	42.6663	39.6557	37.0656	32.8172	26.7444	19.5600
60	98.0183	87.2834	78.1999	70.9677	65.2457	60.4787	56.4088	52.8784	47.0340	38.5733	28.4146

Values of Time Integral for Sucrose Gradient Centrifugation Temperature 0.0 Deg C Particle Density 1.50

WT.PCT. SUCROSE	Z0= 5	Z0= 0	Z0= -5	Z0= -10	Z0= -15	Z0= -20	Z0= -25	Z0= -30	Z0= -40	Z0= -60	Z0= -100
0	0.0	0.0	0.0	0.0	0.0	0.0	0.0	0.0	0.0	0.0	0.0
2	0.0	0.0	0.6181	0.3352	0.2302	0.1754	0.1416	0.1188	0.0898	0.0604	0.0365
4	0.0	1.3713	1.1158	0.6407	0.4507	0.3479	0.2833	0.2390	0.1821	0.1233	0.0750
6	0.0	2.2396	1.5461	0.9271	0.6654	0.5196	0.4264	0.3617	0.2775	0.1894	0.1159
8	2.5713	2.9096	1.9355	1.2018	0.8776	0.6925	0.5723	0.4878	0.3768	0.2591	0.1595
10	3.8688	3.4774	2.2998	1.4701	1.0900	0.8682	0.7222	0.6185	0.4808	0.3329	0.2063
12	4.8074	3.9865	2.6495	1.7364	1.3051	1.0486	0.8775	0.7549	0.5904	0.4117	0.2567
14	5.5808	4.4613	2.9922	2.0046	1.5253	1.2355	1.0398	0.8983	0.7068	0.4962	0.3112
16	6.2656	4.9173	3.3340	2.2780	1.7532	1.4308	1.2107	1.0502	0.8311	0.5873	0.3707
18	6.9013	5.3657	3.6805	2.5603	1.9913	1.6368	1.3921	1.2123	0.9648	0.6863	0.4358
20	7.5120	5.8155	4.0365	2.8550	2.2427	1.8559	1.5863	1.3867	1.1096	0.7945	0.5076
22	8.1150	6.2748	4.4075	3.1660	2.5105	2.0911	1.7960	1.5758	1.2677	0.9135	0.5874
24	8.7236	6.7511	4.7987	3.4980	2.7988	2.3458	2.0242	1.7825	1.4416	1.0455	0.6764
26	9.3501	7.2522	5.2163	3.8559	3.1120	2.6242	2.2748	2.0103	1.6344	1.1929	0.7767
28	10.0061	7.7867	5.6673	4.2460	3.4557	2.9313	2.5524	2.2635	1.8498	1.3589	0.8903
30	10.7044	8.3646	6.1602	4.6757	3.8366	3.2734	2.8627	2.5476	2.0927	1.5472	1.0203
32	11.4590	8.9975	6.7052	5.1543	4.2631	3.6581	3.2131	2.8693	2.3691	1.7629	1.1701
34	12.2870	9.7001	7.3154	5.6935	4.7462	4.0957	3.6130	3.2374	2.6868	2.0123	1.3445
36	13.2112	10.4923	8.0086	6.3097	5.3008	4.5999	4.0752	3.6641	3.0566	2.3042	1.5500
38	14.2588	11.3983	8.8068	7.0231	5.9456	5.1881	4.6160	4.1646	3.4921	2.6499	1.7948
40	15.4665	12.4513	9.7402	7.8613	6.7062	5.8843	5.2578	4.7599	4.0121	3.0649	2.0904
42	16.8083	13.6998	10.8531	8.8651	7.6204	6.7236	6.0336	5.4810	4.6442	3.5719	2.4536
44	18.5951	15.2083	12.2044	10.0890	8.7389	7.7534	6.9876	6.3698	5.4260	4.2019	2.9074
46	20.6825	17.0638	13.8746	11.6074	10.1309	9.0383	8.1808	7.4835	6.4087	4.9975	3.4835
48	23.2861	19.3907	15.9778	13.5263	11.8951	10.6709	9.7001	8.9042	7.6661	6.0200	4.2279
50	26.6051	22.3712	18.6826	16.0020	14.1775	12.7880	11.6742	10.7534	9.3077	7.3605	5.2086
52	30.9405	26.2820	22.2444	19.2720	17.2000	15.5978	14.2993	13.2165	11.5003	9.1582	6.5303
54	36.7379	31.5329	27.0430	23.6901	21.2933	19.4110	17.8682	16.5705	14.4938	11.6221	8.3503
56	44.7507	38.8179	33.7214	29.8552	27.0184	24.7547	22.8782	21.2860	18.7132	15.1081	10.9370
58	56.2146	49.2772	43.3380	38.7548	35.3005	32.4994	30.1509	28.1411	24.8621	20.2064	14.7369
60	73.2083	64.8322	57.6791	52.0576	47.7053	44.1197	41.0801	38.4568	34.1365	27.9230	20.5130

Values of Time Integral for Sucrose Gradient Centrifugation Temperature 0.0 Deg C Particle Density 1.60

WT.PCT. SUCROSE	ZO= 5	ZO=	ZO= -5	ZO= -10	ZO= -15	ZO= -20	ZO= -25	ZO= -30	ZO= -40	ZO= -60	ZO= -100
0	0.0	0.0	0.0	0.0	0.0	0.0	0.0	0.0	0.0	0.0	0.0
2	0.0	0.0	0.6157	0.3339	0.2293	0.1747	0.1411	0.1183	0.0895	0.0601	0.0363
4	0.0	1.3623	1.1101	0.6374	0.4483	0.3460	0.2818	0.2377	0.1811	0.1227	0.0746
6	2.5396	2.2224	1.5363	0.9211	0.6610	0.5161	0.4236	0.3592	0.2756	0.1881	0.1151
8	3.8169	2.9840	1.9236	1.1923	0.8712	0.6868	0.5676	0.4838	0.3736	0.2569	0.1582
10	4.7377	3.4429	2.2794	1.4564	1.0796	0.8598	0.7151	0.6124	0.4760	0.3296	0.2042
12	5.4938	3.9423	2.6224	1.7176	1.2906	1.0368	0.8675	0.7462	0.5836	0.4069	0.2536
14	6.1608	4.4065	2.9574	1.9798	1.5059	1.2194	1.0261	0.8864	0.6973	0.4894	0.3070
16	6.7776	4.8506	3.2904	2.2461	1.7278	1.4097	1.1926	1.0343	0.8184	0.5782	0.3649
18	7.3678	5.2857	3.6265	2.5199	1.9588	1.6095	1.3686	1.1916	0.9481	0.6742	0.4281
20	7.9479	5.7203	3.9706	2.8047	2.2017	1.8212	1.5563	1.3602	1.0880	0.7788	0.4975
22	8.5309	6.1622	4.3275	3.1040	2.4595	2.0475	1.7580	1.5421	1.2402	0.8933	0.5742
24	9.1281	6.6184	4.7022	3.4219	2.7356	2.2915	1.9766	1.7401	1.4067	1.0198	0.6595
26	9.7503	7.0961	5.1003	3.7631	3.0341	2.5559	2.2154	1.9572	1.5905	1.1603	0.7550
28	10.4090	7.6031	5.5280	4.1331	3.3600	2.8482	2.4747	2.1974	1.7948	1.3176	0.8628
30	11.1167	8.1482	5.9930	4.5385	3.7193	3.1708	2.7715	2.4654	2.0239	1.4953	0.9854
32	11.8887	8.7418	6.5042	4.9873	4.1194	3.5317	3.1001	2.7671	2.2832	1.6976	1.1259
34	12.7447	9.3969	7.0730	5.4901	4.5698	3.9396	3.4729	3.1103	2.5794	1.9301	1.2885
36	13.7083	10.1306	7.7151	6.0608	5.0835	4.4066	3.9010	3.5054	2.9218	2.2005	1.4788
38	14.8110	10.9640	8.4493	6.7169	5.6766	4.9477	4.3984	3.9658	3.3224	2.5185	1.7040
40	16.0987	11.9254	9.3015	7.4822	6.3710	5.5833	4.9844	4.5093	3.7972	2.8973	1.9739
42	17.6314	13.0562	10.3094	8.3914	7.1990	6.3435	5.6870	5.1625	4.3697	3.3565	2.3028
44	19.4385	14.4107	11.5229	9.4904	8.2034	7.2682	6.5437	5.9605	5.0717	3.9222	2.7103
46	21.7818	16.0616	13.0088	10.8413	9.4418	8.4113	7.6053	6.9513	5.9460	4.6301	3.2229
48	24.6735	18.1111	14.8614	12.5315	10.9957	9.8493	8.9435	8.2027	7.0535	5.5307	3.8785
50	28.4064	20.7080	17.2179	14.6884	12.9842	11.6939	10.6634	9.8138	8.4837	6.6986	4.7330
52	33.3338	24.0751	20.2847	17.5040	15.5866	14.1131	12.9236	11.9345	10.3715	8.2463	5.8709
54	40.0542	28.5381	24.3631	21.2590	19.0657	17.3540	15.9569	14.7852	12.9158	10.3405	7.4177
56	49.5043	34.4562	29.9591	26.4248	23.8628	21.8315	20.1547	18.7363	16.4512	13.2614	9.5851
58	63.2808	43.2700	37.8916	33.7659	30.6945	28.2199	26.1539	24.3909	21.5232	17.4668	12.7195
60		55.8802	49.5176	44.5501	40.7507	37.6402	35.0138	32.7534	29.0416	23.7223	17.4019

Values of Time Integral for Sucrose Gradient Centrifugation Temperature 0.0 Deg C Particle Density 1.70

WT.PCT. SUCROSE	ZO=5	ZO=0	ZO=-5	ZO=-10	ZO=-15	ZO=-20	ZO=-25	ZO=-30	ZO=-40	ZO=-60	ZO=-100
0	0.0	0.0	0.0	0.0	0.0	0.0	0.0	0.0	0.0	0.0	0.0
2	0.0	0.0	0.6137	0.3328	0.2286	0.1741	0.1406	0.1179	0.0892	0.0599	0.0362
4	0.0	1.3552	1.1055	0.6346	0.4464	0.3445	0.2806	0.2367	0.1803	0.1222	0.0743
6		2.2089	1.5285	0.9162	0.6575	0.5134	0.4213	0.3573	0.2741	0.1871	0.1145
8	2.5160	2.8643	1.9094	1.1849	0.8650	0.6824	0.5639	0.4806	0.3712	0.2552	0.1571
10	3.7784	3.4166	2.2638	1.4459	1.0716	0.8534	0.7097	0.6078	0.4724	0.3271	0.2026
12	4.6863	3.9091	2.6020	1.7035	1.2778	1.0279	0.8600	0.7397	0.5784	0.4032	0.2513
14	5.4300	4.3656	2.9315	1.9613	1.4914	1.2076	1.0160	0.8776	0.6903	0.4845	0.3038
16	6.0845	4.8014	3.2582	2.2226	1.7092	1.3942	1.1793	1.0227	0.8091	0.5716	0.3606
18	6.6880	5.2271	3.5871	2.4906	1.9353	1.5897	1.3516	1.1767	0.9360	0.6655	0.4225
20	7.2640	5.6513	3.9228	2.7684	2.1722	1.7963	1.5347	1.3411	1.0726	0.7675	0.4902
22	7.8284	6.0813	4.2701	3.0597	2.4230	2.0165	1.7310	1.5181	1.2206	0.8790	0.5648
24	8.3940	6.5238	4.6346	3.3681	2.6909	2.2532	1.9430	1.7102	1.3822	1.0016	0.6476
26	8.9715	6.9857	5.0185	3.6981	2.9796	2.5099	2.1740	1.9202	1.5599	1.1375	0.7400
28	9.5711	7.4743	5.4308	4.0546	3.2937	2.7906	2.4277	2.1516	1.7568	1.2892	0.8439
30	10.2037	7.9979	5.8773	4.4439	3.6388	3.1005	2.7089	2.4090	1.9769	1.4598	0.9616
32	10.8810	8.5659	6.3665	4.8734	4.0216	3.4458	3.0234	2.6977	2.2249	1.6534	1.0961
34	11.6168	9.1902	6.9087	5.3526	4.4509	3.8345	3.3787	3.0248	2.5072	1.8750	1.2510
36	12.4293	9.8867	7.5181	5.8943	4.9384	4.2778	3.7850	3.3999	2.8323	2.1316	1.4316
38	13.3399	10.6743	8.2120	6.5144	5.4989	4.7891	4.2551	3.8349	3.2108	2.4321	1.6444
40	14.3772	11.5787	9.0136	7.2343	6.1522	5.3871	4.8063	4.3462	3.6574	2.7885	1.8983
42	15.5827	12.6372	9.9572	8.0854	6.9273	6.0987	5.4641	4.9576	4.1934	3.2184	2.2062
44	17.0101	13.8987	11.0873	9.1089	7.8627	6.9598	6.2619	5.7009	4.8471	3.7452	2.5857
46	18.7300	15.4276	12.4634	10.3600	9.0095	8.0185	7.2450	6.6185	5.6568	4.4007	3.0605
48	20.8415	17.3146	14.1691	11.9161	10.4402	9.3425	8.4771	7.7706	6.6765	5.2299	3.6641
50	23.4872	19.6906	16.3252	13.8896	12.2596	11.0301	10.0508	9.2447	7.9851	6.2985	4.4459
52	26.8797	22.7507	19.1122	16.4484	14.6247	13.2287	12.1048	11.1720	9.7007	7.7051	5.4800
54	31.3258	26.7776	22.7923	19.8365	17.7638	16.1530	14.8417	13.7441	11.9964	9.5946	6.8757
56	37.3370	32.2428	27.8024	24.4616	22.0588	20.1618	18.6001	17.2816	15.1617	12.2097	8.8161
58	45.7334	39.9034	34.8458	30.9797	28.1246	25.8340	23.9267	22.3023	19.6651	15.9437	11.5991
60	57.8558	50.9995	45.0758	40.4691	36.9734	34.1232	31.7228	29.6607	26.2807	21.4480	15.7193

Values of Time Integral for Sucrose Gradient Centrifugation Temperature 0.0 Deg C Particle Density 1.80

WT.PCT. SUCROSE	ZO= 5	ZO= 0	ZO= -5	ZO= -10	ZO= -15	ZO= -20	ZO= -25	ZO= -30	ZO= -40	ZO= -60	ZO= -100
0	0.0	0.0	0.0	0.0	0.0	0.0	0.0	0.0	0.0	0.0	0.0
2	0.0	0.0	0.6119	0.3318	0.2279	0.1736	0.1402	0.1176	0.0889	0.0598	0.0361
4	0.0	1.3492	1.1015	0.6323	0.4447	0.3432	0.2795	0.2358	0.1796	0.1217	0.0740
6	0.0	2.1978	1.5219	0.9122	0.6546	0.5111	0.4194	0.3557	0.2729	0.1862	0.1140
8	2.4972	2.8483	1.8999	1.1788	0.8605	0.6789	0.5609	0.4781	0.3692	0.2538	0.1563
10	3.7480	3.3955	2.2510	1.4374	1.0652	0.8482	0.7054	0.6040	0.4695	0.3250	0.2013
12	4.6460	3.8826	2.5855	1.6922	1.2709	1.0208	0.8540	0.7345	0.5744	0.4004	0.2495
14	5.3803	4.3333	2.9109	1.9467	1.4800	1.1982	1.0080	0.8706	0.6848	0.4806	0.3014
16	6.0253	4.7628	3.2328	2.2042	1.6946	1.3821	1.1690	1.0137	0.8019	0.5664	0.3573
18	6.6190	5.1815	3.5563	2.4678	1.9170	1.5745	1.3384	1.1651	0.9267	0.6588	0.4182
20	7.1843	5.5979	3.8859	2.7406	2.1496	1.7773	1.5182	1.3265	1.0608	0.7590	0.4845
22	7.7373	6.0191	4.2261	3.0259	2.3953	1.9930	1.7105	1.5000	1.2058	0.8682	0.5577
24	8.2901	6.4511	4.5814	3.3273	2.6571	2.2243	1.9177	1.6877	1.3637	0.9880	0.6386
26	8.8533	6.9022	4.9568	3.6491	2.9387	2.4746	2.1430	1.8925	1.5370	1.1206	0.7288
28	9.4368	7.3776	5.3580	3.9960	3.2443	2.7478	2.3898	2.1177	1.7286	1.2681	0.8298
30	10.0508	7.8857	5.7913	4.3739	3.5792	3.0485	2.6628	2.3675	1.9422	1.4337	0.9441
32	10.7064	8.4356	6.2649	4.7897	3.9498	3.3828	2.9677	2.6469	2.1823	1.6211	1.0743
34	11.4167	9.0383	6.7833	5.2523	4.3642	3.7581	3.3102	2.9627	2.4548	1.8350	1.2239
36	12.1989	9.7087	7.3750	5.7737	4.8336	4.1848	3.7013	3.3238	2.7678	2.0821	1.3977
38	13.0729	10.4667	8.0409	6.3689	5.3715	4.6756	4.1525	3.7413	3.1311	2.3705	1.6020
40	14.0654	11.3300	8.8079	7.0577	5.9966	5.2477	4.6799	4.2305	3.5584	2.7115	1.8449
42	15.2150	12.3395	9.7077	7.8693	6.7358	5.9253	5.3072	4.8136	4.0695	3.1214	2.1385
44	16.5714	13.5382	10.7817	8.8420	7.6246	6.7446	6.0654	5.5199	4.6907	3.6221	2.4992
46	18.1999	14.9059	12.0847	10.0266	8.7105	7.7470	6.9962	6.3887	5.4574	4.2427	2.9446
48	20.1914	16.7657	13.6934	11.4943	10.0599	8.9958	8.1583	7.4753	6.4192	5.0248	3.5180
50	22.6767	18.9975	15.7187	13.3480	11.7689	10.5810	9.6364	8.8600	7.6483	6.0285	4.2523
52	25.8496	21.8595	18.3254	15.7412	13.9034	12.6373	11.5575	10.6625	9.2529	7.3441	5.2195
54	29.9888	25.6086	21.7514	18.8955	15.9034	15.3598	14.1056	13.0572	11.3902	9.1032	6.5188
56	35.5581	30.6720	26.3932	23.1805	20.8826	19.0738	17.5876	16.3345	14.3227	11.5260	8.3166
58	43.2970	37.7326	32.8850	29.1882	25.4734	24.3018	22.4971	20.9620	18.4734	14.9675	10.8817
60	54.4086	47.9035	42.2620	37.8863	34.5843	31.8997	29.6431	27.7068	24.5374	20.0129	14.6583

Values of Time Integral for Sucrose Gradient Centrifugation Temperature 0.0 Deg C Particle Density 1.90

WT.PCT. SUCROSE	$Z_0=5$	$Z_0=0$	$Z_0=-5$	$Z_0=-10$	$Z_0=-15$	$Z_0=-20$	$Z_0=-25$	$Z_0=-30$	$Z_0=-40$	$Z_0=-60$	$Z_0=-120$
0	0.0	0.0	0.0	0.0	0.0	0.0	0.0	0.0	0.0	0.0	0.0
2	0.0	0.0	0.6132	0.3309	0.2272	0.1731	0.1398	0.1172	0.0887	0.0596	0.0360
4	0.0	1.3440	1.0978	0.6302	0.4433	0.3421	0.2786	0.2350	0.1790	0.1213	0.0737
6	2.4816	2.1863	1.5152	0.9087	0.6520	0.5091	0.4177	0.3543	0.2718	0.1855	0.1135
8		2.8346	1.8917	1.1736	0.8566	0.6758	0.5534	0.4759	0.3675	0.2527	0.1556
10	3.7230	3.3777	2.2402	1.4302	1.0598	0.8439	0.7017	0.6009	0.4670	0.3233	0.2003
12	4.6130	3.8606	2.5717	1.6827	1.2637	1.0149	0.8490	0.7302	0.5710	0.3980	0.2480
14	5.3398	4.3066	2.8937	1.9346	1.4706	1.1905	1.0015	0.8649	0.6803	0.4774	0.2993
16	5.9773	4.7310	3.2119	2.1892	1.6827	1.3723	1.1606	1.0063	0.7960	0.5622	0.3547
18	6.5632	5.1443	3.5312	2.4493	1.9022	1.5621	1.3278	1.1558	0.9192	0.6534	0.4147
20	7.1203	5.5546	3.8560	2.7181	2.1314	1.7619	1.5049	1.3148	1.0513	0.7521	0.4802
22	7.6644	5.9690	4.1907	2.9988	2.3732	1.9742	1.6941	1.4855	1.1940	0.8595	0.5521
24	8.2075	6.3939	4.5397	3.2949	2.6303	2.2014	1.8977	1.6699	1.3491	0.9773	0.6316
26	8.7597	6.8357	4.9079	3.6105	2.9064	2.4469	2.1186	1.8707	1.5190	1.1072	0.7200
28	9.3309	7.3011	5.3005	3.9601	3.2056	2.7142	2.3602	2.0911	1.7066	1.2517	0.8189
30	9.9308	7.7975	5.7240	4.3192	3.5329	3.0081	2.6269	2.3352	1.9153	1.4135	0.9305
32	10.5702	8.3338	6.1858	4.7242	3.8943	3.3341	2.9236	2.6077	2.1494	1.5962	1.0575
34	11.2615	8.9204	6.6952	5.1749	4.2976	3.6994	3.2576	2.9151	2.4147	1.8044	1.2031
36	12.0212	9.5716	7.2650	5.6814	4.7535	4.1138	3.6375	3.2658	2.7186	2.0444	1.3720
38	12.8682	10.3042	7.9104	6.2582	5.2748	4.5894	4.0746	3.6704	3.0707	2.3239	1.5699
40	13.8279	11.1408	8.6521	6.9242	5.8791	5.1426	4.5847	4.1434	3.4839	2.6536	1.8047
42	14.9368	12.1145	9.5200	7.7071	6.5922	5.7972	5.1898	4.7059	3.9769	3.0490	2.0880
44	16.2420	13.2681	10.5534	8.6430	7.4475	6.5846	5.9193	5.3855	4.5747	3.5308	2.4350
46	17.8049	14.6574	11.8039	9.7799	8.4896	7.5466	6.8127	6.2193	5.3104	4.1264	2.8664
48	19.7110	16.3608	13.3436	11.1846	9.7811	8.7418	7.9249	7.2593	6.2309	4.8749	3.4113
50	22.0827	18.4907	15.2764	12.9537	11.4121	10.2546	9.3355	8.5807	7.4040	5.8328	4.1121
52	25.1016	21.2139	17.7565	15.2307	13.5167	12.2111	11.1633	10.2958	8.9306	7.0845	5.0323
54	29.0276	24.7697	21.0060	18.2225	15.2886	14.7933	13.5801	12.5670	10.9577	8.7529	6.2647
56	34.2920	29.5560	25.3938	22.2729	20.0499	18.3040	16.8716	15.6650	13.7298	11.0431	7.9641
58	41.5818	36.2068	31.5087	27.9319	25.3162	23.2286	21.4960	20.0238	17.6395	14.2849	10.3802
60	52.0095	45.7517	40.3086	36.0947	32.9279	30.3589	28.2022	26.3535	23.3303	19.0197	13.9243

Values of Time Integral for Sucrose Gradient Centrifugation Temperature 5.0 Deg C Particle Density 1.10

WT.PCT. SUCROSE	Z0= 5	Z0= 0	Z0= -5	Z0= -10	Z0= -15	Z0= -20	Z0= -25	Z0= -30	Z0= -40	Z0= -60	Z0= -100
0	0.0	0.0	0.0	0.0	0.0	0.0	0.0	0.0	0.0	0.0	0.0
2	0.0	0.0	0.5523	0.2998	0.2060	0.1559	0.1267	0.1063	0.0804	0.0541	0.0327
4	0.0	1.3098	1.0291	0.5926	0.4173	0.3223	0.2626	0.2216	0.1689	0.1144	0.0696
6	0.0	2.2080	1.4748	0.8894	0.6399	0.5004	0.4110	0.3488	0.2678	0.1830	0.1120
8	2.8093	2.9663	1.9159	1.2007	0.8804	0.6963	0.5763	0.4918	0.3804	0.2619	0.1615
10	4.5142	3.6792	2.3737	1.5380	1.1475	0.9173	0.7649	0.6562	0.5112	0.3549	0.2203
12	5.8442	4.4020	2.8704	1.9164	1.4532	1.1738	0.9857	0.8501	0.6671	0.4669	0.2920
14	7.1163	5.1840	3.4352	2.3585	1.8163	1.4819	1.2533	1.0866	0.8591	0.6062	0.3820
16	8.4736	6.0887	4.1139	2.9016	2.2690	1.8700	1.5929	1.3885	1.1061	0.7874	0.5002
18	10.0844	7.2263	4.9933	3.6184	2.8739	2.3933	2.0540	1.8006	1.4460	1.0391	0.6659
20	12.2288	8.8521	6.2813	4.6848	3.7839	3.1868	2.7575	2.4324	1.9708	1.4312	0.9263
22	16.3557	11.9569	8.7923	6.7927	5.6002	4.7825	4.1804	3.7162	3.0447	2.2405	1.4684

Values of Time Integral for Sucrose Gradient Centrifugation Temperature 5.0 Deg C Particle Density 1.20

WT.PCT. SUCROSE	ZO=5	ZO=0	ZO=-5	ZO=-10	ZO=-15	ZO=-20	ZO=-25	ZO=-30	ZO=-40	ZO=-60	ZO=-100
0	0.0	0.0	0.0	0.0	0.0	0.0	0.0	0.0	0.0	0.0	0.0
2	0.0	0.0	0.5357	0.2906	0.1996	0.1521	0.1228	0.1030	0.0779	0.0524	0.0317
4	0.0	1.2163	0.9776	0.5619	0.3954	0.3053	0.2487	0.2098	0.1598	0.1083	0.0659
6	2.4017	2.0068	1.3695	0.8228	0.5911	0.4618	0.3791	0.3215	0.2468	0.1685	0.1031
8	3.6521	2.6340	1.7341	1.0800	0.7898	0.6236	0.5156	0.4397	0.3398	0.2337	0.1440
10	4.5867	3.1816	2.0856	1.3389	0.9947	0.7932	0.6603	0.5658	0.4401	0.3050	0.1891
12	5.3846	3.6888	2.4340	1.6043	1.2090	0.9730	0.8151	0.7017	0.5494	0.3835	0.2393
14	6.1190	4.1787	2.7876	1.8810	1.4363	1.1659	0.9826	0.8497	0.6695	0.4707	0.2957
16	6.8306	4.6679	3.1544	2.1744	1.6808	1.3754	1.1660	1.0127	0.8029	0.5685	0.3595
18	7.5475	5.1699	3.5423	2.4905	1.9475	1.6061	1.3692	1.1943	0.9526	0.6794	0.4324
20	8.2937	5.6980	3.9603	2.8365	2.2426	1.8634	1.5972	1.3991	1.1227	0.8064	0.5168
22	9.0937	6.2665	4.4195	3.2216	2.5743	2.1546	1.8568	1.6332	1.3185	0.9539	0.6155
24	9.9756	6.8926	4.9339	3.6580	2.9533	2.4896	2.1569	1.9050	1.5471	1.1274	0.7326
26	10.9752	7.5981	5.5218	4.1620	3.3943	2.8816	2.5097	2.2258	1.8186	1.3350	0.8738
28	12.1429	8.4126	6.2092	4.7565	3.9181	3.3497	2.9328	2.6118	2.1470	1.5880	1.0471
30	13.5537	9.3792	7.0336	5.4754	4.5553	3.9219	3.4521	3.0871	2.5534	1.9031	1.2645
32	15.3280	10.5626	8.0528	6.3704	5.3531	4.6415	4.1075	3.6888	3.0704	2.3065	1.5448
34	17.6302	12.0683	9.3606	7.5262	6.3386	5.5794	4.9646	4.4780	3.7516	2.8412	1.9188
36	21.0371	14.0849	11.1254	9.0952	7.8009	6.8634	6.1417	5.5645	4.6934	3.5849	2.4422
38	26.4545	16.9888	13.6842	11.3820	9.8681	8.7495	7.8758	7.1694	6.0900	4.6938	3.2275
40	38.0635	21.7133	17.8728	15.1441	13.2324	11.8749	10.7574	9.8425	8.4251	6.5576	4.5553
42		31.9123	26.9672	23.3498	20.7577	18.7392	17.1031	15.7424	13.5982	10.7081	7.5299

Values of Time Integral for Sucrose Gradient Centrifugation Temperature 5.0 Deg C Particle Density 1.30

WT.PCT. SUCROSE	Z0= 5	Z0= 0	Z0= -5	Z0= -10	Z0= -15	Z0= -20	Z0= -25	Z0= -30	Z0= -40	Z0= -60	Z0= -100
0	0.0	0.0	0.0	0.0	0.0	0.0	0.0	0.0	0.0	0.0	0.0
2	0.0	0.0	0.5297	0.2873	0.1973	0.1503	0.1214	0.1018	0.0770	0.0518	0.0313
4	0.0	1.1861	0.9604	0.5517	0.3881	0.2996	0.2440	0.2059	0.1568	0.1063	0.0646
6	0.0	1.9449	1.3364	0.8020	0.5758	0.4497	0.3691	0.3131	0.2402	0.1640	0.1004
8	2.2693	2.5368	1.6804	1.0447	0.7633	0.6025	0.4980	0.4245	0.3280	0.2255	0.1389
10	3.4281	3.0439	2.0059	1.2844	0.9530	0.7595	0.6319	0.5413	0.4209	0.2915	0.1807
12	4.2762	3.5041	2.3220	1.5251	1.1475	0.9225	0.7723	0.6646	0.5200	0.3627	0.2262
14	4.9841	3.9387	2.6357	1.7706	1.3491	1.0936	0.9209	0.7959	0.6265	0.4401	0.2762
16	5.6194	4.3617	2.9528	2.0243	1.5605	1.2748	1.0794	0.9368	0.7418	0.5246	0.3313
18	6.2176	4.7837	3.2789	2.2899	1.7846	1.4686	1.2502	1.0894	0.8677	0.6178	0.3927
20	6.8012	5.2136	3.6191	2.5715	2.0248	1.6781	1.4358	1.2561	1.0061	0.7212	0.4613
22	7.3869	5.6598	3.9795	2.8738	2.2851	1.9066	1.6395	1.4398	1.1597	0.8369	0.5387
24	7.9890	6.1309	4.3665	3.2021	2.5702	2.1586	1.8653	1.6443	1.3317	0.9675	0.6269
26	8.6209	6.6364	4.7878	3.5632	2.8862	2.4395	2.1181	1.8741	1.5262	1.1162	0.7280
28	9.2970	7.1873	5.2526	3.9653	3.2404	2.7560	2.4042	2.1351	1.7483	1.2872	0.8452
30	10.0339	7.7972	5.7728	4.4188	3.6424	3.1170	2.7317	2.4349	2.0047	1.4860	0.9823
32	10.8516	8.4830	6.3634	4.9374	4.1047	3.5339	3.1115	2.7836	2.3042	1.7197	1.1447
34	11.7754	9.2669	7.0442	5.5391	4.6437	4.0221	3.5576	3.1943	2.6587	1.9980	1.3393
36	12.8399	10.1794	7.8427	6.2489	5.2826	4.6030	4.0900	3.6858	3.0847	2.3343	1.5760
38	14.0911	11.2616	8.7961	7.1009	6.0527	5.3056	4.7360	4.2836	3.6049	2.7473	1.8684
40	15.5948	12.5726	9.9532	8.1446	6.9997	6.1724	5.5352	5.0248	4.2523	3.2640	2.2365
42	17.4484	14.2004	11.4092	9.4534	8.1918	7.2668	6.5467	5.9651	5.0766	3.9251	2.7101
44	19.7954	16.2746	13.2676	11.1365	9.7299	8.6829	7.8587	7.1874	6.1517	4.7915	3.3342
46	22.8514	18.9914	15.7129	13.3597	11.7680	10.5643	9.6058	8.8161	7.5906	5.9565	4.1780
48	26.9650	22.6678	19.0361	16.3916	14.5556	13.1440	12.0065	11.0630	9.5777	7.5723	5.5543
50	32.7251	27.8408	23.7306	20.6887	18.5172	16.8188	15.4332	14.2730	12.4272	9.8943	7.0568
52	41.1957	35.4819	30.6902	27.0785	24.4234	22.3095	20.5630	19.0864	16.7121	13.4126	9.6399
54	54.4584	47.4952	41.6693	37.1872	33.7897	31.0350	28.7297	26.7616	23.5627	19.0516	13.8054
56	77.2105	68.1825	60.6353	54.6965	50.0500	46.2127	42.9600	40.1557	35.5484	28.9546	21.1545
58	122.5723	109.5740	98.5958	89.9221	82.8339	76.8713	71.7522	67.2957	59.8943	49.1436	36.2042
60	253.7656	229.6937	209.4659	192.6932	178.6834	166.6727	156.2236	147.0344	131.5981	108.8210	80.8915

Values of Time Integral for Sucrose Gradient Centrifugation Temperature 5.0 Deg C Particle Density 1.40

WT.PCT. SUCROSE	Z0= 5	Z0= 0	Z0= -5	Z0= -10	Z0= -15	Z0= -20	Z0= -25	Z0= -30	Z0= -40	Z0= -60	Z0= -100
0	0.0	0.0	0.0	0.0	0.0	0.0	0.0	0.0	0.0	0.0	0.0
2	0.0	0.9	0.5262	0.2854	0.1960	0.1493	0.1206	0.1011	0.0765	0.0514	0.0311
4	0.0	1.1703	0.9510	0.5461	0.3842	0.2965	0.2415	0.2037	0.1552	0.1052	0.0639
6	0.0	1.9134	1.3192	0.7913	0.5680	0.4435	0.3640	0.3087	0.2369	0.1617	0.0989
8	2.2059	2.4883	1.6534	1.0269	0.7500	0.5919	0.4892	0.4170	0.3221	0.2215	0.1364
10	3.3222	2.9769	1.9668	1.2578	0.9328	0.7431	0.6181	0.5294	0.4116	0.2850	0.1766
12	4.1319	3.4161	2.2685	1.4876	1.1183	0.8987	0.7521	0.6471	0.5062	0.3530	0.2201
14	4.8011	3.8269	2.5650	1.7196	1.3089	1.0604	0.8926	0.7712	0.6068	0.4261	0.2673
16	5.3953	4.2225	2.8617	1.9569	1.5066	1.2299	1.0408	0.9030	0.7147	0.5052	0.3189
18	5.9485	4.6128	3.1632	2.2025	1.7139	1.4091	1.1988	1.0441	0.8311	0.5913	0.3756
20	6.4817	5.0055	3.4740	2.4598	1.9333	1.6004	1.3683	1.1963	0.9575	0.6857	0.4383
22	7.0097	5.4077	3.7988	2.7322	2.1679	1.8064	1.5519	1.3619	1.0960	0.7900	0.5081
24	7.5445	5.8262	4.1426	3.0239	2.4212	2.0303	1.7524	1.5436	1.2488	0.9060	0.5864
26	8.0970	6.2681	4.5109	3.3396	2.6974	2.2758	1.9734	1.7445	1.4188	1.0360	0.6748
28	8.6778	6.7414	4.9102	3.6649	3.0017	2.5477	2.2192	1.9687	1.6095	1.1829	0.7754
30	9.2987	7.2552	5.3485	3.9992	3.3404	2.8518	2.4952	2.2213	1.8255	1.3504	0.8910
32	9.9730	7.8208	5.8355	4.4947	3.7215	3.1956	2.8083	2.5087	2.0725	1.5431	1.0248
34	10.7166	8.4518	6.3835	4.9790	4.1554	3.5886	3.1674	2.8393	2.3578	1.7671	1.1815
36	11.5506	9.1666	7.0090	5.5350	4.6559	4.0436	3.5845	3.2244	2.6915	2.0305	1.3669
38	12.5011	9.9887	7.7333	6.1823	5.2409	4.5773	4.0752	3.6785	3.0867	2.3442	1.5890
40	13.6040	10.9503	8.5856	6.9477	5.9355	5.2130	4.6613	4.2221	3.5615	2.7232	1.8589
42	14.9092	12.0964	9.6073	7.8692	6.7748	5.9836	5.3734	4.8841	4.1418	3.1886	2.1924
44	16.4850	13.4891	10.8549	8.9992	7.8074	6.9343	6.2543	5.7047	4.8636	3.7703	2.6114
46	18.4242	15.2129	12.4065	10.4098	9.1005	8.1280	7.3628	6.7393	5.7765	4.5094	3.1466
48	20.8620	17.3916	14.3758	12.2065	10.7524	9.6567	8.7853	8.0695	6.9539	5.4668	3.8436
50	23.9993	20.2090	16.9326	14.5467	12.9099	11.6579	10.6515	9.8176	8.5057	6.7340	4.7707
52	28.1417	23.9457	20.3358	17.6712	15.7479	14.3427	13.1597	12.1711	10.6007	8.4516	6.0335
54	33.7658	29.0396	24.9910	21.9572	19.7690	18.0419	16.6220	15.4249	13.5049	10.8420	7.7992
56	41.6538	36.2112	31.5655	28.0064	25.4050	23.3025	21.5540	20.0670	17.6586	14.2738	10.3457
58	53.1235	46.6758	41.1871	36.9306	33.6914	31.0513	28.8306	26.9258	23.8107	19.3748	14.1476
60	70.5283	62.6074	55.8753	50.5556	45.3966	42.9531	40.0246	37.4914	33.3099	27.2785	20.0639

Values of Time Integral for Sucrose Gradient Centrifugation Temperature 5.0 Deg C Particle Density 1.50

WT.PCT. SUCROSE	ZO= 5	ZO= 0	ZO= -5	ZO= -10	ZO= -15	ZO= -20	ZO= -25	ZO= -30	ZO= -40	ZO= -60	ZO= -100
0	0.0	0.0	0.0	0.0	0.0	0.0	0.0	0.0	0.0	0.0	0.0
2	0.0	0.0	0.5237	0.2840	0.1951	0.1486	0.1200	0.1006	0.0761	0.0512	0.0309
4	0.0	1.1601	0.9447	0.5424	0.3816	0.2945	0.2398	0.2023	0.1541	0.1044	0.0635
6	2.1676	1.8934	1.3080	0.7843	0.5629	0.4395	0.3607	0.3059	0.2347	0.1602	0.0980
8	3.2590	2.4581	1.6363	1.0158	0.7417	0.5852	0.4836	0.4122	0.3184	0.2189	0.1348
10	4.0465	2.9357	1.9427	1.2415	0.9203	0.7330	0.6097	0.5221	0.4059	0.2810	0.1741
12	4.6937	3.3629	2.2361	1.4649	1.1008	0.8844	0.7400	0.6366	0.4979	0.3471	0.2164
14	5.2652	3.7602	2.5228	1.6893	1.2851	1.0408	0.8758	0.7566	0.5952	0.4178	0.2621
16	5.7940	4.1407	2.8081	1.9175	1.4753	1.2038	1.0184	0.8833	0.6990	0.4939	0.3117
18	6.3003	4.5137	3.0963	2.1523	1.6734	1.3751	1.1694	1.0182	0.8102	0.5762	0.3659
20	6.7983	4.8866	3.3915	2.3966	1.8817	1.5567	1.3304	1.1628	0.9302	0.6659	0.4254
22	7.2990	5.2659	3.6978	2.6535	2.1029	1.7510	1.5035	1.3190	1.0608	0.7642	0.4912
24	7.8121	5.6577	4.0196	2.9266	2.3401	1.9605	1.6912	1.4890	1.2039	0.8728	0.5645
26	8.3470	6.0682	4.3617	3.2198	2.5966	2.1886	1.8965	1.6756	1.3617	0.9935	0.6466
28	8.9136	6.5040	4.7294	3.5378	2.8768	2.4390	2.1228	1.8821	1.5374	1.1288	0.7393
30	9.5229	6.9729	5.1294	3.8865	3.1859	2.7165	2.3747	2.1126	1.7345	1.2817	0.8447
32	10.1878	7.4839	5.5694	4.2729	3.5303	3.0272	2.6576	2.3723	1.9577	1.4558	0.9657
34	10.9243	8.0481	6.0594	4.7059	3.9182	3.3785	2.9786	2.6679	2.2128	1.6560	1.1057
36	11.7543	8.6798	6.6122	5.1973	4.3605	3.7806	3.3472	3.0081	2.5077	1.8888	1.2696
38	12.7037	9.3973	7.2443	5.7621	4.8711	4.2464	3.7755	3.4044	2.8525	2.1626	1.4634
40	13.8105	10.2250	7.9779	6.4210	5.4689	4.7936	4.2799	3.8723	3.2612	2.4888	1.6958
42	15.1246	11.1969	8.8442	7.2024	6.1806	5.4469	4.8838	4.4337	3.7533	2.8834	1.9785
44	16.7124	12.3583	9.8847	8.1448	7.0418	6.2398	5.6194	5.1180	4.3552	3.3685	2.3279
46	18.6680	13.7698	11.1551	9.2997	8.1005	7.2172	6.5260	5.9651	5.1027	3.9736	2.7661
48	21.1279	15.5175	12.7349	10.7410	9.4256	8.4434	7.6671	7.0322	6.0472	4.7417	3.3252
50	24.2927	17.7265	14.7395	12.5758	11.1172	10.0125	9.1302	8.4027	7.2638	5.7351	4.0521
52	28.4653	20.5813	17.3396	14.9629	13.3236	12.0636	11.0464	10.2007	8.8643	7.0474	5.0168
54	34.1235	24.3605	20.7933	18.1461	16.2697	14.8080	13.6151	12.6147	11.0188	8.8207	6.3267
56	42.0356	29.5047	25.5091	22.4961	20.3123	18.5813	17.1527	15.9444	13.9982	11.2822	8.1532
58	53.5036	36.7235	32.1463	28.6383	25.0283	23.9264	22.1721	20.6755	18.2419	14.8008	10.7757
60		47.2206	41.8241	37.6154	34.3994	31.7681	29.5474	27.6367	24.5004	20.0081	14.6735

Values of Time Integral for Sucrose Gradient Centrifugation Temperature 5.0 Deg C Particle Density 1.80

WT.PCT. SUCROSE	Z0= 5	Z0= 0	Z0= -5	Z0= -10	Z0= -15	Z0= -20	Z0= -25	Z0= -30	Z0= -40	Z0= -60	Z0= -100
0	0.0	0.0	0.0	0.0	0.0	0.0	0.0	0.0	0.0	0.0	0.0
2	0.0	0.0	0.5184	0.2811	0.1931	0.1470	0.1188	0.0996	0.0753	0.0506	0.0306
4	0.0	1.1415	0.9326	0.5353	0.3765	0.2906	0.2367	0.1996	0.1521	0.1030	0.0627
6	2.1059	1.8584	1.2877	0.7718	0.5538	0.4324	0.3548	0.3009	0.2308	0.1575	0.0964
8	2.6890	2.4068	1.6064	0.9965	0.7224	0.5738	0.4741	0.4041	0.3121	0.2146	0.1321
10	3.1585	2.8673	1.9019	1.2141	0.8996	0.7163	0.5957	0.5101	0.3964	0.2744	0.1700
12	3.9124	3.2762	2.1827	1.4280	1.0724	0.8612	0.7204	0.6196	0.4845	0.3377	0.2105
14	4.5274	3.6537	2.4552	1.6412	1.2475	1.0098	0.8494	0.7336	0.5770	0.4044	0.2539
16	5.0660	4.0123	2.7240	1.8562	1.4267	1.1534	0.9838	0.8531	0.6747	0.4765	0.3006
18	5.5603	4.3610	2.9934	2.0757	1.6118	1.3235	1.1249	0.9791	0.7737	0.5535	0.3513
20	6.0294	4.7065	3.2669	2.3020	1.8048	1.4918	1.2741	1.1131	0.8799	0.6366	0.4064
22	6.4866	5.0547	3.5481	2.5379	2.0080	1.6701	1.4330	1.2565	1.0093	0.7269	0.4668
24	6.9419	5.4110	3.8408	2.7862	2.2236	1.8607	1.6037	1.4111	1.1399	0.8256	0.5335
26	7.4038	5.7805	4.1437	3.0501	2.4545	2.0650	1.7885	1.5790	1.2820	0.9343	0.6074
28	7.8802	6.1686	4.4762	3.3334	2.7041	2.2890	1.9901	1.7629	1.4384	1.0547	0.6899
30	8.3792	6.5816	4.8734	3.6404	2.9763	2.5334	2.2118	1.9659	1.6120	1.1893	0.7828
32	8.9095	7.0263	5.2114	3.9767	3.2760	2.8037	2.4561	2.1919	1.8062	1.3209	0.8881
34	9.4809	7.5112	5.6324	4.3488	3.6093	3.1056	2.7340	2.4459	2.0254	1.5129	1.0084
36	10.1060	8.0470	6.1013	4.7656	3.9845	3.4457	3.0466	2.7345	2.2755	1.7104	1.1473
38	10.7997	8.6470	6.6299	5.2380	4.4114	3.8362	3.4047	3.0659	2.5639	1.9293	1.3094
40	11.5818	9.3288	7.2343	5.7807	4.9039	4.2870	3.8203	3.4514	2.9006	2.2030	1.5008
42	12.4792	10.1168	7.9356	6.4142	5.4609	4.8167	4.3099	3.9065	3.2995	2.5280	1.7300
44	13.5267	11.0426	8.7660	7.1654	5.9961	5.4487	4.6954	4.4520	3.7793	2.9146	2.0086
46	14.7896	12.1474	9.7604	8.0695	6.9335	6.2137	5.6058	5.1150	4.3644	3.3633	2.3516
48	16.2709	13.4891	10.9732	9.1759	8.0133	7.1551	6.4818	5.9342	5.0894	3.9779	2.7808
50	18.1202	15.1499	12.4802	10.5553	9.2850	8.3347	7.5817	6.9645	6.0041	4.7247	3.3272
52	20.4465	17.2483	14.3914	12.3099	10.9068	9.8423	8.9902	8.2861	7.1805	5.6892	4.0363
54	23.4400	19.9595	16.8690	14.5910	13.0203	11.8111	10.8329	10.0178	8.7261	6.9614	4.9759
56	27.3935	23.5539	20.1642	17.6328	15.8450	14.4476	13.3047	12.3443	10.8078	8.6812	6.2521
58	32.7660	28.4555	24.6707	21.8034	19.7260	18.0768	16.7128	15.5566	13.6891	11.0702	8.0326
60	40.3130	35.3635	31.0395	27.7110	25.2348	23.2372	21.5662	20.1376	17.8076	14.4969	10.5976

Values of Time Integral for Sucrose Gradient Centrifugation Temperature 5.0 Deg C Particle Density 1.90

WT.PCT. SUCROSE	Z0= 5	Z0= 0	Z0= -5	Z0= -10	Z0= -15	Z0= -20	Z0= -25	Z0= -30	Z0= -40	Z0= -60	Z0= -100
0	0.0	0.0	0.0	0.0	0.0	0.0	0.0	0.0	0.0	0.0	0.0
2	0.0	0.0	0.5169	0.2803	0.1925	0.1456	0.1184	0.0993	0.0751	0.0505	0.0305
4	0.0	1.1371	0.9295	0.5335	0.3753	0.2896	0.2359	0.1990	0.1516	0.1027	0.0624
6	0.0	1.8504	1.2829	0.7688	0.5516	0.4307	0.3534	0.2997	0.2299	0.1569	0.0960
8	2.0929	2.3954	1.5996	0.9921	0.7242	0.5712	0.4720	0.4023	0.3107	0.2136	0.1315
10	3.1376	2.8524	1.8928	1.2081	0.8951	0.7127	0.5924	0.5074	0.3944	0.2730	0.1691
12	3.8849	3.2577	2.1712	1.4201	1.0663	0.8563	0.7163	0.6160	0.4817	0.3357	0.2092
14	4.4937	3.6314	2.4409	1.6311	1.2396	1.0033	0.8440	0.7289	0.5732	0.4022	0.2522
16	5.0261	3.9859	2.7066	1.8437	1.4168	1.1552	0.9768	0.8470	0.6698	0.4730	0.2984
18	5.5140	4.3300	2.9725	2.0603	1.5995	1.3132	1.1161	0.9714	0.7724	0.5490	0.3484
20	5.9764	4.6706	3.2421	2.2834	1.7898	1.4791	1.2631	1.1034	0.8821	0.6309	0.4027
22	6.4263	5.0133	3.5188	2.5155	1.9897	1.6546	1.4195	1.2445	1.0000	0.7197	0.4622
24	6.8736	5.3633	3.8063	2.7594	2.2015	1.8418	1.5872	1.3964	1.1278	0.8167	0.5277
26	7.3267	5.7257	4.1083	3.0183	2.4280	2.0431	1.7684	1.5611	1.2672	0.9233	0.6002
28	7.7931	6.1057	4.4290	3.2956	2.6723	2.2615	1.9658	1.7412	1.4204	1.0413	0.6810
30	8.2808	6.5093	4.7733	3.5958	2.9384	2.5004	2.1826	1.9396	1.5900	1.1728	0.7717
32	8.7981	6.9432	5.1468	3.9238	3.2307	2.7641	2.4227	2.1601	1.7795	1.3206	0.8744
34	9.3544	7.4152	5.5568	4.2861	3.5553	3.0580	2.6913	2.4073	1.9929	1.4882	0.9916
36	9.9617	7.9358	6.0123	4.6910	3.9197	3.3893	2.9950	2.6877	2.2359	1.6800	1.1266
38	10.6342	8.5174	6.5247	5.1489	4.3336	3.7669	3.3422	3.0090	2.5154	1.9019	1.2837
40	11.3907	9.1770	7.1093	5.6739	4.8100	4.2030	3.7442	3.3818	2.8411	2.1618	1.4688
42	12.2567	9.9374	7.7871	6.2853	5.3668	4.7142	4.2167	3.8210	3.2261	2.4706	1.6900
44	13.2651	10.8286	8.5855	7.0084	6.0276	5.3226	4.7803	4.3461	3.6880	2.8428	1.9581
46	14.4585	11.8894	9.5403	7.8764	6.8234	6.0571	5.4624	4.9828	4.2497	3.2976	2.2875
48	15.8961	13.1742	10.7016	8.9359	7.7974	6.9585	6.3013	5.7672	4.9440	3.8621	2.6985
50	17.6619	14.7599	12.1406	10.2530	9.0117	8.0848	7.3515	6.7510	5.8173	4.5753	3.2202
52	19.8766	16.7576	13.9601	11.9234	10.5556	9.5201	8.6924	8.0091	6.9373	5.4935	3.8953
54	22.7174	19.3306	16.3114	14.0883	12.5614	11.3885	10.4412	9.6526	8.4041	6.7008	4.7870
56	26.4571	22.7306	19.4283	16.9655	15.2332	13.8824	12.7792	11.8532	10.3732	8.3276	5.9941
58	31.5212	27.3508	23.6762	20.8966	18.8916	17.3033	15.9911	14.8811	13.0891	10.5795	7.6725
60	38.6089	33.8385	29.6574	26.4448	24.0651	22.1497	20.5498	19.1833	16.9570	13.7976	10.0813

Values of Time Integral for Sucrose Gradient Centrifugation Temperature 5.0 Deg C Particle Density 1.60

WT.PCT. SUCROSE	Z0= 5	Z0= 0	Z0= -5	Z0= -10	Z0= -15	Z0= -20	Z0= -25	Z0= -30	Z0= -40	Z0= -60	Z0= -100
0	0.0	0.0	0.0	0.0	0.0	0.0	0.0	0.0	0.0	0.0	0.0
2	0.0	0.0	0.5216	0.2629	0.1943	0.1480	0.1195	0.1002	0.0758	0.0510	0.0308
4	0.0	1.1526	0.9399	0.5396	0.3796	0.2929	0.2386	0.2013	0.1533	0.1039	0.0632
6	0.0	1.8790	1.2998	0.7792	0.5592	0.4366	0.3583	0.3039	0.2331	0.1591	0.0974
8	2.1413	2.4368	1.6240	1.0078	0.7358	0.5805	0.4797	0.4089	0.3158	0.2171	0.1337
10	3.2158	2.9069	1.9256	1.2300	0.9116	0.7260	0.6038	0.5171	0.4019	0.2783	0.1724
12	3.9886	3.3261	2.2135	1.4493	1.0887	0.8745	0.7317	0.6293	0.4922	0.3431	0.2139
14	4.6216	3.7146	2.4940	1.6687	1.2689	1.0274	0.8645	0.7467	0.5874	0.4122	0.2585
16	5.1784	4.0854	2.7719	1.8910	1.4542	1.1862	1.0034	0.8702	0.6884	0.4853	0.3069
18	5.6917	4.4474	3.0516	2.1189	1.6465	1.3525	1.1499	1.0011	0.7964	0.5662	0.3595
20	6.1812	4.8079	3.3370	2.3551	1.8479	1.5281	1.3056	1.1409	0.9124	0.6529	0.4170
22	6.6605	5.1731	3.6319	2.6024	2.0609	1.7151	1.4722	1.2912	1.0381	0.7476	0.4804
24	7.1404	5.5485	3.9403	2.8641	2.2881	1.9160	1.6522	1.4542	1.1752	0.8517	0.5506
26	7.6298	5.9401	4.2666	3.1437	2.5328	2.1335	1.8479	1.6321	1.3258	0.9668	0.6289
28	8.1375	6.3537	4.6156	3.4456	2.7988	2.3711	2.0627	1.8281	1.4925	1.0952	0.7169
30	8.6724	6.7964	4.9931	3.7747	3.0905	2.6331	2.3005	2.0457	1.6786	1.2395	0.8164
32	9.2443	7.2761	5.4062	4.1375	3.4138	2.9247	2.5660	2.2895	1.8881	1.4029	0.9300
34	9.8647	7.8025	5.8634	4.5415	3.7758	3.2525	2.8656	2.5653	2.1261	1.5898	1.0606
36	10.5481	8.3882	6.3759	4.9971	4.1858	3.6253	3.2073	2.8808	2.3995	1.8056	1.2125
38	11.3119	9.0489	6.9580	5.5172	4.6560	4.0543	3.6017	3.2457	2.7171	2.0577	1.3910
40	12.1798	9.8055	7.6286	6.1195	5.2025	4.5545	4.0628	3.6734	3.0907	2.3559	1.6034
42	13.1836	10.6869	8.4143	6.8282	5.8479	5.1470	4.6105	4.1825	3.5370	2.7138	1.8598
44	14.3655	11.7314	9.3501	7.6757	6.5224	5.8601	5.2712	4.7979	4.0783	3.1500	2.1740
46	15.7805	12.9893	10.4822	8.7050	7.5660	6.7311	6.0800	5.5529	4.7444	3.6893	2.5646
48	17.5062	14.5316	11.8763	9.9768	8.7353	7.8132	7.0869	6.4945	5.5778	4.3670	3.0579
50	19.6538	16.4602	13.6264	11.5787	10.2121	9.1830	8.3643	7.6910	6.6400	5.2344	3.6925
52	22.3850	18.9238	15.8702	13.6387	12.1161	10.9530	10.0179	9.2426	8.0211	6.3668	4.5250
54	25.9403	22.1440	18.7658	16.3481	14.6264	13.2915	12.2065	11.2995	9.8569	7.8778	5.6411
56	30.6948	26.4665	22.7756	20.0061	18.0233	16.4621	15.1791	14.0973	12.3604	9.9460	7.1758
58	37.2420	32.4399	28.2677	25.0886	22.7531	20.8850	19.3325	18.0121	15.8719	12.8576	9.3458
60	46.5717	40.9798	36.1409	32.3918	29.5633	27.2645	25.3325	23.6753	20.9663	17.0938	12.5167

Values of Time Integral for Sucrose Gradient Centrifugation Temperature 5.0 Deg C Particle Density 1.70

WT.PCT. SUCROSE	ZO=5	ZO=0	ZO=-5	ZO=-10	ZO=-15	ZO=-20	ZO=-25	ZO=-30	ZO=-40	ZO=-60	ZO=-100
0	0.0	0.0	0.0	0.0	0.0	0.0	0.0	0.0	0.0	0.0	0.0
2	0.0	0.0	0.5199	0.2820	0.1936	0.1475	0.1191	0.0999	0.0755	0.0508	0.0307
4	0.0	1.1466	0.9360	0.5373	0.3779	0.2917	0.2375	0.2004	0.1527	0.1034	0.0629
6	0.0	1.8677	1.2933	0.7752	0.5562	0.4343	0.3564	0.3022	0.2319	0.1583	0.0968
8	2.1215	2.4203	1.6144	1.0016	0.7312	0.5768	0.4766	0.4062	0.3137	0.2157	0.1328
10	3.1838	2.8850	1.9125	1.2212	0.9050	0.7207	0.5993	0.5132	0.3989	0.2761	0.1711
12	3.9459	3.2984	2.1965	1.4375	1.0796	0.8671	0.7254	0.6239	0.4879	0.3401	0.2120
14	4.5686	3.6806	2.4724	1.6533	1.2569	1.0176	0.8361	0.7394	0.5816	0.4081	0.2559
16	5.1151	4.0445	2.7451	1.8715	1.4387	1.1734	0.9924	0.8606	0.6807	0.4808	0.3033
18	5.6175	4.3988	3.0189	2.0946	1.6269	1.3362	1.1358	0.9887	0.7864	0.5590	0.3548
20	6.0953	4.7507	3.2975	2.3251	1.8236	1.5076	1.2877	1.1251	0.8997	0.6437	0.4110
22	6.5619	5.1062	3.5845	2.5658	2.0309	1.6896	1.4500	1.2715	1.0220	0.7358	0.4727
24	7.0276	5.4705	3.8838	2.8198	2.2514	1.8845	1.6246	1.4296	1.1551	0.8368	0.5408
26	7.5011	5.8493	4.1994	3.0903	2.4881	2.0949	1.8140	1.6018	1.3007	0.9482	0.6166
28	7.9906	6.2481	4.5359	3.3813	2.7445	2.3240	2.0210	1.7907	1.4615	1.0720	0.7014
30	8.5045	6.6735	4.8987	3.6976	3.0249	2.5758	2.2495	1.9998	1.6403	1.2106	0.7970
32	9.0521	7.1327	5.2942	4.0449	3.3344	2.8549	2.5037	2.2332	1.8408	1.3671	0.9057
34	9.6437	7.6347	5.7302	4.4302	3.6795	3.1676	2.7894	2.4962	2.0678	1.5453	1.0303
36	10.2928	8.1911	6.2170	4.8629	4.0690	3.5216	3.1140	2.7958	2.3275	1.7503	1.1746
38	11.0152	8.8159	6.7674	5.3548	4.5136	3.9273	3.4869	3.1409	2.6278	1.9887	1.3434
40	11.8322	9.5282	7.3988	5.9218	5.0281	4.3982	3.9211	3.5436	2.9795	2.2694	1.5434
42	12.7727	10.3540	8.1349	6.5858	5.6329	4.9534	4.4342	4.0206	3.3976	2.6047	1.7836
44	13.8743	11.3276	9.0071	7.3758	6.3548	5.6180	5.0500	4.5943	3.9022	3.0113	2.0765
46	15.1061	12.4937	10.0567	8.3300	7.2295	6.4254	5.7998	5.2941	4.5197	3.5113	2.4386
48	16.7767	13.9152	11.3416	9.5022	8.3072	7.4228	6.7279	6.1620	5.2879	4.1359	2.8933
50	18.7440	15.6819	12.9448	10.9696	9.6600	8.6776	7.8980	7.2580	6.2609	4.9304	3.4745
52	21.2293	17.9237	14.9865	12.8441	11.3926	10.2883	9.4027	8.6699	7.5176	5.9608	4.2321
54	24.4417	20.8333	17.6455	15.2921	13.6608	12.4012	11.3802	10.5284	9.1764	7.3261	5.2405
56	28.7050	24.7093	21.1987	18.5722	16.7067	15.2442	14.0457	13.0371	11.4212	9.1807	6.6166
58	34.5279	30.0219	26.0832	23.0925	20.9133	19.1778	17.7396	16.5188	14.5441	11.7700	8.5465
60	42.7524	37.5500	33.0237	29.5305	26.9166	24.8014	23.0287	21.5110	19.0324	15.5043	11.3418

Values of Time Integral for Sucrose Gradient Centrifugation Temperature 20.0 Deg C Particle Density 1.10

WT.PCT. SUCROSE	Z0= 5	Z0= 0	Z0= -5	Z0= -10	Z0= -15	Z0= -20	Z0= -25	Z0= -30	Z0= -40	Z0= -60	Z0= -100
0	0.0	0.0	0.0	0.0	0.0	0.0	0.0	0.0	0.0	0.0	0.0
2	0.0	0.0	0.3580	0.1943	0.1335	0.1017	0.0821	0.0689	0.0521	0.0350	0.0212
4	0.0	0.8426	0.6646	0.3826	0.2694	0.2080	0.1695	0.1430	0.1090	0.0739	0.0449
6	0.0	1.4150	0.9485	0.5717	0.4112	0.3215	0.2640	0.2241	0.1720	0.1175	0.0720
8	1.8232	1.8930	1.2266	0.7679	0.5628	0.4450	0.3683	0.3142	0.2430	0.1673	0.1031
10	2.8349	2.3368	1.5116	0.9778	0.7290	0.5825	0.4856	0.4165	0.3244	0.2251	0.1397
12	3.6501	2.7797	1.8159	1.2097	0.9163	0.7397	0.6209	0.5353	0.4199	0.2938	0.1836
14	4.4149	3.2497	2.1553	1.4754	1.1345	0.9248	0.7817	0.6774	0.5353	0.3775	0.2378
16	5.2099	3.7796	2.5528	1.7934	1.3996	1.1521	0.9806	0.8542	0.6799	0.4836	0.3070
18	6.1186	4.4212	3.0488	2.1976	1.7407	1.4472	1.2406	1.0866	0.8715	0.6255	0.4004
20	7.2851	5.2813	3.7300	2.7616	2.2219	1.8668	1.6125	1.4206	1.1491	0.8328	0.5380
22	9.1129	6.6757	4.8572	3.7076	3.0369	2.5826	2.2508	1.9964	1.6306	1.1956	0.7810
24	16.5664	12.5413	9.6930	7.8212	5.6161	5.7502	5.0918	4.5719	3.8004	2.8457	1.8967

Values of Time Integral for Sucrose Gradient Centrifugation Temperature 20.0 Deg C Particle Density 1.20

WT.PCT. SUCROSE	ZO= 5	ZO= 0	ZO= -5	ZO= -10	ZO= -15	ZO= -20	ZO= -25	ZO= -30	ZO= -40	ZO= -60	ZO= -100
0	0.0	0.0	0.0	0.0	0.0	0.0	0.0	0.0	0.0	0.0	0.0
2	0.0	0.0	0.3506	0.1902	0.1306	0.0995	0.0804	0.0674	0.0510	0.0343	0.0207
4	0.0	0.7916	0.6381	0.3667	0.2580	0.1992	0.1622	0.1369	0.1043	0.0707	0.0430
6	1.5433	1.3028	0.8915	0.5354	0.3845	0.3004	0.2466	0.2091	0.1605	0.1096	0.0671
8	2.3403	1.7056	1.1257	0.7006	0.5121	0.4043	0.3343	0.2850	0.2202	0.1515	0.0933
10	2.9309	2.0546	1.3496	0.8655	0.6427	0.5124	0.4264	0.3653	0.2842	0.1969	0.1221
12	3.4305	2.3751	1.5698	1.0332	0.7781	0.6260	0.5242	0.4512	0.3532	0.2465	0.1538
14	3.8858	2.6819	1.7912	1.2065	0.9204	0.7467	0.6291	0.5439	0.4284	0.3011	0.1891
16	4.3220	2.9850	2.0185	1.3883	1.0720	0.8766	0.7428	0.6449	0.5111	0.3617	0.2286
18	4.7561	3.2927	2.2563	1.5820	1.2354	1.0180	0.8673	0.7562	0.6028	0.4296	0.2733
20	5.2019	3.6125	2.5094	1.7915	1.4141	1.1737	1.0054	0.8802	0.7058	0.5066	0.3244
22	5.6728	3.9521	2.7837	2.0216	1.6122	1.3477	1.1604	1.0201	0.8228	0.5946	0.3833
24	6.1035	4.3207	3.0864	2.2785	1.8353	1.5449	1.3371	1.1801	0.9573	0.6968	0.4523
26	6.7520	4.7292	3.4269	2.5703	2.0907	1.7719	1.5414	1.3658	1.1145	0.8170	0.5340
28	7.4026	5.1925	3.8178	2.9084	2.3886	2.0381	1.7820	1.5853	1.3013	0.9609	0.6326
30	8.1696	5.7310	4.2771	3.3089	2.7436	2.3569	2.0713	1.8501	1.5277	1.1364	0.7537
32	9.1063	6.3744	4.8312	3.7955	3.1773	2.7481	2.4276	2.1772	1.8088	1.3557	0.9061
34	10.3013	7.1692	5.5216	4.4056	3.7239	3.2432	2.8800	2.5938	2.1683	1.6380	1.1035
36	11.9186	8.1937	6.4182	5.2026	4.4413	3.8954	3.4780	3.1457	2.6467	2.0157	1.3693
38	14.3120	9.5927	7.6508	6.3043	5.4372	4.8040	4.3133	3.9188	3.3195	2.5498	1.7476
40	18.5008	11.6798	9.5011	7.9661	6.9452	6.1844	5.5860	5.0994	4.3508	3.3730	2.3340
42		15.3591	12.7815	10.9255	9.6410	8.6596	7.8741	7.2266	6.2157	4.8690	3.4060
44	32.1487	27.4325	23.6060	20.7354	18.6102	16.9209	15.5310	14.3615	12.4946	9.9328	7.0568

Values of Time Integral for Sucrose Gradient Centrifugation Temperature 20.0 Deg C Particle Density 1.30

WT.PCT. SUCROSE	Z0= 5	Z0= 0	Z0= -5	Z0= -10	Z0= -15	Z0= -20	Z0= -25	Z0= -30	Z0= -40	Z0= -60	Z0= -100
0	0.0	0.0	0.0	0.0	0.0	0.0	0.0	0.0	0.0	0.0	0.0
2	0.0	0.0	0.3477	0.1886	0.1295	0.0987	0.0797	0.0668	0.0505	0.0340	0.0206
4	0.0	0.7748	0.6289	0.3612	0.2541	0.1962	0.1598	0.1348	0.1027	0.0696	0.0423
6	1.4653	1.2676	0.8732	0.5238	0.3760	0.2936	0.2410	0.2044	0.1568	0.1071	0.0655
8	2.2082	1.6496	1.0952	0.6804	0.4970	0.3922	0.3242	0.2763	0.2135	0.1468	0.0904
10	2.7478	1.9746	1.3038	0.8340	0.6186	0.4928	0.4100	0.3511	0.2730	0.1891	0.1172
12	3.1945	2.2674	1.5048	0.9872	0.7423	0.5966	0.4993	0.4296	0.3361	0.2344	0.1461
14	3.5919	2.5416	1.7028	1.1421	0.8695	0.7045	0.5930	0.5124	0.4033	0.2832	0.1777
16	3.9626	2.8062	1.9012	1.3007	1.0017	0.8178	0.6922	0.6006	0.4754	0.3361	0.2122
18	4.3205	3.0677	2.1032	1.4653	1.1406	0.9379	0.7980	0.6951	0.5534	0.3938	0.2501
20	4.6758	3.3313	2.3119	1.6380	1.2879	1.0664	0.9118	0.7973	0.6382	0.4572	0.2922
22	5.0366	3.6019	2.5304	1.8213	1.4457	1.2049	1.0354	0.9087	0.7314	0.5273	0.3392
24	5.4106	3.8843	2.7623	2.0181	1.6166	1.3560	1.1707	1.0313	0.8345	0.6056	0.3920
26	5.8055	4.1835	3.0116	2.2318	1.8036	1.5222	1.3203	1.1673	0.9496	0.6936	0.4519
28	6.2298	4.5052	3.2831	2.4666	2.0105	1.7071	1.4874	1.3197	1.0793	0.7935	0.5203
30	6.6933	4.8564	3.5827	2.7278	2.2420	1.9149	1.6760	1.4924	1.2269	0.9079	0.5993
32	7.2083	5.2452	3.9175	3.0217	2.5040	2.1513	1.8912	1.6900	1.3967	1.0404	0.6913
34	7.7904	5.6822	4.2970	3.3571	2.8044	2.4234	2.1399	1.9189	1.5943	1.1955	0.7998
36	8.4604	6.1811	4.7336	3.7453	3.1538	2.7410	2.4310	2.1877	1.8272	1.3794	0.9292
38	9.2462	6.7606	5.2441	4.2015	3.5661	3.1172	2.7769	2.5077	2.1057	1.6005	1.0858
40	10.1873	7.4457	5.8514	4.7468	4.0610	3.5702	3.1945	2.8951	2.4441	1.8705	1.2781
42	11.3410	8.2721	6.5881	5.4113	4.6662	4.1258	3.7081	3.3725	2.8625	2.2062	1.5185
44	12.7907	9.2918	7.5016	6.2387	5.4223	4.8219	4.3530	3.9733	3.3910	2.6321	1.8253
46	14.6645	10.5805	8.6615	7.2933	6.3891	5.7143	5.1817	4.7468	4.0735	3.1846	2.2255
48	17.1696	12.2551	10.1752	8.6743	7.6588	6.8893	6.2752	5.7693	4.9786	3.9206	2.7613
50	20.6586	14.5048	12.2168	10.5430	9.3816	8.4874	7.7653	7.1652	6.2177	4.9325	3.5016
52	25.7750	17.6521	15.0834	13.1748	11.8142	10.7488	9.8781	9.1476	7.9824	6.3794	4.5654
54	33.8222	22.2864	19.3186	17.0742	15.4272	14.1146	13.0283	12.1082	10.6249	8.5545	6.1721
56	47.8996	29.6031	26.0263	23.2666	21.1777	19.4821	18.0607	16.8449	14.8634	12.0564	8.7708
58	77.9747	42.4478	37.8368	34.1971	31.3502	28.9950	26.9943	25.2656	22.4170	18.3199	13.4396
60		69.9806	63.2236	57.7483	53.3134	49.5707	46.3475	43.5334	38.8424	31.9883	23.6728

Values of Time Integral for Sucrose Gradient Centrifugation Temperature 20.0 Deg C Particle Density 1.40

WT.PCT. SUCROSE	Z0= 5	Z0= 0	Z0= -5	Z0= -10	Z0= -15	Z0= -20	Z0= -25	Z0= -30	Z0= -40	Z0= -60	Z0=-100
0	0.0	0.0	0.0	0.0	0.0	0.0	0.0	0.0	0.0	0.0	0.0
2	0.0	0.0	0.3459	0.1876	0.1289	0.0982	0.0793	0.0665	0.0503	0.0338	0.0204
4	0.0	0.7658	0.6238	0.3582	0.2520	0.1945	0.1584	0.1336	0.1018	0.0690	0.0419
6	1.4276	1.2494	0.8634	0.5177	0.3715	0.2901	0.2381	0.2019	0.1549	0.1058	0.0647
8	2.1451	1.6213	1.0796	0.6701	0.4893	0.3861	0.3190	0.2719	0.2100	0.1444	0.0889
10	2.6618	1.9352	1.2810	0.8185	0.6067	0.4832	0.4019	0.3442	0.2675	0.1853	0.1148
12	3.0855	2.2155	1.4735	0.9651	0.7251	0.5825	0.4874	0.4193	0.3279	0.2286	0.1425
14	3.4586	2.4756	1.6612	1.1120	0.8458	0.6849	0.5763	0.4978	0.3916	0.2749	0.1724
16	3.8029	2.7240	1.8475	1.2610	0.9699	0.7913	0.6694	0.5806	0.4593	0.3245	0.2048
18	4.1314	2.9668	2.0351	1.4138	1.0989	0.9028	0.7677	0.6684	0.5317	0.3781	0.2401
20	4.4534	3.2088	2.2266	1.5723	1.2341	1.0207	0.8721	0.7622	0.6097	0.4363	0.2787
22	4.7759	3.4540	2.4247	1.7384	1.3771	1.1463	0.9841	0.8632	0.6941	0.4999	0.3213
24	5.1052	3.7064	2.6320	1.9143	1.5299	1.2813	1.1050	0.9727	0.7862	0.5698	0.3685
26	5.4471	3.9698	2.8515	2.1024	1.6945	1.4276	1.2367	1.0924	0.8875	0.6473	0.4211
28	5.8079	4.2484	3.0865	2.3058	1.8736	1.5877	1.3814	1.2244	0.9998	0.7338	0.4804
30	6.1941	4.5470	3.3412	2.5278	2.0704	1.7644	1.5412	1.3712	1.1253	0.8311	0.5475
32	6.6135	4.8709	3.6201	2.7727	2.2887	1.9613	1.7211	1.5358	1.2668	0.9415	0.6242
34	7.0758	5.2268	3.9292	3.0459	2.5334	2.1829	1.9236	1.7223	1.4277	1.0678	0.7125
36	7.5929	5.6231	4.2760	3.3541	2.8108	2.4351	2.1548	1.9357	1.6127	1.2138	0.8153
38	8.1800	6.0703	4.6700	3.7062	3.1291	2.7255	2.4217	2.1827	1.8276	1.3845	0.9361
40	8.8574	6.5822	5.1237	4.1136	3.4988	3.0639	2.7337	2.4721	2.0804	1.5862	1.0798
42	9.6525	7.1770	5.6539	4.5919	3.9344	3.4638	3.1033	2.8157	2.3816	1.8277	1.2529
44	10.6017	7.8796	6.2834	5.1620	4.4554	3.9434	3.5477	3.2296	2.7457	2.1212	1.4642
46	11.7562	8.7235	7.0429	5.8525	5.0884	4.5277	4.0903	3.7361	3.1925	2.4830	1.7262
48	13.1889	9.7552	7.9755	6.7033	5.8706	5.2516	4.7639	4.3660	3.7501	2.9363	2.0563
50	15.0069	11.0418	9.1430	7.7719	6.8558	6.1655	5.6161	5.1642	4.4586	3.5149	2.4796
52	17.3706	12.6817	10.6366	9.1432	8.1232	7.3437	6.7168	6.1970	5.3780	4.2687	3.0338
54	20.5284	14.8226	12.5930	10.9445	9.7921	8.8983	8.1719	7.5645	6.5985	5.2733	3.7758
56	24.8789	17.6935	15.2249	13.3740	12.0482	11.0041	10.1461	9.4227	8.2612	6.6469	4.7951
58	31.0874	21.6627	18.8743	16.7513	15.1911	13.9431	12.9060	12.0241	10.5946	8.5816	6.2370
60		27.3456	24.1135	21.6112	19.7229	18.1883	16.8987	15.7926	13.9827	11.4006	8.3471

Values of Time Integral for Sucrose Gradient Centrifugation Temperature 20.0 Deg C Particle Density 1.50

WT.PCT. SUCROSE	Z0= 5	Z0= 0	Z0= -5	Z0= -10	Z0= -15	Z0= -20	Z0= -25	Z0= -30	Z0= -40	Z0= -60	Z0= -100
0	0.0	0.0	0.0	0.0	0.0	0.0	0.0	0.0	0.0	0.0	0.0
2	0.0	0.0	0.3446	0.1869	0.1284	0.0978	0.0790	0.0662	0.0501	0.0337	0.0204
4	0.0	0.7599	0.6203	0.3561	0.2505	0.1933	0.1574	0.1328	0.1012	0.0686	0.0417
6	1.4046	1.2376	0.8570	0.5137	0.3686	0.2878	0.2362	0.2003	0.1537	0.1049	0.0642
8	2.1071	1.6035	1.0696	0.6636	0.4844	0.3822	0.3158	0.2692	0.2079	0.1429	0.0880
10	2.6105	1.9108	1.2668	0.8088	0.5994	0.4773	0.3969	0.3399	0.2642	0.1829	0.1133
12	3.0211	2.1838	1.4543	0.9517	0.7147	0.5740	0.4802	0.4130	0.3230	0.2251	0.1403
14	3.3807	2.4358	1.6362	1.0940	0.8316	0.6732	0.5663	0.4891	0.3847	0.2700	0.1693
16	3.7105	2.6752	1.8157	1.2375	0.9512	0.7757	0.6561	0.5689	0.4500	0.3178	0.2005
18	4.0233	2.9079	1.9954	1.3840	1.0748	0.8826	0.7502	0.6530	0.5193	0.3692	0.2343
20	4.3278	3.1383	2.1778	1.5349	1.2035	0.9948	0.8496	0.7423	0.5935	0.4246	0.2711
22	4.6307	3.3702	2.3651	1.6920	1.3388	1.1136	0.9555	0.8378	0.6733	0.4847	0.3113
24	4.9375	3.6072	2.5598	1.8571	1.4822	1.2403	1.0691	0.9406	0.7599	0.5504	0.3556
26	5.2536	3.8527	2.7643	2.0325	1.6356	1.3767	1.1918	1.0522	0.8543	0.6226	0.4047
28	5.5842	4.1102	2.9816	2.2204	1.8012	1.5247	1.3255	1.1742	0.9581	0.7025	0.4595
30	5.9348	4.3838	3.2150	2.4239	1.9815	1.6866	1.4725	1.3087	1.0731	0.7917	0.5210
32	6.3118	4.6779	3.4682	2.6462	2.1797	1.8653	1.6353	1.4582	1.2015	0.8919	0.5906
34	6.7227	4.9977	3.7460	2.8917	2.3996	2.0645	1.8173	1.6257	1.3461	1.0054	0.6700
36	7.1769	5.3499	4.0542	3.1657	2.6462	2.2887	2.0228	1.8154	1.5105	1.1352	0.7614
38	7.6859	5.7428	4.4002	3.4749	2.9257	2.5437	2.2572	2.0324	1.6993	1.2851	0.8675
40	8.2650	6.1865	4.7936	3.8282	3.2463	2.8371	2.5277	2.2833	1.9184	1.4599	0.9920
42	8.9339	6.6950	5.2468	4.2369	3.6186	3.1789	2.8436	2.5769	2.1759	1.6664	1.1399
44	9.7190	7.2862	5.7765	4.7167	4.0570	3.5825	3.2175	2.9253	2.4822	1.9133	1.3178
46	10.6558	7.9841	6.4046	5.2877	4.5805	4.0658	3.6663	3.3441	2.8518	2.2125	1.5345
48	11.7937	8.8212	7.1613	5.9781	5.2152	4.6531	4.2129	3.8552	3.3042	2.5803	1.8022
50	13.2035	9.8631	8.0886	6.8268	5.9976	5.3789	4.8897	4.4892	3.8670	3.0399	2.1385
52	14.9872	11.1147	9.2468	7.8901	6.9804	6.2925	5.7432	5.2900	4.5798	3.6244	2.5681
54	17.2975	12.7303	10.7232	9.2468	8.2398	7.4657	6.8412	6.3219	5.5008	4.3824	3.1281
56	20.3689	14.8307	12.6486	11.0269	9.8904	9.0063	8.2856	7.6814	6.7172	5.3874	3.8738
58	24.5734	17.6329	15.2250	13.4111	12.1091	11.0810	10.2339	9.5178	8.3644	6.7531	4.8916
60		21.4814	18.7730	16.7022	15.1781	13.9559	12.9377	12.0698	10.6588	8.6620	6.3205

Values of Time Integral for Sucrose Gradient Centrifugation Temperature 20.0 Deg C Particle Density 1.60

WT.PCT. SUCROSE	Z0= 5	Z0= 0	Z0= -5	Z0= -10	Z0= -15	Z0= -20	Z0= -25	Z0= -30	Z0= -40	Z0= -60	Z0= -100
0	0.0	0.0	0.0	0.0	0.0	0.0	0.0	0.0	0.0	0.0	0.0
2	0.0	0.0	0.3435	0.1863	0.1279	0.0974	0.0787	0.0660	0.0499	0.0336	0.0203
4	0.0	0.7555	0.6176	0.3545	0.2493	0.1924	0.1567	0.1322	0.1007	0.0682	0.0415
6	1.3888	1.2291	0.8522	0.5107	0.3664	0.2861	0.2348	0.1991	0.1527	0.1043	0.0638
8	2.0811	1.5907	1.0624	0.6589	0.4809	0.3794	0.3135	0.2672	0.2063	0.1418	0.0873
10	2.5756	1.8936	1.2567	0.8020	0.5942	0.4731	0.3934	0.3368	0.2618	0.1812	0.1123
12	2.9776	2.1618	1.4409	0.9423	0.7075	0.5681	0.4752	0.4087	0.3195	0.2227	0.1388
14	3.3284	2.4085	1.6190	1.0816	0.8219	0.6652	0.5595	0.4832	0.3800	0.2666	0.1672
16	3.6490	2.6421	1.7940	1.2217	0.9386	0.7652	0.6471	0.5610	0.4437	0.3133	0.1976
18	3.9518	2.8682	1.9687	1.3640	1.0587	0.8691	0.7386	0.6428	0.5111	0.3632	0.2305
20	4.2455	3.0913	2.1453	1.5101	1.1833	0.9777	0.8349	0.7292	0.5829	0.4168	0.2661
22	4.5363	3.3149	2.3259	1.6616	1.3138	1.0923	0.9369	0.8213	0.6599	0.4748	0.3049
24	4.8296	3.5425	2.5128	1.8202	1.4515	1.2140	1.0460	0.9201	0.7429	0.5379	0.3474
26	5.1303	3.7771	2.7083	1.9878	1.5981	1.3443	1.1633	1.0267	0.8332	0.6069	0.3944
28	5.4431	4.0221	2.9150	2.1665	1.7556	1.4851	1.2905	1.1427	0.9319	0.6829	0.4464
30	5.7731	4.2810	3.1359	2.3591	1.9263	1.6383	1.4295	1.2700	1.0407	0.7673	0.5047
32	6.1259	4.5577	3.3742	2.5683	2.1128	1.8065	1.5828	1.4107	1.1616	0.8616	0.5702
34	6.5081	4.8571	3.6342	2.7981	2.3186	1.9929	1.7531	1.5675	1.2969	0.9678	0.6445
36	6.9278	5.1847	3.9208	3.0529	2.5480	2.2014	1.9442	1.7439	1.4499	1.0886	0.7294
38	7.3948	5.5477	4.2406	3.3387	2.8063	2.4371	2.1609	1.9444	1.6243	1.2270	0.8275
40	7.9222	5.9549	4.6016	3.6628	3.1004	2.7063	2.4091	2.1746	1.8254	1.3875	0.9418
42	8.5265	6.4179	5.0143	4.0351	3.4394	3.0176	2.6968	2.4421	2.0598	1.5755	1.0765
44	9.2297	6.9520	5.4928	4.4684	3.8355	3.3822	3.0346	2.7567	2.3366	1.7986	1.2371
46	10.0608	7.5771	6.0554	4.9799	4.3043	3.8150	3.4365	3.1319	2.6676	2.0665	1.4312
48	11.0603	8.3199	6.7268	5.5924	4.8675	4.3361	3.9214	3.5853	3.0690	2.3929	1.6688
50	12.2849	9.2174	7.5412	6.3379	5.5547	4.9736	4.5158	4.1422	3.5632	2.7965	1.9641
52	13.8160	10.3220	8.5473	7.2616	6.4084	5.7672	5.2573	4.8378	4.1825	3.3042	2.3373
54	15.7730	11.7087	9.8145	8.4282	7.4494	6.7742	6.1997	5.7235	4.9730	3.9549	2.8179
56	18.3374	13.4880	11.4456	9.9339	8.8876	8.0792	7.4232	6.8751	6.0034	4.8061	3.4496
58	21.7925	15.8276	13.5967	11.9246	10.7401	9.8115	9.0499	8.4084	7.3787	5.9464	4.2994
60		18.9901	16.5122	14.6291	13.2619	12.1738	11.2717	10.5054	9.2640	7.5151	5.4735

Values of Time Integral for Sucrose Gradient Centrifugation Temperature 20.0 Deg C Particle Density 1.70

WT.PCT. SUCROSE	ZO= 5	ZO= 0	ZO= -5	ZO= -10	ZO= -15	ZO= -20	ZO= -25	ZO= -30	ZO= -40	ZO= -60	ZO= -100
0	0.0	0.0	0.0	0.0	0.0	0.0	0.0	0.0	0.0	0.0	0.0
2	0.0	0.0	0.3425	0.1857	0.1276	0.0972	0.0785	0.0658	0.0498	0.0335	0.0202
4	0.0	0.7519	0.6153	0.3532	0.2484	0.1917	0.1561	0.1317	0.1003	0.0680	0.0413
6		1.2224	0.8484	0.5083	0.3647	0.2847	0.2336	0.1981	0.1520	0.1037	0.0635
8	1.3768	1.5808	1.0566	0.6552	0.4782	0.3772	0.3116	0.2656	0.2051	0.1410	0.0868
10	2.0616	1.8804	1.2488	0.7967	0.5902	0.4699	0.3907	0.3345	0.2600	0.1800	0.1115
12	2.5497	2.1451	1.4306	0.9352	0.7020	0.5636	0.4714	0.4054	0.3170	0.2209	0.1377
14	2.9455	2.3880	1.6060	1.0724	0.8147	0.6593	0.5545	0.4788	0.3765	0.2641	0.1656
16	3.2901	2.6174	1.7779	1.2099	0.9293	0.7575	0.6404	0.5552	0.4390	0.3100	0.1955
18	3.6042	2.8390	1.9491	1.3494	1.0470	0.8593	0.7301	0.6353	0.5051	0.3589	0.2277
20	3.9001	3.0569	2.1216	1.4922	1.1687	0.9654	0.8242	0.7198	0.5752	0.4113	0.2625
22	4.1863	3.2749	2.2976	1.6398	1.2959	1.0770	0.9237	0.8095	0.6503	0.4678	0.3003
24	4.4688	3.4960	2.4792	1.7939	1.4297	1.1953	1.0296	0.9055	0.7310	0.5290	0.3416
26	4.7530	3.7233	2.6686	1.9562	1.5717	1.3215	1.1432	1.0088	0.8184	0.5959	0.3871
28	5.0433	3.9598	2.8682	2.1288	1.7238	1.4574	1.2661	1.1208	0.9137	0.6693	0.4374
30	5.3444	4.2090	3.0808	2.3141	1.8880	1.6049	1.3999	1.2433	1.0185	0.7505	0.4934
32	5.6609	4.4744	3.3093	2.5148	2.0669	1.7663	1.5468	1.3782	1.1344	0.8409	0.5562
34	5.9979	4.7604	3.5577	2.7343	2.2635	1.9443	1.7096	1.5280	1.2637	0.9425	0.6272
36	6.3617	5.0722	3.8305	2.9768	2.4818	2.1428	1.8915	1.6960	1.4092	1.0573	0.7081
38	6.7594	5.4162	4.1336	3.2477	2.7266	2.3661	2.0968	1.8860	1.5745	1.1886	0.8010
40	7.2002	5.8005	4.4742	3.5535	3.0042	2.6202	2.3310	2.1032	1.7643	1.3400	0.9089
42	7.6955	6.2354	4.8619	3.9032	3.3226	2.9125	2.6012	2.3544	1.9845	1.5166	1.0354
44	8.2604	6.7346	5.3091	4.3083	3.6928	3.2533	2.9169	2.6485	2.2432	1.7251	1.1855
46	8.9142	7.3158	5.8322	4.7838	4.1287	3.6557	3.2906	2.9973	2.5509	1.9742	1.3660
48	9.6827	8.0026	6.4530	5.3502	4.6494	4.1376	3.7390	3.4166	2.9220	2.2760	1.5857
50	10.6014	8.8276	7.2016	6.0354	5.2812	4.7236	4.2854	3.9284	3.3764	2.6470	1.8571
52	11.7200	9.8366	8.1206	6.8791	6.0609	5.4484	4.9627	4.5639	3.9420	3.1108	2.1980
54	13.1089	11.0946	9.2702	7.9375	7.0416	6.3620	5.8176	5.3674	4.6591	3.7010	2.6340
56	14.8715	12.6971	10.7392	9.2936	8.3008	7.5373	6.9196	6.4045	5.5872	4.4677	3.2029
58	17.1632	14.7879	12.6615	11.0725	9.9563	9.0853	8.3733	7.7747	6.8161	5.4867	3.9623
60	20.2248	17.5902	15.2450	13.4689	12.1909	11.1786	10.3420	9.6329	8.4868	6.8766	5.0027

Values of Time Integral for Sucrose Gradient Centrifugation Temperature 20.0 Deg C Particle Density 1.80

WT.PCT. SUCROSE	Z0=5	Z0=0	Z0=-5	Z0=-10	Z0=-15	Z0=-20	Z0=-25	Z0=-30	Z0=-40	Z0=-60	Z0=-100
0	0.0	0.0	0.0	0.0	0.0	0.0	0.0	0.0	0.0	0.0	0.0
2	0.0	0.0	0.3416	0.1852	0.1272	0.0969	0.0783	0.0656	0.0496	0.0334	0.0202
4	0.0	0.7489	0.6133	0.3520	0.2475	0.1910	0.1556	0.1312	0.1000	0.0677	0.0412
6	1.3673	1.2168	0.8450	0.5063	0.3632	0.2836	0.2327	0.1973	0.1514	0.1033	0.0632
8	2.0462	1.5727	1.0518	0.6521	0.4759	0.3753	0.3101	0.2643	0.2041	0.1403	0.0864
10	2.5292	1.8696	1.2424	0.7924	0.5869	0.4673	0.3885	0.3326	0.2585	0.1789	0.1108
12	2.9203	2.1316	1.4223	0.9295	0.6976	0.5601	0.4684	0.4028	0.3149	0.2194	0.1368
14	3.2602	2.3717	1.5955	1.0650	0.8089	0.6545	0.5505	0.4753	0.3737	0.2621	0.1643
16	3.5694	2.5979	1.7652	1.2007	0.9220	0.7514	0.6352	0.5507	0.4354	0.3074	0.1938
18	3.8603	2.8160	1.9337	1.3380	1.0378	0.8516	0.7235	0.6295	0.5004	0.3555	0.2255
20	4.1409	3.0302	2.1032	1.4783	1.1575	0.9559	0.8160	0.7125	0.5694	0.4070	0.2597
22	4.4174	3.2439	2.2758	1.6230	1.2821	1.0654	0.9135	0.8005	0.6429	0.4624	0.2968
24	4.6940	3.4603	2.4535	1.7738	1.4131	1.1811	1.0172	0.8944	0.7219	0.5224	0.3373
26	4.9777	3.6822	2.6385	1.9323	1.5518	1.3044	1.1281	0.9953	0.8073	0.5876	0.3816
28	5.2704	3.9127	2.8329	2.1005	1.6999	1.4368	1.2478	1.1045	0.9002	0.6592	0.4306
30	5.5772	4.1549	3.0395	2.2806	1.8596	1.5801	1.3779	1.2231	1.0020	0.7381	0.4851
32	5.9032	4.4123	3.2611	2.4752	2.0330	1.7366	1.5203	1.3543	1.1143	0.8258	0.5460
34	6.2540	4.6888	3.5013	2.6874	2.2237	1.9088	1.6777	1.4992	1.2394	0.9239	0.6147
36	6.6365	4.9895	3.7644	2.9213	2.4337	2.1002	1.8532	1.6611	1.3797	1.0347	0.6926
38	7.0591	5.3204	4.0559	3.1818	2.6691	2.3149	2.0506	1.8439	1.5387	1.1610	0.7820
40	7.5325	5.6888	4.3825	3.4751	2.9352	2.5585	2.2752	2.0522	1.7206	1.3062	0.8854
42	8.0706	6.1045	4.7530	3.8093	3.2396	2.8380	2.5335	2.2923	1.9311	1.4750	1.0063
44	8.6913	6.5801	5.1790	4.1952	3.5922	3.1626	2.8342	2.5724	2.1775	1.6735	1.1494
46	9.4182	7.1318	5.6756	4.6466	4.0061	3.5446	3.1890	2.9035	2.4697	1.9101	1.3207
48	10.2838	7.7811	6.2628	5.1823	4.4986	4.0004	3.6131	3.3001	2.8207	2.1955	1.5285
50	11.3333	8.5587	6.9681	5.8279	5.0938	4.5525	4.1279	3.7823	3.2488	2.5450	1.7842
52	12.6309	9.5054	7.8304	6.6195	5.8254	5.2326	4.7633	4.3786	3.7795	2.9802	2.1041
54	14.1700	10.6807	8.9044	7.6083	6.7415	6.0860	5.5620	5.1292	4.4495	3.5316	2.5114
56	16.3907	12.1709	10.2704	8.8693	7.9126	7.1790	6.5868	6.0937	5.3124	4.2445	3.0404
58	19.2090	14.1056	12.0493	10.5155	9.4445	8.6115	7.9319	7.3616	6.4497	5.1875	3.7431
60		16.6853	14.4276	12.7216	11.5016	10.5385	9.7443	9.0722	7.9876	6.4670	4.7009

388

Values of Time Integral for Sucrose Gradient Centrifugation Temperature 20.0 Deg C Particle Density 1.90

WT.PCT. SUCROSE	ZO= 5	ZO= 0	ZO= -5	ZO= -10	ZO= -15	ZO= -20	ZO= -25	ZO= -30	ZO= -40	ZO= -60	ZO= -100
0	0.0	0.0	0.0	0.0	0.0	0.0	0.0	0.0	0.0	0.0	0.0
2	0.0	0.0	0.3407	0.1848	0.1269	0.0967	0.0781	0.0655	0.0495	0.0333	0.0201
4	0.0	0.7462	0.6114	0.3509	0.2468	0.1905	0.1551	0.1308	0.0997	0.0675	0.0411
6	0.0	1.2119	0.8421	0.5044	0.3619	0.2825	0.2318	0.1966	0.1508	0.1029	0.0630
8	1.3593	1.5657	1.0477	0.6494	0.4739	0.3738	0.3088	0.2632	0.2032	0.1397	0.0860
10	2.0334	1.8605	1.2369	0.7888	0.5842	0.4650	0.3866	0.3310	0.2572	0.1781	0.1103
12	2.5124	2.1203	1.4153	0.9246	0.6939	0.5571	0.4659	0.4006	0.3132	0.2182	0.1360
14	2.8997	2.3580	1.5868	1.0589	0.8042	0.6506	0.5471	0.4724	0.3714	0.2605	0.1633
16	3.2359	2.5818	1.7546	1.1931	0.9160	0.7464	0.6310	0.5469	0.4324	0.3052	0.1925
18	3.5413	2.7972	1.9210	1.3286	1.0304	0.8454	0.7181	0.6248	0.4966	0.3528	0.2238
20	3.8281	3.0084	2.0882	1.4670	1.1484	0.9482	0.8093	0.7067	0.5646	0.4036	0.2575
22	4.1044	3.2189	2.2581	1.6095	1.2711	1.0560	0.9054	0.7933	0.6371	0.4581	0.2940
24	4.3762	3.4316	2.4329	1.7578	1.3999	1.1698	1.0073	0.8856	0.7147	0.5171	0.3338
26	4.6486	3.6494	2.6144	1.9134	1.5360	1.2908	1.1162	0.9847	0.7985	0.5811	0.3774
28	4.9257	3.8753	2.8049	2.0782	1.6812	1.4205	1.2335	1.0916	0.8895	0.6517	0.4254
30	5.2120	4.1122	3.0070	2.2543	1.8373	1.5607	1.3607	1.2081	0.9891	0.7284	0.4786
32	5.5116	4.3634	3.2234	2.4443	2.0066	1.7135	1.4998	1.3358	1.0988	0.8140	0.5381
34	5.8292	4.6329	3.4514	2.6511	2.1919	1.8813	1.6532	1.4770	1.2206	0.9097	0.6050
36	6.1704	4.9254	3.7133	2.8786	2.3967	2.0674	1.8238	1.6345	1.3571	1.0175	0.6809
38	6.5416	5.2465	3.9962	3.1314	2.6252	2.2759	2.0154	1.8118	1.5115	1.1400	0.7676
40	6.9509	5.6033	4.3125	3.4154	2.8829	2.5117	2.2329	2.0135	1.6876	1.2806	0.8677
42	7.4083	6.0049	4.6705	3.7383	3.1770	2.7818	2.4824	2.2455	1.8910	1.4436	0.9845
44	7.9270	6.4633	5.0811	4.1103	3.5168	3.0947	2.7723	2.5155	2.1285	1.6351	1.1224
46	8.5238	6.9938	5.5586	4.5443	3.9148	3.4620	3.1134	2.8339	2.4094	1.8625	1.2871
48	9.2209	7.6168	6.1217	5.0580	4.3871	3.8990	3.5201	3.2142	2.7461	2.1362	1.4864
50	10.0487	8.3601	6.7962	5.6755	4.9563	4.4270	4.0125	3.6754	3.1554	2.4705	1.7309
52	11.0495	9.2629	7.6105	6.4303	5.6540	5.0756	4.6184	4.2440	3.6615	2.8854	2.0360
54	12.2832	10.3803	8.6396	7.3704	6.5250	5.8870	5.3778	4.9576	4.2985	3.4097	2.4232
56	13.8365	11.7925	9.9342	8.5655	7.6347	6.9228	6.3489	5.8716	5.1163	4.0853	2.9246
58	15.8395	13.6199	11.6143	10.1203	9.0816	8.2758	7.6194	7.0692	6.1905	4.9759	3.5883
60	18.4921	16.0478	13.5527	12.1966	11.0177	10.0894	9.3252	8.6791	7.6379	6.1802	4.4897

Appendix D

Gradient Shapes

NOTE ON EXPONENTIAL APPROXIMATION

Although gradients are ideally generated through fully programmable devices, the cost and availability of these instruments usually force us to accept approximations. The exponential generators, as a class, are inexpensive and function effectively for both swinging bucket and zonal rotors.

Although one may construct exponential approximations of specific gradient shapes by hand (cf. Noll, 1967), it is no more difficult and usually more precise to employ computer programs.

In the tables which follow, the parameters of the exponential approximations are indicated by three quantities corresponding to Eq. (5.4) and Fig. 5.6: (a) c_s is the concentration of the starting solution; this solution should fully occupy the mixing chamber, with no air space; (b) c_L is the concentration of the limiting solution; this solution is placed in the reservoir; (c) v_M is the volume of the mixing chamber.

D1. PARAMETERS FOR ISOKINETIC GRADIENTS OF SUCROSE FOR TWO IEC ROTORS[a]

Particle density (gm/cm³)	Rotor temperature (°C)	Rotor IEC SB-405 4.0 ml gradient volume 5.43–9.61 cm radius Concentration % w/v				Rotor IEC SB-283 12.0 ml gradient volume 6.74–14.3 cm radius Concentration % w/v			
		Top = c_s	Bottom	v_M (cm³)	c_L (% w/v)	Top = c_s	Bottom	v_M (cm³)	c_L (% w/v)
1.3	2	0	12.3	4.30	20.4	0	15.6	11.2	22.5
1.3	2	5	16.1	4.85	24.8	5	19.4	12.5	28.4
1.3	2	10	20.5	6.54	32.9	10	23.5	13.3	32.8
1.3	2	15	24.9	5.36	33.9	15	27.7	11.9	35.0
1.3	2	20	29.2	5.42	37.5	20	31.8	12.7	39.4
1.3	2	25	33.4	5.22	40.7	25	35.9	12.9	43.1
1.3	6	0	12.5	5.73	24.8	0	15.8	11.2	23.9
1.3	6	5	16.6	4.41	24.5	5	19.9	11.4	27.9
1.3	6	10	20.7	6.03	32.1	10	23.8	13.1	32.9
1.3	6	15	25.1	5.69	35.1	15	27.9	12.3	35.8
1.3	6	20	29.4	5.22	37.5	20	32.0	12.0	39.0
1.3	6	25	33.5	5.10	40.7	25	36.1	12.8	43.3
1.4	2	0	13.3	4.19	21.6	0	16.8	11.2	24.3
1.4	2	5	17.1	4.98	26.9	5	20.7	12.8	30.8
1.4	2	10	21.4	6.54	35.0	10	24.7	13.2	34.7
1.4	2	15	25.9	5.27	35.5	15	28.9	11.9	36.9
1.4	2	20	30.1	5.50	39.6	20	33.0	12.6	41.2
1.4	2	25	34.4	5.26	42.6	25	37.2	13.1	45.3
1.4	6	0	13.4	5.38	25.6	0	17.0	10.9	25.6
1.4	6	5	17.6	4.52	26.5	5	21.2	11.6	30.2

Continued

Particle density (gm/cm³)	Rotor temperature (°C)	Rotor IEC SB-405 4.0 ml gradient volume 5.43–9.61 cm radius Concentration % w/v				Rotor IEC SB-283 12.0 ml gradient volume 6.74–14.3 cm radius Concentration % w/v			
		Top = c_s	Bottom	v_M (cm³)	c_L (% w/v)	Top = c_s	Bottom	v_M (cm³)	c_L (% w/v)
1.4	6	10	21.7	5.92	34.0	10	25.1	13.1	35.1
1.4	6	15	26.1	5.61	36.8	15	29.2	12.1	37.7
1.4	6	20	30.4	5.20	39.3	20	33.2	11.8	40.7
1.4	6	25	34.5	5.22	42.7	25	37.4	13.0	45.5
1.5	2	0	13.9	4.12	22.3	0	17.7	10.3	25.6
1.5	2	5	17.7	5.08	28.3	5	21.5	12.9	32.3
1.5	2	10	22.0	6.43	36.0	10	25.5	12.9	35.7
1.5	2	15	26.5	5.19	36.3	15	29.7	11.9	38.2
1.5	2	20	30.7	5.49	40.7	20	33.7	12.4	42.0
1.5	2	25	35.0	5.40	44.0	25	37.9	12.9	46.2
1.5	6	0	14.1	5.15	26.1	0	17.9	11.9	26.8
1.5	6	5	18.3	4.57	27.8	5	22.1	11.7	31.6
1.5	6	10	22.3	5.93	35.1	10	25.9	12.9	36.3
1.5	6	15	26.7	5.53	37.7	15	30.0	11.9	38.7
1.5	6	20	30.9	5.14	40.2	20	33.9	11.6	41.6
1.5	6	25	35.1	5.35	44.2	25	38.1	12.9	46.6
1.6	2	0	14.3	4.06	22.9	0	18.2	10.4	26.6
1.6	2	5	18.2	5.14	29.3	5	22.0	12.9	33.2
1.6	2	10	22.5	6.35	36.7	10	25.9	12.8	36.3
1.6	2	15	26.8	5.12	36.8	15	30.2	11.9	38.9

1.6	2	20	31.1	5.46	41.3	20	34.1	12.2	42.6
1.6	2	25	35.3	5.44	44.8	25	38.3	12.7	46.8
1.6	6	0	14.5	4.99	26.3	0	18.5	10.9	27.7
1.6	6	5	18.7	4.59	28.6	5	22.6	11.7	32.6
1.6	6	10	22.8	5.91	35.9	10	26.4	12.8	37.0
1.6	6	15	27.1	5.43	38.3	15	30.5	11.8	39.3
1.6	6	20	31.3	5.09	40.7	20	34.4	11.5	42.2
1.6	6	25	35.5	5.40	45.0	25	38.5	12.9	47.3
1.7	2	0	14.7	4.02	23.2	0	18.7	10.4	27.3
1.7	2	5	18.5	5.17	30.0	5	22.4	12.9	33.9
1.7	2	10	22.8	6.28	37.1	10	26.4	12.7	36.7
1.7	2	15	27.1	5.06	37.2	15	30.5	11.8	39.4
1.7	2	20	31.3	5.43	41.7	20	34.5	12.0	42.9
1.7	2	25	35.6	5.45	45.3	25	38.6	12.6	47.1
1.7	6	0	14.9	4.88	26.5	0	18.9	10.9	28.3
1.7	6	5	19.1	4.61	29.3	5	23.1	11.8	33.3
1.7	6	10	23.1	5.89	36.5	10	26.8	12.7	37.5
1.7	6	15	27.4	5.35	38.6	15	30.9	11.7	39.7
1.7	6	20	31.6	5.05	41.1	20	34.7	11.5	42.8
1.7	6	25	35.7	5.41	45.5	25	38.8	12.8	47.7
1.8	2	0	14.9	3.98	23.5	0	19.0	10.4	27.8
1.8	2	5	18.7	5.19	30.6	5	22.7	12.9	34.4
1.8	2	10	23.0	6.23	37.4	10	26.6	12.6	37.0
1.8	2	15	27.3	5.01	37.4	15	30.8	11.8	39.7
1.8	2	20	31.5	5.40	42.0	20	34.7	12.0	43.3
1.8	2	25	35.8	5.44	45.7	25	38.8	12.5	47.3
1.8	6	0	15.1	4.79	26.7	0	19.3	10.9	28.8
1.8	6	5	19.3	4.61	29.7	5	23.4	11.8	33.8
1.8	6	10	23.3	5.86	36.9	10	27.1	12.6	37.8
1.8	6	15	27.6	5.29	38.8	15	31.1	11.6	40.0
1.8	6	20	31.7	5.01	41.4	20	34.9	11.5	43.2
1.8	6	25	35.9	5.42	45.9	25	39.0	12.7	47.9

Noll, H. (1969). Polysomes: Analysis of structure and function. *In* "Techniques in Protein Biosyntheses" (P. N. Campbell and J. R. Sargent, eds.), pp. 101–179. Academic Press, New York.

D2. PARAMETERS FOR ISOKINETIC GRADIENTS IN SUCROSE FOR FOUR SPINCO ROTORS*

Particle density (gm/cm³)	Rotor temperature (°C)	c_s = top (% w/v)	Rotor SW 39 or 50L Delivery vol. 5.0 ml 5.61–9.80 cm		Rotor SW 25.1 Delivery vol. 30 ml 6.49–12.90 cm		Rotor SW 25.2 Delivery vol. 58 ml 7.50–15.3 cm		Rotor SW 25.3 Delivery vol. 16.5 ml 7.55–16.19 cm	
			v_M (cm³)	c_L (% w/v)	v_M (cm³)	c_L (% w/v)	v_M (cm³)	c_L (% w/v)	v_M (cm³)	c_L (% w/v)
1.33	5	5	6.07	23.7	30.2	24.8	56.5	25.0	14.5	25.5
1.33	5	10	6.30	27.1	31.4	28.1	58.5	28.2	14.9	28.6
1.33	5	15	6.50	30.4	32.2	31.2	60.2	31.5	15.3	31.8
1.33	20	5	6.00	24.8	29.7	26.0	55.5	26.2	14.2	26.6
1.33	20	10	6.17	28.0	30.7	29.1	56.6	30.4	14.6	29.7
1.33	20	15	6.37	31.4	31.6	32.3	59.1	32.5	15.1	32.9
1.41	5	5	6.00	24.6	29.9	25.8	55.9	26.0	14.3	26.5
1.41	5	10	6.23	28.0	31.0	29.0	57.9	29.2	14.8	29.6
1.41	5	15	6.47	31.4	31.9	32.3	59.6	32.5	15.2	32.8
1.41	20	5	5.90	25.8	29.4	27.0	54.9	27.3	14.0	27.8
1.41	20	10	6.10	29.0	30.3	30.1	55.9	31.2	14.5	30.8
1.41	20	15	6.30	32.4	31.4	33.3	58.6	33.6	15.0	34.0
1.51	5	5	5.93	25.4	28.1	25.7	55.2	26.8	14.1	27.3
1.51	5	10	6.17	28.7	30.6	29.8	57.2	30.0	14.6	30.4
1.51	5	15	6.37	32.0	31.6	33.0	59.0	33.2	15.1	33.6
1.51	20	5	5.80	26.6	28.9	27.9	54.1	28.2	13.8	28.7
1.51	20	10	6.00	29.8	29.9	31.0	54.6	32.3	14.3	31.7
1.51	20	15	6.23	33.1	31.0	34.2	57.9	34.4	14.8	34.8

1.77	5	5	5.77	26.3	28.9	27.7	53.8	27.9	13.8	28.4
1.77	10	5	6.03	29.6	29.9	30.8	55.9	31.0	14.3	31.4
1.77	15	5	6.23	32.9	30.9	33.9	57.7	34.1	14.8	34.5
1.77	5	20	5.67	27.7	28.2	29.0	52.7	29.3	13.5	29.8
1.77	10	20	5.87	30.8	29.2	32.1	54.4	32.4	14.0	32.8
1.77	15	20	6.10	33.1	30.3	35.0	56.7	35.4	14.5	35.9
1.81	5	5	5.77	26.4	28.7	27.7	53.7	28.0	13.7	28.5
1.81	10	5	6.00	29.7	29.9	30.9	55.8	31.1	14.3	31.5
1.81	15	5	6.23	33.0	30.8	34.0	57.6	34.2	14.7	34.6
1.81	5	20	5.63	27.8	28.1	29.1	52.5	29.4	13.5	30.0
1.81	10	20	5.83	30.9	29.1	32.2	52.2	29.6	13.9	32.0
1.81	15	20	6.07	34.2	30.2	35.3	56.5	35.5	14.5	36.0
1.89	5	5	5.73	26.6	28.6	27.9	53.4	28.2	13.7	28.7
1.89	10	5	5.97	29.8	29.7	31.0	55.5	31.2	14.2	31.7
1.89	15	5	6.20	33.1	30.7	34.1	57.3	34.4	14.6	34.8
1.89	5	20	5.60	28.0	27.9	29.3	54.2	32.6	13.4	30.1
1.89	10	20	5.83	31.1	28.9	32.3	54.2	32.6	13.9	33.1
1.89	15	20	6.07	34.3	30.1	35.5	56.3	35.7	14.4	36.1

* McCarty, D. S., Stafford, D., and Brown, O. (1968). Resolution and fractionation of macromolecules by isokinetic sucrose density gradient sedimentation. *Anal. Biochem.* **24**, 314–329.

D3. EQUIVOLUMETRIC GRADIENTS OF SUCROSE FOR OAK RIDGE B-XIV ROTORS[a,b]

Volume (cm³)	Volumetric mixing fraction			
	$\rho_p = 1.10$ (gm/cm³)	$\rho_p = 1.15$ (gm/cm³)	$\rho_p = 1.20$ (gm/cm³)	$\rho_p = 1.40$ (gm/cm³)
0	0.0	0.0	0.0	0.0
25	0.191	0.177	0.170	0.167
50	0.325	0.303	0.291	0.286
75	0.426	0.398	0.385	0.377
100	0.506	0.475	0.460	0.451
125	0.570	0.538	0.522	0.512
150	0.623	0.591	0.575	0.565
175	0.669	0.637	0.621	0.610
200	0.708	0.677	0.661	0.651
225	0.742	0.713	0.697	0.686
250	0.772	0.744	0.729	0.719
275	0.799	0.772	0.758	0.748
300	0.823	0.798	0.784	0.775
325	0.844	0.821	0.809	0.800
350	0.864	0.843	0.831	0.823
375	0.881	0.863	0.852	0.844
400	0.898	0.881	0.871	0.864
425	0.913	0.898	0.889	0.883
450	0.926	0.913	0.906	0.901
475	0.939	0.928	0.922	0.917
500	0.951	0.942	0.936	0.933
525	0.962	0.955	0.951	0.948
550	0.973	0.967	0.964	0.962
575	0.982	0.979	0.976	0.975
600	0.991	0.900	0.988	0.988
625	1.000	1.000	1.000	1.000
c_f (% w/w)	19.8	26.1	30.4	37.3
v_M (cm³)	150	163	176	184
c_s (% w/w)	5	5	5	5
c_L (% w/w)	19.4	25.6	30.1	37.3

[a] From Eikenberry, E. F. (1973). Generation of density gradients. Approximation to equivolumetric gradients from zonal rotors. *Anal. Biochem.* **55**, 338–357.

[b] Normalized equivolumetric gradients of sucrose at 4°C are expressed as the fractional volumetric mixing ratio. The numbers in the body of the table represent the fraction between the initial and the final concentration and would correspond to the height of a template on a mechanically programmed generator (cf. Section 5.3). The values of c_f are the actual concentrations of sucrose in % w/w of the final solutions. The concentration of the initial solution is uniformly 5% w/w. Other values of c_i and c_f are easily obtained from the same template (cf. Eikenberry, 1973). v_M, c_s, and c_L are the constants for the exponential approximations to each of these gradients.

The sample should be pumped sufficiently far into the rotor (≥ 33 cm³ of overlay) to clear the pyramidal ramp of the core (cf. Appendix E).

See Fig. D.1 for a comparison of normalized equivolumetric gradients.

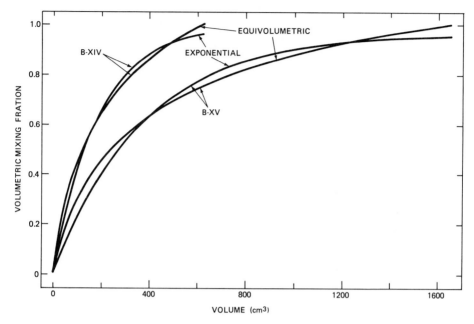

Fig. D.1. Comparison of normalized equivolumetric gradients of sucrose for the B-XIV and XV rotors with the best-fit exponential approximations (Eikenberry, 1973).

D4. EQUIVOLUMETRIC GRADIENTS OF SUCROSE FOR OAK RIDGE B-XV ROTORS[a,b]

Volume (cm³)	Volumetric mixing fraction			
	$\rho_p = 1.10$ (gm/cm³)	$\rho_p = 1.15$ (gm/cm³)	$\rho_p = 1.20$ (gm/cm³)	$\rho_p = 1.40$ (gm/cm³)
0	0.0	0.0	0.0	0.0
50	0.220	0.198	0.188	0.182
100	0.360	0.328	0.311	0.301
150	0.460	0.422	0.402	0.389
200	0.536	0.495	0.472	0.458
250	0.596	0.553	0.530	0.514
300	0.645	0.602	0.578	0.562
350	0.685	0.643	0.618	0.602
400	0.719	0.678	0.654	0.638
450	0.749	0.709	0.685	0.669
500	0.774	0.736	0.713	0.697

Continued

D4.   Continued

Volume (cm³)	Volumetric mixing fraction			
	$\rho_p = 1.10$ (gm/cm³)	$\rho_p = 1.15$ (gm/cm³)	$\rho_p = 1.20$ (gm/cm³)	$\rho_p = 1.40$ (gm/cm³)
550	0.797	0.760	0.738	0.723
600	0.817	0.782	0.761	0.746
650	0.835	0.802	0.782	0.767
700	0.851	0.820	0.800	0.787
750	0.866	0.837	0.818	0.805
800	0.879	0.852	0.834	0.822
850	0.891	0.866	0.849	0.837
900	0.902	0.879	0.863	0.852
950	0.912	0.891	0.877	0.866
1000	0.922	0.902	0.889	0.879
1050	0.931	0.913	0.901	0.892
1100	0.939	0.923	0.912	0.903
1150	0.946	0.932	0.922	0.915
1200	0.953	0.941	0.932	0.925
1250	0.960	0.949	0.941	0.935
1300	0.966	0.957	0.950	0.945
1350	0.972	0.964	0.959	0.954
1400	0.978	0.971	0.967	0.963
1450	0.983	0.978	0.975	0.972
1500	0.988	0.985	0.982	0.980
1550	0.993	0.991	0.989	0.988
1600	0.997	0.997	0.996	0.995
1650	1.002	1.002	1.002	1.003
c_f (% w/w)	21.1	28.5	33.7	41.0
v_M (cm³)	276	318	348	368
c_s (% w/w)	5	5	5	5
c_L (% w/w)	20.3	27.4	32.4	39.8

[a] From Eikenberry, E. F. (1973). Generation of density gradients. Approximation to equivolumetric gradients from zonal rotors. *Anal. Biochem.* **55,** 338–357.

[b] Same as Appendix D3, but for the B-XV rotor. The volume of overlay required is ≥ 48 cm³. The value of c_i is uniformly 5% w/w.

D5. CONSTRUCTION OF HYPERBOLIC GRADIENT FOR THE SEPARATION OF RIBOSOMES[a,b]

Volume (ml)	Radius (cm)	Density at 5°C (gm/cm³)[a]	Sucrose concentration at 5°C (% w/w)	Computed factor for gradient generator[d]
0 to 708	1.9 to 6.0	1.0	0.0	0
750[c]	6.15	1.013[b]	3.4	0.077
800[c]	6.32	1.028[c]	7.1	0.164
808	6.34	1.029	7.4	—
850	6.49	1.042	10.4	0.244
900	6.66	1.055	13.4	0.318
950	6.82	1.067	16.1	0.387
1000	6.98	1.078	18.6	0.451
1050	7.13	1.088	20.9	0.511
1100	7.28	1.098	23.0	0.566
1150	7.42	1.107	24.9	0.619
1200	7.57	1.115	26.7	0.669
1250	7.71	1.124	28.5	0.711
1300	7.85	1.131	30.0	0.763
1350	7.98	1.139	31.5	0.805
1400	8.12	1.146	32.9	0.846
1450	8.25	1.152	34.2	0.886
1500	8.38	1.159	35.5	0.924
1550	8.52	1.165	36.8	0.962
1600	8.66	1.171	38.0	1.000
1650	8.88	1.208	45.0	—

[a] From Eikenberry, E. F., Bickle, T. A. Traut, R. R., and Price, C. A. (1970). Separation of large quantities of ribosomal subunits by zonal ultracentrifugation. *Eur. J. Biochem.* **12**, 113–116.

[b] Gradient computed for the separation of particles of 1.56 gm/cm³ in a B-XV zonal rotor.

[c] These figures computed for the hyperbolical gradient are listed for reference only since in operation this region is normally occupied by the sample zone.

[d] Volumetric fraction of 38% (w/w) sucrose required to achieve desired density.

D6. ACCELERATION GRADIENT[*]

Acceleration gradients exploit a peculiar property of CsCl solutions, especially in D_2O, of viscosity *decreasing* with concentration over a wide concentration range. The result is that more rapidly sedimenting particle zones "run away" from less rapid ones. Since zone widths are about the same as in isokinetic gradients, there is a net increase in resolution.

In the gradients described here, the ratio of the distances (Δr_1 and Δr_2) moved by two particles is related to their sedimentation coefficients (s_1 and s_2) by

$$\frac{\Delta r_1}{\Delta r_2} = \frac{e^{(s_1/s_2)[\ln(1 + k\Delta r_2)]} - 1}{k\Delta r_2}$$

where k is a gradient constant.

Acceleration gradients suitable for the separation of ribosomes or ribosomal subunits in IEC SB283 or Spinco SW40Ti rotors can be constructed in an exponential gradient maker (cf. Section 5.3) as follows:

   Buffer: 10 mM Tris–HCl pH 7.4, 10 mM magnesium acetate, 0.1 mg/cm^3 gelatin, in D_2O.

   Starting (mixing) solution: 0% CsCl in buffer.

   Limiting solution: 20% w/w CsCl in buffer.

The volumes in cm^3 of starting and limiting solutions required are equal to 12.5 times the number of gradients desired. The D_2O remaining in the mixing chamber may be recovered by distillation.

D7. SHAPES OF SUCROSE AND NACl GRADIENTS AT SEDIMENTATION–DIFFUSION EQUILIBRIUM[†]

The distribution of sucrose (Fig. D.2) or NaCl (Fig. D.3) in sedimentation–diffusion equilibrium is calculated for the indicated swinging-bucket rotors and speeds at 25°C from Eq. (4.3) and tabulated values of $\beta°$ (Appendix C16). The initial or mean concentrations of solutes are indicated in the figures as z_e. The geometries of the rotors are shown in Table 6.1.

   * Kaempfer, R., and Meselson, M. (1971). Sedimentation velocity analysis in accelerating gradients. *In* "Methods in Enzymology," Vol. XX, Part C, pp. 521–528.
   † C. R. McEwen (1967). Computation of density distributions in solutions at sedimentation equilibrium. *Anal. Biochem.* **19**, 23–39.

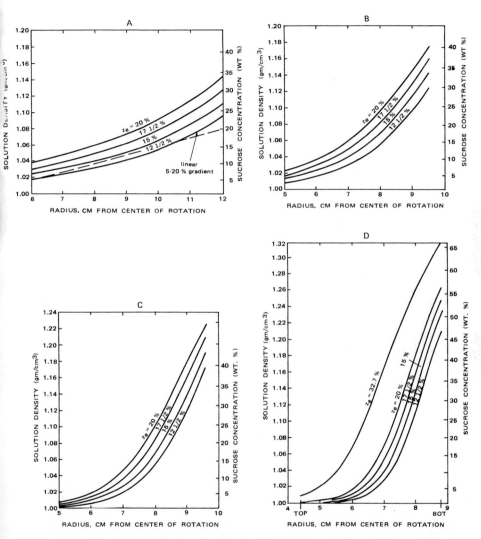

Fig. D.2. Sedimentation-diffusion equilibrium gradients of sucrose in swinging bucket rotors. (A) SW 25.1 at 25,000 rpm, (B) SW 39 at 39,000 rpm, (C) SW 50 at 50,000 rpm, and (D) SW 65 at 65,000 rpm (McEwen, 1967).

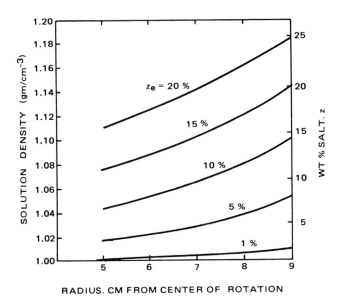

Fig. D.3. Sedimentation-diffusion equilibrium gradients of NaCl in the SW 65 rotor at 65,000 rpm (McEwen, 1967).

Appendix E

Zonal Rotors

404

E1. ORNL DESIGNATIONS FOR ZONAL ROTORS

Series	No.	Material	Capacity (cm³)	RPM (max)	g (max)	Drive	Comments
A	I	Pyrex tubes	2–68	3,000	2,500	PR-2	
A	II	Pyrex bottles	6–250	2,200	1,100	PR-2	
A	III	Aluminum	4,000	2,000	939	PR-2	
A	IV	Aluminum	625	18,000	23,545	Spinco K	
A	V	Lucite	1,300	1,000	152	PR-2	
A	VI	Aluminum	3,000	6,000	7,100	PR-2	
A	VII	Lucite	127	3,000	292	PR-2	
A	VIII	Aluminum	1,450	6,000	2,817	PR-2	
A	IX	Lucite	1,300	4,000	3,200	PR-2	
A	X	Lucite	300	4,000	3,200	PR-2	Core for A-IX
A	XI	Aluminum-steel	Two 20-cm³ cells	6,000	7,100	PR-2	
A	XII	Aluminum-steel	1,300	6,000	3,200	PR-2	Commercial
A	XIII	Aluminum-steel	350	6,000	3,200	PR-2	
A	XIV	No rotor built					
A	XV	No rotor built					
A	XVI	Brass-polycarbonate	672	5,000	1,300	PR-2	
B	I[a]	Aluminum	1,450	40,000	125,216	Spinco L	
B	II[a]	Aluminum	1,625	20,000	22,738	Spinco L	
B	III	Aluminum	1,450	1,500	176	Spinco L	
B	IV	Aluminum	1,685	40,000	90,952	Spinco L-4	New top bearing
B	V	Aluminum	150	40,000	90,952	Spinco L-4	Continuous flow
B	VI	Aluminum	1,338	35,000	69,635	Spinco L-4	New top bearing
B	VII	Aluminum	1,012	35,000	69,635	Spinco L-4	New top bearing
B	VIII	Aluminum	952	35,000	69,635	Spinco L-4	Continuous flow
B	IX	Aluminum	754	35,000	69,635	Spinco L-4	Design stage

B	X	Aluminum	600			Design stage, removable seals, Spinco L
B	XI	Aluminum	1,500			Design stage, removable seals, Spinco L
B	XII	Steel	1,700	50,000	142,000	Spinco L
B	XIII	No rotor				
B	XIV	Titanium	640	37,000	102,000	Spinco L Commercial, removable seal
B	XV	Titanium	1,665	28,000	77,000	Spinco L Commercial, removable seal
B	XVI	Aluminum	750	40,000	90,952	Spinco L-4 B-IV Type, Continuous flow
B	XVII	Aluminum	750	40,000	90,952	Spinco L-4 B-XVI Type, floater trap
B	XVIII	No rotor built				B-XIV continuous flow
B	XIX	No rotor built				B-XV continuous flow
B	XX	No rotor built				
B	XXI	Stainless steel		2,000		Gradient distribution head for Spinco #30 rotor
B	XXII	Stainless steel				Same as above for Spinco #40 rotor
B	XXIII	Titanium	1,665	28,000	77,000	Spinco L Edge unloading B-XV
B	XXIV	Titanium	1,665	28,000	77,000	Spinco L B-XV with large flow lines to edge for viscous sucrose
B	XXV	Titanium	1,665	28,000	77,000	Spinco L B-XV with large flow lines to center for DNA
B	XXVI	Aluminum	754	35,000	69,635	Spinco L B-IX for reorienting gradient
B	XXVII	Titanium	640	37,000	102,000	Spinco L B-XIV for pelleting last 0.5 cm
B	XXVIII	Titanium	1,665	28,000	77,000	Spinco L B-XV with no vanes for preclean-out of influenza virus
B	XXIX	Titanium	1,450	28,000	77,000	Spinco L Improved B-XXIII
B	XXX	Titanium	No rotor built			B-XXIX but B-XIV size
B	XXXI	Titanium	1,450	28,000	77,000	Spinco L 3-pass seal and core
B	XXXII					
B	XXXIII	Titanium	1,450	28,000	77,000	Spinco L Reorienting DNA
B	XXXIV	Titanium	1,400	47,500	128,257	Spinco L Flotation fractionation of lipoproteins

Continued

E1. Continued

Series	No.	Material	Capacity (ml)	RPM (mag)	g (max)	Drive	Comments
K	I	Aluminum	3.6 l	35,000	83,000		Continuous flow with banding
K	II	Titanium	3.2 l	35,000	98,000		K-II
K	III	Aluminum	6.8 l	35,000	98,000		Rate core for dynamic loading and unloading in K-II shell
K	V	Aluminum	6.8 l	35,000	98,000		Rate core for static loading and unloading in K-II shell
K	VI	Aluminum	3.6 l	35,000	83,000		K-II with center debris trap
K	VII	Titanium					Same as K-IV but using K-III shell
K	VIII	Titanium	8.5 l	35,000			Same as K-V but using K-III shell
K	IX	Titanium					Same as K-VI but using K-III shell
K	X	Aluminum	6.7 l	35,000	83,000		Continuous flow with pelleting
K	XI	Titanium	385 cm^3	35,000	98,000		Core and cap modification for flow improvement
K	XII	Aluminum	3.6 l	35,000	83,000		
J	I	Titanium	800 cm^3	60,000	178,880		Research model of K-II

[a] Courtesy of N. G. Anderson.

Figures E.1.–E.11. indicate rotor volume as a function of distance.

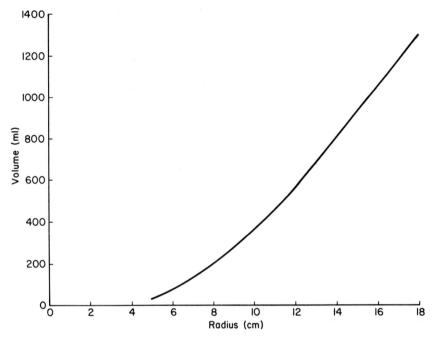

Fig. E.1.   A-XII zonal rotor.

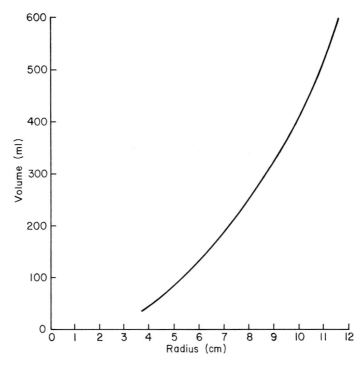

Fig. E.2.   HS zonal rotor.

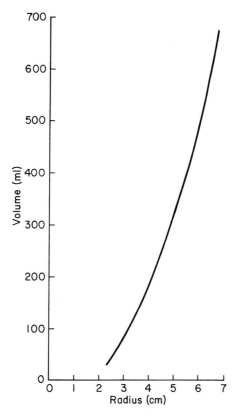

Fig. E.3.   B-XIV zonal rotor.

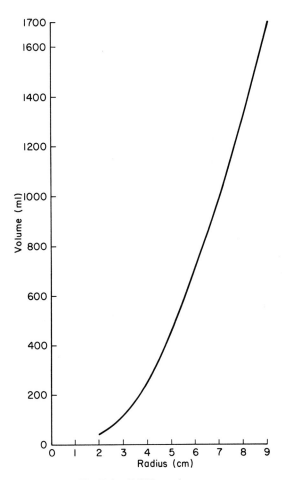

Fig. E.4.   B-XV zonal rotor.

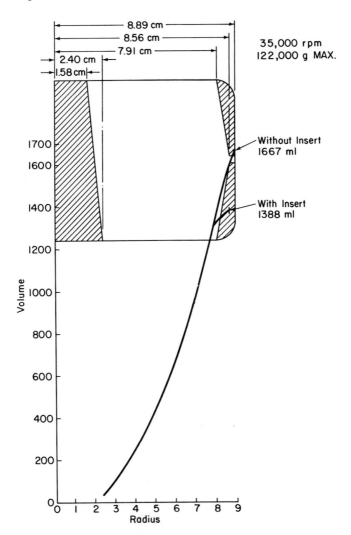

Fig. E.5.   B-29-A (B-15) zonal rotor.

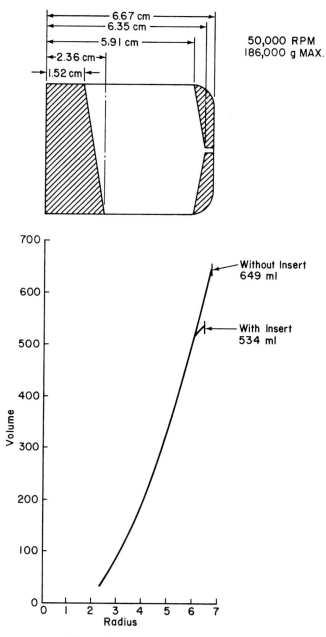

Fig. E.6.   B-30-A (B-14) zonal rotor.

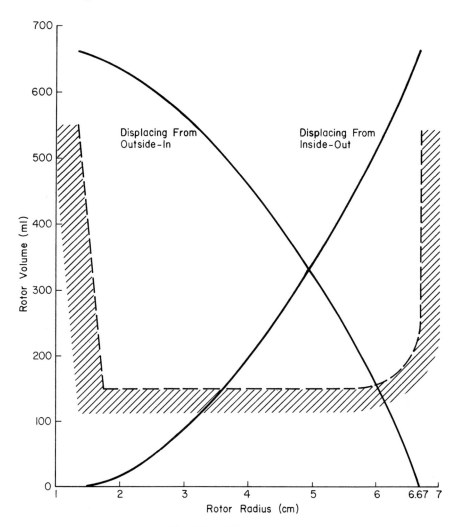

Fig. E.7.   Al/Ti-14 rotor.

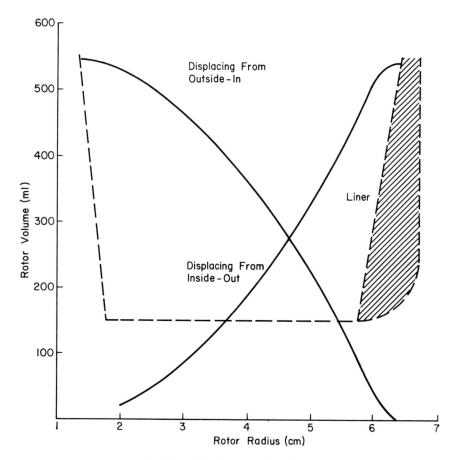

Fig. E.8.   Al/Ti-14 rotor with 29 liner.

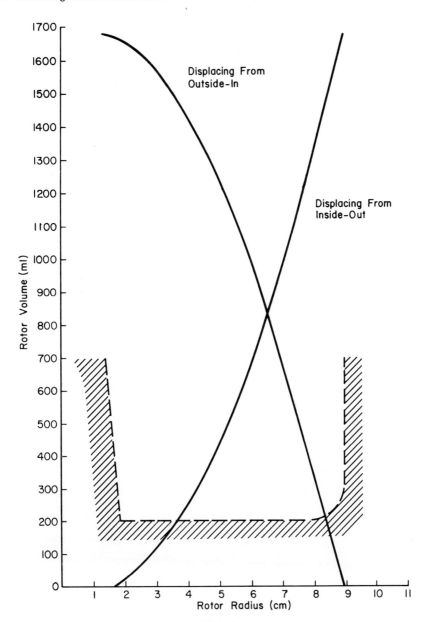

Fig. E.9. Al/Ti-15 rotor.

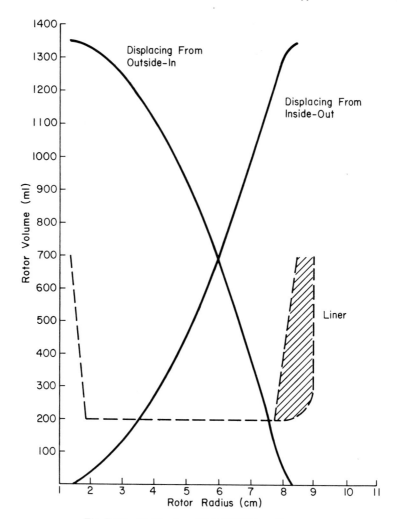

Fig. E.10. Tl-15 rotor with B-XXIX type liner.

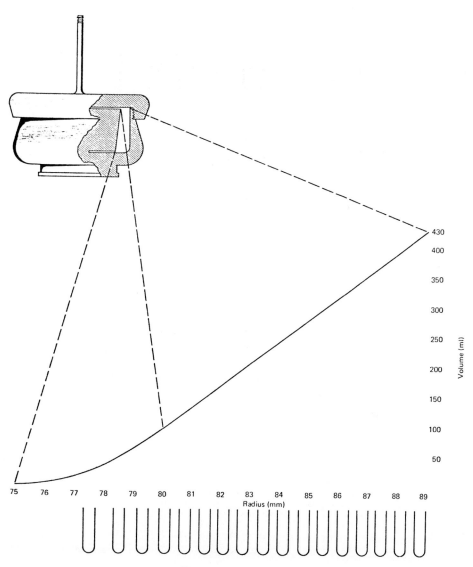

Fig. E.11.   CF-32 rotor

Appendix F

Chemical Resistance of Various Plastics

The following table was compiled for plastics marketed by Nalgene Labware Division, Nalge Company. The resistance of other brands of the same nominal plastics may differ significantly.

1st letter: at 20°C → EG ← 2nd letter: at 50°C

CHEMICAL	CPE	LPE	PP	PMP	FEP/TFE	PC	PVC
Acetaldehyde	GN	GF	GN	GN	EE	FN	GN
Acetamide, Sat.	EE	EE	EE	EE	EE	NN	NN
Acetic Acid, 5%	EE	EE	EE	EE	EE	EG	EE
Acetic Acid, 50%	EE	EE	EE	EE	EE	EG	EG
Acetone	EE	EE	EE	EE	EE	NN	FN
Adipic Acid	EG	EE	EE	EE	EE	EE	EG
Alanine	EE	EE	EE	EE	EE	NN	NN
Allyl Alcohol	EE	EE	EE	EG	EE	EG	GF
Aluminum Hydroxide	EG	EE	EG	EG	EE	FN	EG
Aluminum Salts	EE	EE	EE	EE	EE	EG	EE
Amino Acids	EE	EE	EE	EE	EE	EE	EE
Ammonia	EE	EE	EE	EE	EE	NN	EG
Ammonium Acetate, Sat.	EE	EE	EE	EE	EE	EE	EE
Ammonium Glycolate	EG	EE	EG	EG	EE	GF	EE
Ammonium Hydroxide, 5%	EE	EE	EE	EE	EE	FN	EE
Ammonium Hydroxide,	EG	EE	EE	EG	EE	NN	EG
Ammonium Oxalate	EG	EE	EE	EG	EE	EE	EE
Ammonium Salts	EE	EE	EE	EE	EE	EG	EG
n-Amyl Acetate	GF	EG	GF	GF	EE	NN	NN
Amyl Chloride	NN	FN	NN	NN	EE	NN	NN
Aniline	EG	EG	GF	GF	EE	FN	NN
Benzaldehyde	EG	EE	EG	EG	EE	FN	NN
Benzene	FN	GG	GF	GF	EE	NN	NN
Benzoic Acid, Sat.	EE	EE	EG	EG	EE	EG	EG
Benzyl Acetate	EG	EE	EG	EG	EE	FN	FN
Benzyl Alcohol	NN	FN	NN	NN	EE	GF	GF
Bromine	NN	NN	NN	NN	EE	FN	GN
Bromobenzene	NN	FN	NN	NN	EE	NN	NN
Bromoform	NN	NN	NN	NN	EE	NN	NN
Butadiene	NN	FN	NN	NN	EE	NN	FN
n-Butyl Acetate	GF	EG	GF	GF	EE	NN	NN
n-Butyl Alcohol	EE	EE	EE	EG	EE	GF	GF
sec-Butyl Alcohol	EG	EE	EE	EG	EE	GF	GG
tert-Butyl Alcohol	EG	EE	EE	EG	EE	GF	EG
Butyric Acid	NN	FN	NN	NN	EE	FN	GN
Calcium Hydroxide, Conc.	EE	EE	EE	EE	EE	NN	EE
Calcium Hypochlorite, Sat.	EE	EE	EE	EG	EE	FN	GF
Carbazole	EE	EE	EE	EE	EE	NN	NN
Carbon Disulfide	NN	NN	NN	FN	EE	NN	NN
Carbon Tetrachloride	FN	GF	GF	NN	EE	NN	GF
Cedarwood Oil	NN	FN	NN	NN	EE	EG	FN
Cellosolve Acetate	EG	EE	EG	EG	EE	FN	FN
Chlorine, 10% in Air	GN	EF	GN	GN	EE	EG	EE
Chlorine, 10% (Moist)	GN	GF	GN	GN	EE	GF	EG
Chloroacetic Acid	EE	EE	EG	EG	EE	FN	FN
p-Chloroacetophenone	EE	EE	EE	EE	EE	NN	NN
Chloroform	FN	GF	GF	FN	FN	NN	NN
Chromic Acid, 10%	EE	EE	EE	EE	EE	GF	EG
Chromic Acid, 50%	EE	EE	EG	EG	EE	FN	EF
Cinnamon Oil	NN	FN	NN	NN	EE	GF	NN
Citric Acid, 10%	EE	EE	EE	EE	EE	EG	EG
Cresol	NN	FN	GF	GF	EE	NN	NN
Cyclohexane	GF	EG	GF	NN	EE	EG	GF
Decalin	GF	EG	GF	FN	EE	NN	EG
o-Dichlorobenzene	FN	FF	FN	FN	EE	NN	GN
p-Dichlorobenzene	FN	GF	GF	GF	EE	NN	NN
Diethyl Benzene	NN	FN	NN	NN	EE	FN	NN
Diethyl Ether	NN	FN	NN	NN	EE	FN	FN
Diethyl Ketone	GF	GG	GG	GF	EE	NN	NN
Diethyl Malonate	EE	EE	EE	EG	EE	FN	GN
Diethylene Glycol	EE	EE	EE	EE	EE	GF	FN
Diethylene Glycol Ethyl Ether	EE	EE	EE	EE	EE	GF	FN
Dimethyl Formamide	EE	EE	EE	EE	EE	NN	FN
Dimethylsulfoxide	EE	EE	EE	EE	EE	NN	NN
1,4-Dioxane	GF	GG	GF	GF	EE	GF	FN
Dipropylene Glycol	EE	EE	EE	EE	EE	GF	GF
Ether	NN	FN	NN	NN	EE	NN	FN
Ethyl Acetate	EE	EE	EE	EG	EE	NN	FN
Ethyl Alcohol	EG	EE	EG	EG	EE	EG	EG
Ethyl Alcohol, 40%	EG	EE	EG	EG	EE	EG	EE
Ethyl Benzene	FN	GF	FN	FN	EE	NN	NN
Ethyl Benzoate	FF	GG	GF	GF	EE	NN	NN
Ethyl Butyrate	GN	GF	GN	FN	EE	NN	NN
Ethyl Chloride, Liquid	FN	FF	FN	FN	EE	NN	NN
Ethyl Cyanoacetate	EE	EE	EE	EE	EE	FN	FN
Ethyl Lactate	EE	EE	EE	EE	EE	FN	FN
Ethylene Chloride	GN	GF	FN	NN	EE	NN	NN
Ethylene Glycol	EE	EE	EE	EE	EE	GF	EE
Ethylene Glycol Methyl Ether	EE	EE	EE	EE	EE	FN	FN
Ethylene Oxide	FF	GF	FF	FN	EE	FN	FN
Fluorides	EE	EE	EE	EE	EE	EE	EE
Fluorine	FN	GN	FN	FN	EG	GF	EG
Formaldehyde, 10%	EE	EE	EE	EG	EE	EG	EG
Formaldehyde, 40%	EG	EE	EG	EG	EE	EG	GF
Formic Acid, 3%	EG	EE	EG	EG	EE	EG	GF
Formic Acid, 50%	EG	EE	EG	EG	EE	EG	GF
Formic Acid, 98-100%	EG	EE	EG	EF	EE	EF	FN
Fuel Oil	FN	GF	EG	GF	EE	EG	EE
Gasoline	FN	GG	GF	GF	EE	FF	GN
Glacial Acetic Acid	EG	EE	EG	EG	EE	GF	EG
Glycerine	EE	EE	EE	EE	EE	EE	EE
n-Heptane	FN	GF	FF	FF	EE	EG	FN
Hexane	NN	GF	GF	FN	EE	FN	GN
Hydrochloric Acid, 1-5%	EE	EE	EE	EG	EE	EE	EE
Hydrochloric Acid, 20%	EE	EE	EE	EG	EE	GF	EG
Hydrochloric Acid, 35%	EE	EE	EG	EG	EE	NN	GF
Hydrofluoric Acid, 4%	EG	EE	EG	EG	EE	GF	GF
Hydrofluoric Acid, 48%	EE	EE	EE	EE	EE	NN	GF
Hydrogen Peroxide, 3%	EE	EE	EE	EE	EE	EE	EE
Hydrogen Peroxide, 30%	EG	EE	EG	EG	EE	EE	EE
Hydrogen Peroxide, 90%	EG	EE	EG	EG	EE	EE	EE
Isobutyl Alcohol	EE	EE	EE	EG	EE	EG	EG
Isopropyl Acetate	GF	EG	GF	GF	EE	NN	NN
Isopropyl Alcohol	EE	EE	EE	EE	EE	EE	EG
Isopropyl Benzene	FN	GF	FN	NN	EE	NN	NN
Kerosene	FN	GG	GF	GF	EE	GF	EE
Lactic Acid, 3%	EG	EE	EG	EG	EE	EG	GF
Lactic Acid, 85%	EE	EE	EG	EG	EE	NN	GF
Methoxyethyl Oleate	EG	EE	EG	EG	EE	FN	NN
Methyl Alcohol	EE	EE	EE	EE	EE	GF	EF
Methyl Ethyl Ketone	EE	EE	EG	EE	EE	NN	NN
Methyl Isobutyl Ketone	GF	EG	GF	FF	EE	NN	NN
Methyl Propyl Ketone	GF	GG	GF	FF	EE	NN	NN
Methylene Chloride	GF	GF	FN	FN	EE	NN	NN
Mineral Oil	GN	EE	FN	EG	EE	EG	EG
Nitric Acid, 1-10%	EE	EE	EE	EE	EE	EG	EG
Nitric Acid, 50%	GG	GN	FN	GN	EE	GF	GF
Nitric Acid, 70%	NN	GN	FN	GN	EE	FN	GN
Nitrobenzene	NN	FN	NN	NN	EE	NN	NN
n-Octane	EE	EE	EE	EE	EE	GF	FN
Orange Oil	FN	GF	GF	FF	EE	FF	FN
Ozone	EG	EE	EG	EE	EE	EG	EG
Perchloric Acid	GN	GN	GN	GN	GF	NN	GN
Perchloroethylene	NN	NN	NN	NN	EE	NN	NN
Phenol, Crystals	GN	GF	GN	FN	EE	EN	FN
Phosphoric Acid, 1-5%	EE	EE	EE	EE	EE	EE	EE
Phosphoric Acid, 85%	EE	EE	EG	EG	EE	EG	EG
Pine Oil	GN	GG	EG	GF	EE	GF	FN
Potassium Hydroxide, 1%	EE	EE	EE	EE	EE	FN	EE
Potassium Hydroxide, Conc.	NN	FN	NN	NN	EE	FN	FN
Propane Gas	NN	FN	NN	NN	EE	NN	EG
Propylene Glycol	EE	EE	EE	EE	EE	GF	FN
Propylene Oxide	EE	EE	EG	EG	EE	GF	FN
Resorcinol, Sat.	EE	EE	EE	EE	EE	GF	FN
Resorcinol, 5%	EE	EE	EE	EE	EE	GF	GN
Salicylaldehyde	EG	EE	EG	EG	EE	GF	FN
Salicylic Acid, Powder	EE	EE	EE	EE	EE	EG	GF
Salicylic Acid, Sat.	EE	EE	EE	EE	EE	EG	GF
Salt Solutions, Metallic	EE	EE	EE	EE	EE	EE	EE
Silver Acetate	EE	EE	EE	EE	EE	EG	GG
Silver Salts	EG	EE	EG	EE	EE	EG	EG
Sodium Acetate, Sat.	EE	EE	EE	EE	EE	EG	GF
Sodium Hydroxide, 1%	EE	EE	EE	EE	EE	NN	EE
Sodium Hydroxide, 50% to Sat.	EE	EE	EE	EE	EE	NN	EG
Sodium Hypochlorite, 15%	EE	EE	EE	EE	EE	GF	EE
Stearic Acid, Crystals	EE	EE	EE	EE	EE	EE	EG
Sulfuric Acid, 1-6%	EE	EE	EE	EE	EE	EE	EE
Sulfuric Acid, 20%	EE	EE	EE	EE	EE	EG	EG
Sulfuric Acid, 60%	EG	EE	EG	EG	EE	GF	EG
Sulfuric Acid, 98%	GG	GG	GG	GG	EE	NN	NN
Sulfur Dioxide, Liq., 46 psi	NN	FN	NN	NN	EE	GN	FN
Sulfur Dioxide, Wet or Dry	EE	EE	EE	EE	EE	EE	EG
Sulfur Salts	FN	GF	FN	FN	EE	NN	NN
Tartaric Acid	EE	EE	EE	EE	EE	EG	EG
Tetrahydrofuran	FN	GF	GF	FF	EE	NN	NN
Thionyl Chloride	NN	NN	NN	NN	EE	NN	NN
Toluene	FN	GG	GF	FF	EE	FN	FN
Tributyl Citrate	GF	EG	GF	GF	EE	FN	NN
Trichloroethane	NN	FN	NN	NN	EE	NN	NN
Trichloroethylene	NN	FN	NN	NN	EE	NN	NN
Triethylene Glycol	EE	EE	EE	EE	EE	EG	GF
Tripropylene Glycol	EE	EE	EE	EE	EE	GF	FN
Turpentine	FN	GG	GF	FF	EE	FN	GF
Undecyl Alcohol	EF	EG	EG	EG	EE	GF	EF
Urea	EE	EE	EE	EE	EE	NN	GN
Vinylidene Chloride	NN	FN	NN	NN	EE	NN	NN
Xylene	GN	GF	FN	FN	EE	NN	NN
Zinc Stearate	EE	EE	EE	EE	EE	EE	EG

Key: CPE   conventional (low density) polyethylene
      LPE   linear (high density) polyethylene
       PP   polypropylene
      PMP   polymethylpentene
      FEP   fluorinated ethylene propylene, Teflon
      TFE   Teflon tetrafluoroethylene
     ETFE   ethylene-tetrafluoroethylene, Tefzel
       PC   polycarbonate
      PVC   polyvinyl chloride, Tygon

Appendix G

Addresses of Some Manufacturers

Anton Paar K.G.
A-8054
Graz, Austria

Beckman, see Spinco

Buchler Instruments
Division of Haake, Inc.
244 Saddle River Road
Saddle Brook, New Jersey 07662

Canadian Scientific
Box 131
Winnepeg, Manitoba, Canada R3 C 2G1

R. P. Cargille Laboratories, Inc.
Cedar Grove, New Jersey 07009

Chemag, A. G.
Maennedorf/ZH, Switzerland

Coulter Electronics, Inc.
590 West 20th St.
Hialeah, Florida 33010

Duke Scientific Corp.
445 Sherman Avenue
Palo Alto, California 94306

E. I. du Pont de Nemours & Co., Inc
Industrial and Biochemicals Department
Wilmington, Delaware 19898

Edmund Scientific Co.
7082 Edscorp Bldg.
Barrington, New Jersey 08007

Gilson Medical Electronics
Middleton, Wisconsin, 53562

Hoefer Scientific Instruments
650 Fifth Avenue
San Francisco, California 94107

(IEC)
Damon/IEC Division
300 Second Avenue
Needham Heights, Massachusetts 02194

ISCO
5624 Seward Avenue
Lincoln, Nebraska 68507

IKB-Produkter. AB
P. O. Box 76
Stockholm-Bromma 1, Sweden
or in U.S.A.
LKB Instruments Inc.
12221 Parklawn Drive
Rockville, Maryland 20852

420

Mettler Instrument Corporation
Box 100
Princeton, New Jersey 08540

MSE
25-28 Buckingham Gate
London, WW1, England

Nygaard AS
Oslo 4, Norway
or in U.S.A.
Accurate Chemical & Scientific Corp.
300 Shames Drive
Westbury, New York 11590

Particle Information Service
P. O. Box 702
Grants Pass, Oregon 97526

Pharmacia Fine Chemicals
Stockholm, Sweden
or in U.S.A.
800 Centennial Avenue
Piscataway, New Jersey 08854

Pressure Chemical Co.
3419 Smallman St.
Pittsburgh, Pennsylvania 15201

Searle Instruments
West Road

Harlow, Essex, CM20 2AG England
or in U.S.A., see Buchler

Small Parts, Inc.
6901 N. E. Third Avenue
Miami, Florida 33138

Sorvall
du Pont Instruments/Sorvall
Biomedical Division
Peck's Lane
Newton, Connecticut 06470

Spinco Division
Beckman Instruments, Inc.
1117 California Avenue
Palo Alto, California 94304

Techne, Inc.
3700 Brunswick Pike
Princeton, New Jersey 08854

Waters Associates
Millipore Corp.
34 Maple St.
Milford, Massachusetts 01757

Winthrop Laboratories
90 Park Avenue
New York, New York, 10016

Index